Gastrointestinal Diseases and Disorders

SOURCEBOOK

Fourth Edition

Health Reference Series

Fourth Edition

Gastrointestinal Diseases and Disorders SOURCEBOOK

Basic Consumer Health Information about the Upper and Lower Gastrointestinal (GI) Tract, Including the Esophagus, Stomach, Intestines, Rectum, Liver, and Pancreas, with Facts about Gastroesophageal Reflux Disease, Gastritis, Hernias, Ulcers, Celiac Disease, Diverticulitis, Irritable Bowel Syndrome, Hemorrhoids, Gastrointestinal Cancers, and Other Diseases and Disorders Related to the Digestive Process

Along with Information about Commonly Used Diagnostic and Surgical Procedures, Statistics, Reports on Current Research Initiatives and Clinical Trials, a Glossary, and Resources for Additional Help and Information

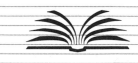

OMNIGRAPHICS

615 Griswold, Ste. 901, Detroit, MI 48226

Bibliographic Note

Because this page cannot legibly accommodate all the copyright notices, the Bibliographic Note portion of the Preface constitutes an extension of the copyright notice.

* * *

OMNIGRAPHICS

Angela L. Williams, *Managing Editor*

***

Library of Congress Cataloging-in-Publication Data

Names: Omnigraphics, Inc., issuing body.

Title: Gastrointestinal diseases and disorders sourcebook: basic consumer health information about the upper and lower gastrointestinal (GI) tract, including the esophagus, stomach, intestines, rectum, liver, and pancreas, with facts about gastroesophageal reflux disease, gastritis, hernias, ulcers, celiac disease, diverticulitis, irritable bowel syndrome, hemorrhoids, gastrointestinal cancers, and other diseases and disorders related to the digestive process; along with information about commonly used diagnostic and surgical procedures, statistics, reports on current research initiatives and clinical trials, a glossary, and resources for additional help and information.

Description: Fourth edition. | Detroit, MI: Omnigraphics, Inc., [2018] | Series: Health reference series | Includes bibliographical references and index.

Identifiers: LCCN 2018034653 (print) | LCCN 2018034843 (ebook) | ISBN 9780780816510 (ebook) | ISBN 9780780816503 (hard cover)

Subjects: LCSH: Gastrointestinal system--Diseases--Popular works.

Classification: LCC RC806 (ebook) | LCC RC806.G37 2018 (print) | DDC 616.3/3--dc23

LC record available at https://lccn.loc.gov/2018034653

Table of Contents

Part VI: Cancers of the Gastrointestinal Tract

Part VII: Food Intolerances and Infectious Disorders of the Gastrointestinal Tract

Preface

About This Book

The gastrointestinal tract includes the stomach, intestines, and other organs related to digestion—the process by which food and drink are changed into molecules of nutrients that can be carried to the body's cells. Disorders that interfere with this process affect an estimated 60 to 70 million Americans and account for more than 48.3 million doctor visits every year. According to the National Institute of Diabetes and Digestive and Kidney Diseases (NIDDK), researchers have only recently begun to understand many gastrointestinal diseases and disorders. As a result, the process of helping people set aside common misconceptions about the causes of symptoms and turn to scientifically based treatments instead of folkloric remedies is progressing only gradually.

Gastrointestinal Diseases and Disorders Sourcebook, Fourth Edition provides readers with updated health information about the causes, symptoms, diagnosis, and treatment of diseases and disorders affecting the esophagus, stomach, intestines, appendix, gallbladder, liver, and pancreas. It also describes how the gastrointestinal tract can be affected by food intolerances, infectious diseases, and various cancers. The structure and function of the digestive system, common diagnostic methods, medical treatments, surgical procedures, and current research initiatives are described. The book concludes with a glossary of related terms and directory of resources for further help and information.

How to Use This Book

This book is divided into parts and chapters. Parts focus on broad areas of interest. Chapters are devoted to single topics within a part.

Part I: Introduction to the Digestive System begins with a look at the anatomy and physiology of the digestive system. The part focuses on common gastrointestinal symptoms, cyclic vomiting syndrome, and discusses how the gastrointestinal tract can be impacted by tobacco use or by frequently used medications.

Part II: Diagnostic and Surgical Procedures Used for Gastrointestinal Disorders provides a detailed look at endoscopic procedures and other types of tests used to diagnose gastrointestinal disorders. It also explains ostomy, colectomy, and other surgical procedures.

Part III: Disorders of the Upper Gastrointestinal Tract looks at disorders of the esophagus and the stomach. It talks about swallowing disorders, peptic ulcers, Whipple disease, dyspepsia, Barrett esophagus, gastroparesis, gastroesophageal reflux disease (GERD), and also other diseases of the upper gastrointestinal tract.

Part IV: Disorders of the Lower Gastrointestinal Tract describes the risk factors, symptoms, and treatment options for disorders affecting the large and small intestines, appendix, gallbladder, anus, and rectum. It focuses on anatomic problems of the lower gastrointestinal tract also.

Part V: Disorders of the Digestive System's Solid Organs: The Liver and Pancreas offers information about the risk factors, symptoms, and treatment options for pancreatitis, hepatitis, cirrhosis of the liver, and other liver disorders.

Part VI: Cancers of the Gastrointestinal Tract provides a detailed look at different cancers that affect the gastrointestinal tract. Each chapter focuses on risk factors, symptoms, diagnostic methods, staging information, and treatment options.

Part VII: Food Intolerances and Infectious Disorders of the Gastrointestinal Tract discusses lactose intolerance, celiac disease, and diseases transmitted by viral, bacterial, or parasitic contamination of food or drinking water.

Part VIII: Additional Help and Information provides a glossary of gastrointestinal terms and a directory of organizations that can provide further information.

Bibliographic Note

This volume contains documents and excerpts from publications issued by the following U.S. government agencies: Centers for Disease Control and Prevention (CDC); Genetic and Rare Diseases Information Center (GARD); Genetics Home Reference (GHR); National Cancer Institute (NCI); National Heart, Lung, and Blood Institute (NHLBI); National Institute of Diabetes and Digestive and Kidney Diseases (NIDDK); National Institutes of Health (NIH); National Institute on Deafness and Other Communication Disorders (NIDCD); *NIH News in Health*; Office on Women's Health (OWH); and U.S. Department of Veterans Affairs (VA).

It may also contain original material produced by Omnigraphics and reviewed by medical documents.

About the Health Reference Series

The *Health Reference Series* is designed to provide basic medical information for patients, families, caregivers, and the general public. Each volume takes a particular topic and provides comprehensive coverage. This is especially important for people who may be dealing with a newly diagnosed disease or a chronic disorder in themselves or in a family member. People looking for preventive guidance, information about disease warning signs, medical statistics, and risk factors for health problems will also find answers to their questions in the *Health Reference Series*. The *Series*, however, is not intended to serve as a tool for diagnosing illness, in prescribing treatments, or as a substitute for the physician/patient relationship. All people concerned about medical symptoms or the possibility of disease are encouraged to seek professional care from an appropriate healthcare provider.

A Note about Spelling and Style

Health Reference Series editors use *Stedman's Medical Dictionary* as an authority for questions related to the spelling of medical terms and the *Chicago Manual of Style* for questions related to grammatical structures, punctuation, and other editorial concerns. Consistent adherence is not always possible, however, because the individual volumes within the *Series* include many documents from a wide variety of different producers, and the editor's primary goal is to present material from each source as accurately as is possible. This sometimes means that information in different chapters or sections may follow other guidelines and alternate spelling authorities. For example, occasionally a copyright holder may require that eponymous terms be shown in possessive forms (Crohn's disease vs. Crohn disease) or that British spelling norms be retained (leukaemia vs. leukemia).

Medical Review

Omnigraphics contracts with a team of qualified, senior medical professionals who serve as medical consultants for the *Health Reference Series*. As necessary, medical consultants review reprinted and originally written material for currency and accuracy. Citations including the phrase "Reviewed (month, year)" indicate material reviewed by this team. Medical consultation services are provided to the *Health Reference Series* editors by:

Dr. Vijayalakshmi, MBBS, DGO, MD
Dr. Senthil Selvan, MBBS, DCH, MD
Dr. K. Sivanandham, MBBS, DCH, MS (Research), PhD

Our Advisory Board

We would like to thank the following board members for providing initial guidance on the development of this series:

- Dr. Lynda Baker, Associate Professor of Library and Information Science, Wayne State University, Detroit, MI

- Nancy Bulgarelli, William Beaumont Hospital Library, Royal Oak, MI

- Karen Imarisio, Bloomfield Township Public Library, Bloomfield Township, MI

- Karen Morgan, Mardigian Library, University of Michigan-Dearborn, Dearborn, MI

- Rosemary Orlando, St. Clair Shores Public Library, St. Clair Shores, MI

Health Reference Series *Update Policy*

The inaugural book in the *Health Reference Series* was the first edition of *Cancer Sourcebook* published in 1989. Since then, the *Series* has been enthusiastically received by librarians and in the medical community. In order to maintain the standard of providing high-quality health information for the layperson the editorial staff at Omnigraphics felt it was necessary to implement a policy of updating volumes when warranted.

Medical researchers have been making tremendous strides, and it is the purpose of the *Health Reference Series* to stay current with the most recent advances. Each decision to update a volume is made on an individual basis. Some of the considerations include how much new information is available and the feedback we receive from people who use the books. If there is a topic you would like to see added to the update list, or an area of medical concern you feel has not been adequately addressed, please write to:

Managing Editor
Health Reference Series
Omnigraphics
615 Griswold, Ste. 901
Detroit, MI 48226

Part One

Introduction to the Digestive System

Chapter 1

Your Digestive System and How It Works

What Is the Digestive System?

The digestive system is made up of the gastrointestinal tract—also called the GI tract or digestive tract—and the liver, pancreas, and gallbladder. The GI tract is a series of hollow organs joined in a long, twisting tube from the mouth to the anus. The hollow organs that make up the GI tract are the mouth, esophagus, stomach, small intestine, large intestine, and anus. The liver, pancreas, and gallbladder are the solid organs of the digestive system. The small intestine has three parts. The first part is called the duodenum. The jejunum is in the middle and the ileum is at the end. The large intestine includes the appendix, cecum, colon, and rectum. The appendix is a finger-shaped pouch attached to the cecum. The cecum is the first part of the large intestine. The colon is next. The rectum is the end of the large intestine.

Bacteria in your GI tract, also called gut flora or microbiome, help with digestion. Parts of your nervous and circulatory systems also help. Working together, nerves, hormones, bacteria, blood, and the organs of your digestive system digest the foods and liquids you eat or drink each day.

This chapter includes text excerpted from "Your Digestive System and How It Works," National Institute of Diabetes and Digestive and Kidney Diseases (NIDDK), December 2017.

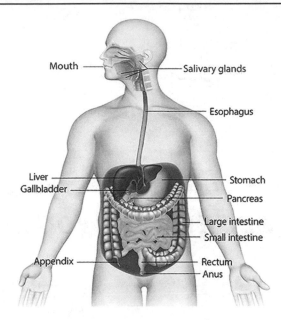

Figure 1.1. *The Digestive System*

Why Is Digestion Important?

Digestion is important because your body needs nutrients from food and drink to work properly and stay healthy. Proteins, fats, carbohydrates, vitamins, minerals, and water are nutrients. Your digestive system breaks nutrients into parts small enough for your body to absorb and use for energy, growth, and cell repair.

- Proteins break into amino acids.
- Fats break into fatty acids and glycerol.
- Carbohydrates break into simple sugars.

How Does My Digestive System Work?

Each part of your digestive system helps to move food and liquid through your GI tract, break food and liquid into smaller parts, or both. Once foods are broken into small enough parts, your body can absorb and move the nutrients to where they are needed. Your large intestine absorbs water, and the waste products of digestion become stool. Nerves and hormones help control the digestive process.

Table 1.1. The Digestive Process

Organ	Movement
Mouth	Chewing
Esophagus	Peristalsis
Stomach	Upper muscle in stomach relaxes to let food enter, and lower muscle mixes food with digestive juice
Small intestine	Peristalsis
Pancreas	None
Liver	None
Large intestine	Peristalsis

How Does Food Move through My Gastrointestinal (GI) Tract?

Food moves through your GI tract by a process called peristalsis. The large, hollow organs of your GI tract contain a layer of muscle that enables their walls to move. The movement pushes food and liquid through your GI tract and mixes the contents within each organ. The muscle behind the food contracts and squeezes the food forward, while the muscle in front of the food relaxes to allow the food to move.

Mouth. Food starts to move through your GI tract when you eat. When you swallow, your tongue pushes the food into your throat. A small flap of tissue, called the epiglottis, folds over your windpipe to prevent choking and the food passes into your esophagus.

Esophagus. Once you begin swallowing, the process becomes automatic. Your brain signals the muscles of the esophagus and peristalsis begins.

Lower esophageal sphincter. When food reaches the end of your esophagus, a ringlike muscle—called the lower esophageal sphincter—relaxes and lets food pass into your stomach. This sphincter usually stays closed to keep what's in your stomach from flowing back into your esophagus.

Stomach. After food enters your stomach, the stomach muscles mix the food and liquid with digestive juices. The stomach slowly empties its contents, called chyme, into your small intestine.

Small intestine. The muscles of the small intestine mix food with digestive juices from the pancreas, liver, and intestine, and push the mixture forward for further digestion. The walls of the small intestine absorb water and the digested nutrients into your bloodstream. As peristalsis continues, the waste products of the digestive process move into the large intestine.

Large intestine. Waste products from the digestive process include undigested parts of food, fluid, and older cells from the lining of your GI tract. The large intestine absorbs water and changes the waste from liquid into stool. Peristalsis helps move the stool into your rectum.

Rectum. The lower end of your large intestine, the rectum, stores stool until it pushes stool out of your anus during a bowel movement.

How Does My Digestive System Break Food into Small Parts My Body Can Use?

As food moves through your GI tract, your digestive organs break the food into smaller parts using:

- Motion, such as chewing, squeezing, and mixing
- Digestive juices, such as stomach acid, bile, and enzymes

Mouth. The digestive process starts in your mouth when you chew. Your salivary glands make saliva, a digestive juice, which moistens food so it moves more easily through your esophagus into your stomach. Saliva also has an enzyme that begins to break down starches in your food.

Esophagus. After you swallow, peristalsis pushes the food down your esophagus into your stomach.

Stomach. Glands in your stomach lining make stomach acid and enzymes that break down food. Muscles of your stomach mix the food with these digestive juices.

Pancreas. Your pancreas makes a digestive juice that has enzymes that break down carbohydrates, fats, and proteins. The pancreas delivers the digestive juice to the small intestine through small tubes called ducts.

Liver. Your liver makes a digestive juice called bile that helps digest fats and some vitamins. Bile ducts carry bile from your liver to your gallbladder for storage, or to the small intestine for use.

Gallbladder. Your gallbladder stores bile between meals. When you eat, your gallbladder squeezes bile through the bile ducts into your small intestine.

Small intestine. Your small intestine makes digestive juice, which mixes with bile and pancreatic juice to complete the breakdown of proteins, carbohydrates, and fats. Bacteria in your small intestine make some of the enzymes you need to digest carbohydrates. Your small intestine moves water from your bloodstream into your GI tract to help break down food. Your small intestine also absorbs water with other nutrients.

Large intestine. In your large intestine, more water moves from your GI tract into your bloodstream. Bacteria in your large intestine help break down remaining nutrients and make vitamin K. Waste products of digestion, including parts of food that are still too large, become stool.

What Happens to the Digested Food?

The small intestine absorbs most of the nutrients in your food, and your circulatory system passes them on to other parts of your body to store or use. Special cells help absorbed nutrients cross the intestinal lining into your bloodstream. Your blood carries simple sugars, amino acids, glycerol, and some vitamins and salts to the liver. Your liver stores, processes, and delivers nutrients to the rest of your body when needed. The lymph system, a network of vessels that carry white blood cells and a fluid called "lymph" throughout your body to fight infection, absorbs fatty acids and vitamins. Your body uses sugars, amino acids, fatty acids, and glycerol to build substances you need for energy, growth, and cell repair.

How Does My Body Control the Digestive Process?

Your hormones and nerves work together to help control the digestive process. Signals flow within your GI tract and back and forth from your GI tract to your brain.

Hormones

Cells lining your stomach and small intestine make and release hormones that control how your digestive system works. These hormones tell your body when to make digestive juices and send signals

7

to your brain that you are hungry or full. Your pancreas also makes hormones that are important to digestion.

Nerves

You have nerves that connect your central nervous system—your brain and spinal cord—to your digestive system and control some digestive functions. For example, when you see or smell food, your brain sends a signal that causes your salivary glands to "make your mouth water" to prepare you to eat.

You also have an enteric nervous system (ENS)—nerves within the walls of your GI tract. When food stretches the walls of your GI tract, the nerves of your ENS release many different substances that speed up or delay the movement of food and the production of digestive juices. The nerves send signals to control the actions of your gut muscles to contract and relax to push food through your intestines.

Chapter 2

Keeping Your Gut in Check

Your digestive system is busy. When you eat something, your food takes a twisty trip that starts with being chewed up and ends with you going to the bathroom. A lot happens in between. The health of your gut plays a key role in your overall health and well-being. You can make choices to help your body stay on track.

Your digestive, or gastrointestinal (GI), tract is a long, muscular tube that runs from your mouth to your anus. It's about 30 feet long and works with other parts of your digestive system to break food and drink down into smaller molecules of nutrients. The blood absorbs these and carries them throughout the body for cells to use for energy, growth, and repair.

With such a long GI highway, it's common to run into bumps in the road. About 60–70 million Americans are affected by digestive diseases, like gastroesophageal reflux disease (GERD) or irritable bowel syndrome (IBS). GERD happens when your stomach acid and/or contents come back up into your esophagus (swallowing tube) or throat. This causes uncomfortable symptoms like heartburn and indigestion. IBS is a group of symptoms that includes pain in the abdomen and changes in bowel habits. People with IBS may have constipation, diarrhea, or both. Many more people have other digestive problems, like bloating and stomach pain.

"There are many factors that can impact gut health," says Dr. Lin Chang, a GI expert at the University of California, Los Angeles

This chapter includes text excerpted from "Keeping Your Gut in Check," *NIH News in Health*, National Institutes of Health (NIH), May 2017.

(UCLA). How your body's built, your family and genetic history, how you manage stress, and what you eat can all affect your gut.

"I see a lot of lifestyle-related GI issues, and there are often no quick fixes for that," she says. "In general, people do well when they create a more routine schedule, eat a healthy diet, and smaller more frequent meals, add in some exercise, and get a good amount of sleep."

Chang studies the connection between stress and IBS. Her research group has found that people who have early life stress are more likely to develop IBS. "However, this increased risk for IBS went down when people confided in someone they trust about the stress they experienced," she explains. "Finding healthy ways to manage stress is important for GI health, and your health overall."

What you eat can help or hurt your digestive system, and influence how you feel. "Increasing fiber is really important for constipation," says Chang. "Most Americans do not eat a lot of fiber so you have to gradually increase the fiber in your diet. Otherwise, you might get gas and more bloating, and won't stick with (the changes)."

Chang says you should eat at least 20–30 grams of fiber a day for constipation. You can spread out your fiber in small amounts throughout the day. Start with small servings and gradually increase them to avoid gas, bloating, and discomfort.

Try to eat fruits and vegetables at every meal. A variety of fruits, vegetables, whole grains, and nuts can provide a healthy mix of different fibers and nutrients to your diet. An added benefit is that the more fiber and whole foods you eat, the less room you'll have for less healthy options.

But some fiber-rich foods, called high Fermentable Oligosaccharides, Disaccharides, Monosaccharides, and Polyols (FODMAP) foods, can be hard to digest. Examples include certain fruits and vegetables, dairy products, and wheat and rye products. If you have IBS, your doctor may recommend a diet low in FODMAP.

Researchers are coming to understand the complex community of bacteria and other microbes that live in the human GI tract. Called gut flora or microbiota, these microbes help with our digestion. But evidence has been growing that gut microbes may influence our health in other ways too. Studies suggest that they may play roles in obesity, type 2 diabetes, IBS, and colon cancer. They might also affect how the immune system functions. This can affect how your body fights illness and disease. Studies have found that microbes' effects on the immune system may impact the development of conditions such as allergy, asthma, and rheumatoid arthritis.

You might have heard that probiotics—live microbes that are similar to those found in the human gut—can improve your gut health. These are also called "friendly bacteria" or "good bacteria." Probiotics are available in dietary supplements and in certain foods, such as yogurt.

There is some evidence that probiotics may be helpful in preventing diarrhea associated with antibiotics and improving symptoms of IBS, but more needs to be learned. Researchers still don't know which probiotics are helpful and which aren't. They also don't know how much of the probiotics people would have to take or who would most likely benefit from them.

Certain food additives called emulsifiers are something else that may affect your gut health. Emulsifiers are added to many processed foods to improve texture and extend shelf life. But studies show they can affect our gut flora.

"Our work and other research indicate that emulsifiers and other food additives can negatively impact the microbiota and promote inflammatory diseases," says Georgia State University's (GSU) Dr. Andrew Gewirtz. His group has been studying the relationships between food additives, gut bacteria, and disease in mice. The team also plans to examine how different food additives may affect people.

Based on what his team and others have found, Gewirtz advises, "The take home message: Eat a balanced diet and less processed foods."

Chapter 3

Common Gastrointestinal Symptoms

Chapter Contents

Section 3.1

Bleeding in the Digestive Tract

This section includes text excerpted from "Gastrointestinal (GI)
Bleeding," National Institute of Diabetes and Digestive and
Kidney Diseases (NIDDK), July 2016.

What Is Gastrointestinal (GI) Bleeding?

Gastrointestinal (GI) bleeding is any type of bleeding that starts in
your GI tract, also called your digestive tract. GI bleeding is a symptom of a disease or condition, rather than a disease or condition itself.
Acute GI bleeding is sudden and can sometimes be severe. Chronic GI
bleeding is slight bleeding that can last a long time or may come and
go. GI bleeding is also called bleeding in the digestive tract, upper GI
bleeding, or lower GI bleeding. The upper GI tract and lower GI tract
are different areas of your GI tract.

How Common Is GI Bleeding?

Every year, about 100,000 people in the United States go to the
hospital for upper GI bleeding. About 20–33 percent of GI bleeding
episodes in Western countries are in the lower GI tract.

Who Is More Likely to Have GI Bleeding?

Men are twice as likely as women to have upper GI bleeding.

What Are the Symptoms of GI Bleeding?

Symptoms of gastrointestinal (GI) bleeding may include:

- Black or tarry stool
- Bright red blood in vomit
- Cramps in the abdomen
- Dark or bright red blood mixed with stool
- Dizziness or faintness
- Feeling tired
- Paleness
- Shortness of breath

- Vomit that looks like coffee grounds

- Weakness

What Causes GI Bleeding

Many conditions can cause GI bleeding. A doctor can try to find the cause of your bleeding by finding its source. The following conditions, which are listed in alphabetical order, include possible causes of GI bleeding:

- **Angiodysplasia.** Angiodysplasia is when you have abnormal or enlarged blood vessels in your GI tract. These blood vessels can become fragile and bleed.

- **Benign tumors and cancer.** Benign tumors and cancer in the esophagus, stomach, colon, or rectum may cause bleeding when they weaken the lining of the GI tract. A benign tumor is an abnormal tissue growth that is not cancerous.

- **Colitis.** Ulcers in the large intestine are a complication of colitis. Ulcerative colitis is an inflammatory bowel disease (IBD) that can cause GI bleeding.

- **Colon polyps.** Colon polyps can cause GI bleeding. You can have more than one colon polyp at a time. Some types of polyps may be cancerous or can become cancerous.

- **Diverticular disease.** Diverticular disease can cause GI bleeding when small pouches, or sacs, form and push outward through weak spots in your colon wall.

- **Esophageal varices.** Esophageal varices can cause GI bleeding. Esophageal varices are usually related to a chronic liver condition called cirrhosis.

- **Esophagitis.** The most common cause of esophagitis is gastroesophageal reflux (GER). GER happens when your lower esophageal sphincter is weak or relaxes when it should not. Stomach acid can damage your esophagus and cause sores and bleeding.

- **Gastritis**. Some common causes of gastritis include:

  - The use of nonsteroidal anti-inflammatory drugs (NSAIDs) and other medicines

  - Infections

- Crohn disease
- Serious illnesses
- Severe injuries

If untreated, gastritis can lead to ulcers or worn-away areas of the stomach lining that can bleed in your GI tract.

- **Hemorrhoids or anal fissures.** Hemorrhoids can cause GI bleeding. Constipation and straining during bowel movements cause hemorrhoids to swell. Hemorrhoids cause itching, pain, and sometimes bleeding in your anus or lower rectum. Anal fissures are small tears that also can cause itching, tearing, or bleeding in your anus.

- **Mallory-Weiss tears.** Severe vomiting may cause Mallory-Weiss tears, which can cause GI bleeding. You can have more than one Mallory-Weiss tear at a time.

- **Peptic ulcers.** The bacteria *Helicobacter pylori* (*H. pylori*) and use of NSAIDs can cause peptic ulcers. Peptic ulcers can wear away your mucosa and cause GI bleeding.

How Do Doctors Diagnose GI Bleeding?

To diagnose gastrointestinal (GI) bleeding, a doctor will first find the site of the bleeding based on your medical history—including what medicines you are taking—and family history, a physical exam, and diagnostic tests.

Physical Exam

During a physical exam, a doctor most often:

- Examines your body
- Listens to sounds in your abdomen using a stethoscope
- Taps on specific areas of your body

Diagnostic Tests

Depending on your symptoms, your doctor will order one or more diagnostic tests to confirm whether you have GI bleeding and, if so, to help find the source of the bleeding.

What Tests Do Doctors Use to Diagnose GI Bleeding?

Your doctor may perform the following tests to help diagnose the cause of your GI bleeding.

Lab Tests

Lab tests to help diagnose the cause of your GI bleeding include:

- Stool tests
- Blood tests

Gastric Lavage

A gastric lavage is a procedure in which a doctor passes a tube through your nose or mouth into your stomach to remove your stomach contents to determine the possible location of your GI bleeding. A doctor may also use gastric lavage to help prepare for another diagnostic test or, most often, for acute, severe bleeding. The doctor performs this procedure in an outpatient center or a hospital. You most often receive a liquid anesthetic to numb your throat.

Endoscopy

Endoscopy procedures involve a doctor examining a hollow passage in your body using a special instrument. An endoscopy procedure may help your doctor see if and where you have GI bleeding and the bleeding's cause. Doctors most often use upper GI endoscopy and colonoscopy to test for acute GI bleeding in the upper and lower GI tracts.

Imaging Tests

To help find the cause of your GI bleeding, your doctor may order one or more of the following imaging tests. You do not need anesthesia for these tests.

- Abdominal CT scan
- Lower GI series
- Upper GI series
- Angiogram
- Radionuclide scan

17

Procedures to Examine the GI Tract

If none of the other tests help your doctor diagnose the source of your GI bleeding, a surgeon may perform one of the following operations to examine your GI tract:

- Laparotomy
- Laparoscopy

How Do Doctors Treat GI Bleeding?

Treatment of gastrointestinal (GI) bleeding depends on the cause and location of your bleeding.

Treatment during a Diagnostic Procedure

During an upper GI endoscopy, a lower GI endoscopy, a colonoscopy, a flexible sigmoidoscopy, or a laparotomy, a doctor can stop the bleeding in your GI tract. He or she can stop the bleeding by inserting tools through an endoscope, colonoscope, or sigmoidoscope to:

- Inject medicines into the bleeding site
- Treat the bleeding site and surrounding tissue with a heat probe, an electric current, or a laser
- Close affected blood vessels with a band or clip

During an angiogram, a radiologist can inject medicines or other materials into blood vessels to stop some types of bleeding.

Medicines

When infections or ulcers cause bleeding in your GI tract, healthcare professionals prescribe medicines to treat the problem.

Surgery

When a person has severe acute bleeding or bleeding that does not stop, a surgeon may need to perform a laparoscopy or a laparotomy to stop the bleeding.

How Can I Prevent GI Bleeding?

Doctors can prevent GI bleeding by treating the conditions that cause the bleeding. You can prevent some of the causes of bleeding in your GI tract by:

- Limiting the amount of nonsteroidal anti-inflammatory drugs (NSAIDs) you take or by talking with your healthcare professional about other medicine options

- Following your doctor's recommendations for treatment of gastroesophageal reflux (GER)

What Should I Eat If I Have GI Bleeding?

If you have a history of gastrointestinal (GI) bleeding from diverticular disease, anal fissures, or hemorrhoids, you should follow the diet your healthcare professional recommends.

What Should I Avoid If I Have GI Bleeding?

If you have had bleeding from peptic ulcers or gastritis, you can help prevent GI bleeding by avoiding alcoholic drinks and smoking. Alcohol and smoking can increase stomach acids and lead to ulcers. Do not drink alcoholic beverages or smoke if you have GI bleeding.

Section 3.2

Gas in the Digestive Tract

This section includes text excerpted from "Gas in the Digestive Tract," National Institute of Diabetes and Digestive and Kidney Diseases (NIDDK), July 2016.

What Is Gas?

Gas is air in your digestive tract. Gas leaves your body through your mouth when you burp or through your anus when you pass gas. Flatulence is excess gas in your stomach or intestines that can cause bloating and flatus. Flatus, gas that leaves your body through your anus, can contain small amounts of sulfur. Flatus that contains more sulfur has more of an odor.

How Common Is Gas?

Everyone has gas. People may think that they burp or pass gas too often and that they have too much gas. Having too much gas is uncommon.

Who Is More Likely to Get Gas?

Certain conditions may cause you to have more gas or to have more symptoms when you have a normal amount of gas in your digestive tract. People who swallow more air or eat certain foods may be more likely to have more gas.

What Are the Symptoms of Gas?

The most common gas symptoms include burping, passing gas, bloating, and pain or discomfort in your abdomen. Gas symptoms vary from person to person.

Burping

Burping, or belching, once in a while, especially during and after meals, is normal. If you burp a lot, you may be swallowing too much air and releasing it before the air enters your stomach.

Passing Gas

Passing gas around 13–21 times a day is normal.

Bloating

Bloating is a feeling of fullness or swelling in your abdomen. Bloating most often occurs during or after a meal.

Pain or Discomfort in Your Abdomen

You may feel pain or discomfort in your abdomen when gas does not move through your intestines normally.

When Should I Talk with a Doctor about My Gas Symptoms?

You should talk with your doctor if:

- Gas symptoms bother you

- Your symptoms change suddenly
- You have other symptoms with gas—such as constipation, diarrhea, or weight loss

What Causes Gas

Gas normally enters your digestive tract when you swallow air and when bacteria in your large intestine break down certain undigested foods. You may have more gas in your digestive tract if you swallow more air or eat certain foods.

Swallowed Air

Everyone swallows a small amount of air when eating and drinking. You swallow more air when you:

- Chew gum
- Drink carbonated, or fizzy, drinks
- Eat or drink too fast
- Smoke
- Suck on hard candy
- Wear loose-fitting dentures

Swallowed air that doesn't leave your stomach by burping moves into your intestines and passes through your anus.

Bacteria in Your Large Intestine

Your stomach and small intestine don't fully digest some of the carbohydrates—sugars, starches, and fiber—in the food you eat. Undigested carbohydrates will pass to your large intestine, which contains bacteria. These bacteria break down undigested carbohydrates and create gas in the process.

What Foods, Drinks, or Products Cause Gas?

A variety of foods, drinks, and products can cause gas. See the following table for examples.

Table 3.1. Examples of Foods, Drinks, and Products That Can Cause Gas

Foods		
Vegetables	**Fruits**	**Milk Products**
Asparagus	Apples	Cheese
Artichokes	Peaches	Ice cream
Black beans	Pears	Yogurt
Broccoli	**Whole Grains**	**Packaged Foods with Lactose**
Brussels Sprouts	Bran	Bread
Cabbage	Whole wheat	Cereal
Cauliflower		Salad dressing
Kidney beans		
Mushrooms		
Navy beans		
Onions		
Pinto beans		
Drinks		
Apple juice	Carbonated drinks	Fruit drinks (such as fruit punch)
Pear juice	Drinks with high-fructose Corn syrup	Milk
Products		
Sugar-Free Products with Sorbitol, Mannitol, or Xylitol		
Candies		
Gum		
Dietary Supplements and Additives		
Certain types of fiber, such as inulin and fructo-oligosaccharide, that may be added to processed foods to replace fat or sugar fiber supplements		

What Conditions Cause Excess Gas or Increase Gas Symptoms?

Some conditions can cause you to have more gas than usual or have more symptoms when you have gas. These conditions include the following:

Small Intestinal Bacterial Overgrowth

Small intestinal bacterial overgrowth is an increase in the number of bacteria or a change in the type of bacteria in your small intestine. These bacteria can produce extra gas and may also cause diarrhea and weight loss. Small intestinal bacterial overgrowth is most often a complication of other conditions.

Irritable Bowel Syndrome (IBS)

Irritable bowel syndrome (IBS) is a group of symptoms—including pain or discomfort in your abdomen and changes in your bowel movement patterns—that occur together. IBS can affect how gas moves through your intestines. You may also feel bloated due to increased sensitivity to normal amounts of gas.

Gastroesophageal Reflux Disease (GERD)

Gastroesophageal reflux disease (GERD) is a chronic condition that occurs when stomach contents flow back up into your esophagus. People with GERD may burp a lot to relieve discomfort.

Problems Digesting Carbohydrates

Problems digesting carbohydrates that can lead to gas and bloating include:

- Lactose intolerance, a condition in which you have digestive symptoms such as bloating, gas, or diarrhea after eating or drinking milk or milk products

- Dietary fructose intolerance, a condition in which you have digestive symptoms such as bloating, gas, or diarrhea after consuming foods that contain fructose

- Celiac disease, an immune disorder in which you cannot tolerate gluten, a protein found in wheat, rye, barley, and some products such as lip balm and cosmetics. If you have celiac disease, gluten damages the lining of your small intestine.

Conditions That Affect How Gas Moves through Your Intestines

Conditions that affect how gas moves through your intestines can lead to problems with gas and bloating. These conditions include dumping syndrome, abdominal adhesions, abdominal hernias, and conditions that can cause an intestinal obstruction such as colon cancer or ovarian cancer.

How Do Doctors Diagnose the Cause of Gas?

Doctors may diagnose the causes of excess gas or increased gas symptoms with a medical history and physical exam. If your doctor thinks you may have a condition that causes excess gas or increases gas symptoms, he or she may order more tests.

Medical History

For a medical history, your doctor will ask about:

- Your symptoms
- Your eating habits
- Prescription and over-the-counter (OTC) medicines you take
- Current and past medical conditions

Your doctor may ask you to keep a diary of the food you eat and when your gas symptoms occur. Your diary may show specific foods that are causing gas. Reviewing your diary may also help your doctor find out if you have more gas or are more sensitive to normal amounts of gas.

Physical Exam

During a physical exam, a doctor typically

- checks for bloating or swelling in your abdomen
- listens to sounds within your abdomen using a stethoscope
- taps on your abdomen to check for tenderness or pain

How Can I Reduce or Prevent Excess Gas?

To reduce or prevent excess gas and gas symptoms, your doctor may suggest the following:

Swallow Less Air

Your doctor may suggest that you take steps to swallow less air. For example, eat more slowly, avoid gum and hard candies, and don't use a straw. If you wear dentures, check with your dentist to make sure they fit correctly. Swallowing less air may help ease gas symptoms, especially if you burp a lot.

Quit Smoking

If you smoke, quit smoking. Your doctor can help you find ways to quit smoking. Studies show that people who get help quitting have a better chance of succeeding.

Change Your Diet

To reduce gas, your doctor may suggest you eat smaller, more frequent meals and eat less of the foods that give you gas.

Take Medicines

Some OTC medicines may reduce gas or gas symptoms:

- Alpha-galactosidase (Beano, Gas-Zyme 3x) contains the enzyme the body lacks to digest sugars in beans, grains, and many vegetables. You can take this enzyme just before eating to break down gas-producing sugars. Doctors recommend the enzyme for adults and for children ages 12 and older.

- Simethicone (Gas-X, Mylanta Gas) can relieve gas-related bloating and pain or discomfort in your abdomen by helping gas pass through your digestive tract. Doctors may recommend simethicone for infants and children.

- Lactase tablets and drops are available for people with lactose intolerance. The lactase enzyme digests the lactose in the food or drink and reduces the chances of developing symptoms such as bloating, gas, or diarrhea. Lactose-free and lactose-reduced milk and milk products are available at most supermarkets and are identical nutritionally to regular milk and milk products. Check with your doctor before using lactase products. Some people, such as children younger than age 3 and pregnant and breastfeeding women, may not be able to take these products.

For safety reasons, talk with your doctor before using supplements or any complementary or alternative medicines or medical practices. Your doctor may prescribe medicines to help reduce gas or gas symptoms, especially if you have small intestinal bacterial overgrowth or irritable bowel syndrome.

What Should I Avoid Eating to Reduce Gas?

You may be able to reduce gas by avoiding or eating less of the foods that give you gas. You can keep a food diary to help figure out which foods give you gas and how much of the gas-producing foods you can handle.

You may try avoiding or limiting:

- Carbonated, or fizzy, drinks

- Fried and high-fat foods

- High-fiber foods for a few weeks and then slowly increasing your daily fiber intake

- Sugar

If your doctor diagnoses you with celiac disease, your doctor will recommend a gluten-free diet. Most people with celiac disease see a big improvement in their symptoms when they follow a gluten-free diet. If your doctor diagnoses you with lactose intolerance, your doctor may recommend limiting how much lactose you eat or drink. Many people can manage the symptoms of lactose intolerance by changing their diet.

If your doctor diagnoses you with irritable bowel syndrome, your doctor may recommend trying a special diet—called Low Fermentable Oligosaccharides, Disaccharides, Monosaccharides, and Polyols or FODMAP. If you follow this diet, you avoid or eat less of certain foods— called high FODMAP foods—that contain carbohydrates that are hard to digest. Examples of high FODMAP foods include certain fruits and vegetables, dairy products, wheat and rye products, and foods that contain certain types of sweeteners.

Section 3.3

Abdominal Pain

"Abdominal Pain," © 2016 Omnigraphics.
Reviewed September 2018.

Commonly known as stomach pain, tummy ache, belly ache, or cramps, abdominal pain refers to a minor or major ache or discomfort in the stomach area (from below the chest to the pelvic area). It is quite common, and most adults have experienced abdominal pain at some point in their lives. However, abdominal pain is also among the most misdiagnosed conditions in emergency rooms. Stomach discomfort encompasses a wide variety of symptoms that can indicate more than one condition and thus can be misleading. For instance, a severe pain or feeling of bloating in the belly may have a cause that is relatively harmless, such as indigestion or menstrual cramping. On the other hand, a minor ache may disguise a serious condition, such as appendicitis. Therefore, it is important to distinguish between the different kinds of abdominal pain and seek medical care when required.

What Are the Types of Abdominal Pain?

There are several different types of abdominal pain, each of which may indicate a different set of possible medical conditions.

Sharp and Local Pain

This type of pain is probably the most serious and may require immediate medical attention. It occurs as an intense ache in a particular part of the stomach and may result from inflammation or trauma to an internal organ. Among the common conditions that cause sharp, localized pain are appendicitis, pancreatitis, diverticulitis, hernia, and colon cancer.

Dull Ache

This type of pain is common and usually felt over a large part of the belly. The likely causes include indigestion, gas, or a stomach virus.

Cramping

This type of pain is usually a result of gas in the intestinal tract and is not generally worrisome unless it persists for a few days or is accompanied by diarrhea, vomiting, or fever. In this case, it may be food poisoning or gastroenteritis—intestinal inflammation caused by a virus, bacterium, or parasite.

Pain That Comes and Goes

This kind of pain mostly occurs in the upper abdomen. It is usually intense and may start and stop suddenly. Possible causes include kidney stones or gallstones, which require immediate medical attention.

What Are the Causes of Abdominal Pain?

A host of conditions can result in abdominal pain. Many of the possible causes are simple problems like overeating, constipation, gas, or nerves, and the symptoms may disappear by themselves over a short period of time. Sometimes, however, abdominal pain may signal a critical condition that warrants urgent medical attention. Some of the more serious causes of abdominal pain may include food allergies, appendicitis, pancreatitis, diverticulitis, irritable bowel syndrome (IBS), kidney stones, gallstones, ulcers, colon cancer, or pregnancy-related complications. Abdominal pain occasionally may be related to problems outside the abdomen. Stomach aches can be a symptom of heart attack, pneumonia, or problems in the pelvis or groin.

It can be difficult to determine whether abdominal pain is symptomatic of a more serious medical condition. A person who experiences any of the following conditions should contact their medical practitioner:

- Your belly feels rigid and is overly sensitive to touch. You also have a fever and are vomiting blood, passing dark, tarry stools, or have bloody diarrhea. These symptoms could be a sign of appendicitis, diverticulitis, or bowel obstruction.

- You have sudden, intense pain in the back that slowly descends to the groin. It could be a sign of a kidney- or bladder-related complication.

- You are pregnant and have abdominal pain along with bleeding or vaginal discharge. You may be having a miscarriage or a tubal pregnancy.

- You have pain in the lower right abdomen and are passing stools tinged with blood or mucus. It may be due to inflammation of the colon or large intestine.

- Your pain starts in the upper abdomen and moves around to the back, or the pain is more pronounced after a fatty meal. These symptoms may indicate gallstones.

- You have mild pain in the lower abdomen and discomfort or a burning sensation while urinating. These could be signs of a urinary tract infection called cystitis.

- You are a woman and have a constant, dull ache in the lower abdomen along with vaginal discharge. These symptoms may indicate pelvic inflammatory disease (PID), an infection surrounding the ovaries, uterus, and fallopian tubes.

- You have diarrhea along with fever, nausea, or vomiting that lasts more than two days. It may be a case of gastroenteritis. Although most people recover without treatment, prolonged gastroenteritis can lead to dehydration, especially in children.

What Is the Diagnosis of Abdominal Pain?

To diagnose a patient suffering from abdominal pain, a medical practitioner will take a medical history, perform a physical examination, and conduct investigative tests based on presenting symptoms in order to determine the underlying cause.

When taking the patient's history, the physician will inquire about the nature of the pain (sharp or dull, localized or general), its location, timing (before or after a meal, or related to a particular activity), and duration, past occurrences and symptoms, and factors that aggravate or alleviate the pain. It is important that patients provide accurate information in their case histories.

During the physical examination, the physician will feel the patient's abdomen for signs of tenderness or rigidity. The pelvis and rectum may also be examined for blood or other abnormalities. Next, the physician may order diagnostic tests to pinpoint or rule out certain conditions. Some of the tests that may be conducted include ultrasound, X-ray, computed tomography (CT) scan, endoscopy, colonoscopy, blood tests, urine or stool examination, electrocardiogram (ECG), or barium enema.

Special Cases of Abdominal Pain

The diagnosis and treatment of abdominal pain may vary depending on the patient's age, gender, and underlying health conditions. Some circumstances that can affect the causes and symptoms of abdominal pain include:

- **During pregnancy:** Most pregnant women feel some kind of abdominal pain as a consequence of the physiological and hormonal changes that occur during pregnancy. Although it is usually mild and harmless, severe or prolonged pain—or pain accompanied by bleeding—could be an indication of a life-threatening complication such as preeclampsia, miscarriage, or ectopic pregnancy. Immediate medical attention is required in such cases.

- **In infants:** Abdominal pain with gas may be a result of colic. Other signs of colic include fussiness, inconsolable crying, and pulling the legs up to the abdomen. Though distressful, colic is a relatively harmless condition that goes away as the child gets older. It is important to consult a pediatrician, however, to rule out any other causes of abdominal pain.

- **In children:** Stomach aches are quite common among young children and are usually a result of minor ailments like constipation, gas, or stomach flu. In these cases, the symptoms generally go away on their own within a few days. However, if the pain worsens with time, or if the child also has fever and nausea, it could be a sign of something more serious that warrants medical attention.

- **In teenage girls:** Sharp pain or dull aches in the lower abdomen or lower back may be related to menstrual cramps.

- **In cancer patients:** People undergoing chemotherapy for cancer treatment may often feel cramping or dull aches in the abdomen because chemotherapy affects the working of the intestines. It can either slow down or speed up the passage of stool through the bowel, thereby causing constipation or diarrhea and resulting in cramping. Chemotherapy also affects digestion and can cause gas. Some cancer medications can also cause ulcers or other abdominal complications. Cancer patients should seek medical attention if the pain is severe and prolonged, and accompanied by other symptoms like fever, vomiting, or sudden swelling of the abdomen.

- **Peritonitis:** A serious condition involving inflammation or infection of the tissue lining the inner wall of the abdominal cavity. It can be caused by the perforation or rupture of an abdominal organ or the leakage of bodily fluids like blood, urine, or gastric juices into the peritoneal cavity. Left untreated, peritonitis can cause potentially fatal damage to the liver, kidneys, and other organs. Symptoms of peritonitis include constant, severe abdominal pain that is aggravated by a slight touch or impact.

How to Prevent and Treat Abdominal Pain

To prevent indigestion and abdominal pain, it is important to drink plenty of water and limit the consumption of carbonated beverages. Since dietary fiber aids in digestion and helps prevent constipation, a diet rich in whole grains, fruits, and vegetables can also help people avoid stomach aches. Other tips include eating small meals at regular intervals rather than overeating at a single meal, and limiting the intake of fatty, greasy, and high-sodium foods.

There are a variety of home remedies and over-the-counter (OTC) medications available to provide relief from abdominal pain caused by indigestion or constipation. Additional treatments include lying down and taking deep breaths, placing a heating pad or hot water bottle on the belly, and eating mild foods like bananas, rice, applesauce, and toast. It is important to avoid taking aspirin or other anti-inflammatory drugs, unless prescribed by a doctor, as they may irritate the stomach and worsen symptoms.

References

1. "Abdominal Pain, Short-term," FamilyDoctor.org, American Academy of Family Physicians (AAFP), 1996.

2. "Abdominal Pain," MedlinePlus, U.S. National Library of Medicine (NLM), 2014.

Section 3.4

Diarrhea

This section includes text excerpted from "Diarrhea," National Institute of Diabetes and Digestive and Kidney Diseases (NIDDK), November 2016.

What Is Diarrhea?

Diarrhea is loose, watery stools three or more times a day. Diarrhea may be acute, persistent, or chronic:

- Acute diarrhea is a common problem that typically lasts one or two days and goes away on its own.
- Persistent diarrhea lasts longer than two weeks and less than four weeks.
- Chronic diarrhea lasts at least four weeks. Chronic diarrhea symptoms may be continual or may come and go.

How Common Is Diarrhea?

Diarrhea is a common problem. Acute diarrhea is more common than persistent or chronic diarrhea. Researchers estimate that about

179 million cases of acute diarrhea occur in the United States each year.

What Are the Complications of Diarrhea?
Dehydration

Diarrhea may cause dehydration, which means your body lacks enough fluid and electrolytes to work properly. Your body loses more fluid and electrolytes in loose stools than solid stools.

Malabsorption

Diarrhea may cause malabsorption. If people do not absorb enough nutrients from the food they eat, they may become malnourished. Certain conditions that cause chronic diarrhea—such as infections, food allergies and intolerances, and certain digestive tract problems—may also cause malabsorption.

What Are the Symptoms of Diarrhea?

The main symptom of diarrhea is passing loose, watery stools three or more times a day. People with diarrhea may also have one or more of the following symptoms:

- An urgent need to use the bathroom
- Cramping
- Loss of control of bowel movements
- Nausea
- Pain in the abdomen

People with diarrhea caused by some infections may also have one or more of the following symptoms:

- Bloody stools
- Fever and chills
- Light-headedness and dizziness
- Vomiting

Diarrhea may cause dehydration and malabsorption.

How Do Doctors Find the Cause of Diarrhea?

Doctors do not typically need to find a cause of acute diarrhea. If your diarrhea lasts longer than four days or you have symptoms such as fever or bloody stools, your doctor may need to find the cause. Your doctor may use information from your medical and family history, a physical exam, or tests to find the cause of your diarrhea.

Medical and Family History

Your doctor will ask for information about your symptoms, such as:

- How long you have had diarrhea
- How much stool you have passed
- How often you have diarrhea
- How your stool looks, such as color or consistency
- Whether you have other symptoms along with diarrhea

Your doctor will ask about the foods you eat and the beverages you drink. If your doctor suspects you have a food allergy or intolerance, he or she may recommend that you change what you eat to see if your symptoms improve.

Your doctor will also ask about:

- Current and past medical conditions
- Prescription and over-the-counter (OTC) medicines
- Recent contact with other people who are sick
- Recent travel to developing countries

Your doctor may ask whether anyone in your family has a history of conditions that cause chronic diarrhea, such as celiac disease, Crohn disease, irritable bowel syndrome (IBS), lactose intolerance, and ulcerative colitis (UC).

Physical Exam

During a physical exam, your doctor may:

- check your blood pressure and pulse for signs of dehydration
- examine your body for signs of fever or dehydration

33

- use a stethoscope to listen to sounds in your abdomen

- tap on your abdomen to check for tenderness or pain

Sometimes, doctors perform a digital rectal exam. Your doctor will have you bend over a table or lie on your side while holding your knees close to your chest. After putting on a glove, the doctor will slide a lubricated finger into your anus to check for blood in your stool.

What Tests Do Doctors Use to Find the Cause of Diarrhea?

Your doctor may use the following tests to help find the cause of your diarrhea:

- Stool test

- Blood tests

- Hydrogen breath test (HBT)

- Fasting tests

- Endoscopy

How Do Doctors Treat Diarrhea?

Doctors may prescribe antibiotics and medicines that target parasites to treat bacterial or parasitic infections. Doctors may also prescribe medicines to treat some of the conditions that cause chronic diarrhea, such as Crohn disease, irritable bowel syndrome, or ulcerative colitis. How doctors treat chronic diarrhea in children also depends on the cause. Doctors may recommend probiotics. Probiotics are live microorganisms, most often bacteria, that are similar to microorganisms you normally have in your digestive tract. Researchers are still studying the use of probiotics to treat diarrhea. For safety reasons, talk with your doctor before using probiotics or any other complementary or alternative medicines or practices. If your doctor recommends probiotics, talk with him or her about how much probiotics you should take and for how long.

How Can I Prevent Diarrhea?

You can prevent certain types of diarrhea, such as those caused by infections—including rotavirus and traveler's diarrhea—and foodborne illnesses.

Infections

You can reduce your chances of getting or spreading infections that can cause diarrhea by washing your hands thoroughly with soap and warm water for 15–30 seconds:

- After using the bathroom
- After changing diapers
- Before and after handling or preparing food

Rotavirus, which causes viral gastroenteritis, was the most common cause of diarrhea in infants before rotavirus vaccines became available. The vaccines have reduced the number of cases of rotavirus and hospitalizations due to rotavirus among children in the United States.

Two oral vaccines are approved to protect children from rotavirus infections:

- Rotavirus vaccine, live, oral, pentavalent (RotaTeq). Doctors give infants this vaccine in three doses: At two months of age, four months of age, and six months of age.
- Rotavirus vaccine, live, oral (Rotarix). Doctors give infants this vaccine in two doses: At two months of age and at four months of age.

For the rotavirus vaccine to be effective, infants should receive all doses by 8 months of age. Infants 15 weeks of age or older who have never received the rotavirus vaccine should not start the series.

Parents or caregivers of infants should discuss rotavirus vaccination with a doctor.

Travelers' Diarrhea

To reduce the chances of getting travelers' diarrhea when traveling to developing countries, avoid:

- drinking tap water
- using tap water to make ice, prepare foods or drinks, or brush your teeth
- drinking juice or milk or eating milk products that have not been pasteurized—heated to kill harmful microbes: viruses, bacteria, and parasites
- eating food from street vendors

- eating meat, fish, or shellfish that is raw, undercooked, or not served hot

- eating raw vegetables and most raw fruits

You can drink bottled water, soft drinks, and hot drinks such as coffee or tea made with boiling water. If you are worried about travelers' diarrhea, talk with your doctor before traveling. Doctors may recommend taking antibiotics before and during a trip to help prevent travelers' diarrhea. Early treatment with antibiotics can shorten a case of travelers' diarrhea.

Foodborne Illnesses

You can prevent foodborne illnesses that cause diarrhea by properly storing, cooking, cleaning, and handling foods.

What Should I Eat If I Have Diarrhea?

If you have diarrhea, you may lose your appetite for a short time. In most cases, when your appetite returns, you can go back to eating your normal diet. Parents and caretakers should give children with diarrhea their usual age-appropriate diet and give infants breast milk or formula. Your doctor may recommend changing your diet to treat some causes of chronic diarrhea, such as lactose intolerance or celiac disease.

What Should I Avoid Eating If I Have Diarrhea?

You should avoid foods that may make your diarrhea worse, such as:

- Alcoholic beverages
- Drinks and foods containing caffeine
- Dairy products such as milk, cheese, and ice cream
- Fatty and greasy foods
- Drinks and foods containing fructose
- Fruits such as apples, peaches, and pears
- Spicy foods
- Diet drinks and sugarless gum and candies containing sweeteners such as sorbitol, mannitol, and xylitol

Research shows that following a restricted diet does not help treat diarrhea in most cases. Most experts do not recommend fasting or following a restricted diet when you have diarrhea.

Section 3.5

Constipation

This section includes text excerpted from "Constipation," National Institute of Diabetes and Digestive and Kidney Diseases (NIDDK), May 2018.

What Is Constipation?

Constipation is a condition in which you may have:

- Fewer than three bowel movements a week
- Stools that are hard, dry, or lumpy
- Stools that are difficult or painful to pass
- A feeling that not all stool has passed

However, people can have different bowel movement patterns, and only you know what's normal for you. Constipation is not a disease, but may be a symptom of another medical problem. Constipation may last for a short or long time.

How Common Is Constipation?

Constipation is common among all ages and populations in the United States. About 16 out of 100 adults have symptoms of constipation. About 33 out of 100 adults ages 60 and older have symptoms of constipation.

Who Is More Likely to Become Constipated?

Certain people are more likely to become constipated, including:

- Women, especially during pregnancy or after giving birth

- Older adults
- Non-Caucasians
- People who eat little to no fiber
- People who take certain medicines or dietary supplements
- People with certain health problems, including functional gastrointestinal disorders

What Are the Complications of Constipation?

People who have constipation that lasts for a short time usually do not have complications. However, long-lasting constipation may have complications, including:

- Hemorrhoids
- Anal fissures
- Rectal prolapse
- Fecal impaction

What Are the Symptoms of Constipation?

Symptoms of constipation may include:

- Fewer than three bowel movements a week
- Stools that are hard, dry, or lumpy
- Stools that are difficult or painful to pass
- A feeling that not all stool has passed

When Should I See a Doctor?

You should see a doctor if your symptoms do not go away with self-care or you have a family history of colon or rectal cancer. You should see a doctor right away if you have constipation and any of the following symptoms:

- Bleeding from your rectum
- Blood in your stool
- Constant pain in your abdomen
- Inability to pass gas

- Vomiting

- Fever

- Lower back pain

- Losing weight without trying

What Causes Constipation

You may be constipated for many reasons, and constipation may have more than one cause at a time. Causes of constipation may include:

- Slow movement of stool through your colon

- Delayed emptying of the colon from pelvic floor disorders, especially in women, and colon surgery

- Functional gastrointestinal disorders, such as irritable bowel syndrome

Certain Medicines and Dietary Supplements

Medicines and dietary supplements that can make constipation worse include:

- Antacids that contain aluminum and calcium

- Anticholinergics and antispasmodics

- Anticonvulsants—used to prevent seizures

- Calcium channel blockers

- Diuretics

- Iron supplements

- Medicines used to treat Parkinson disease (PD)

- Narcotic pain medicines

- Some medicines used to treat depression

Life Changes or Daily Routine Changes

Constipation can happen when your life or daily routine changes. For example, your bowel movements can change:

- if you become pregnant

- as you get older

- when you travel
- when you ignore the urge to have a bowel movement
- if you change your medicines
- if you change how much and what you eat

Certain Health and Nutrition Problems

Certain health and nutrition problems can cause constipation. They are:

- not eating enough fiber
- not drinking enough liquids or dehydration
- not getting enough physical activity
- celiac disease
- disorders that affect your brain and spine, such as Parkinson disease
- spinal cord or brain injuries
- conditions that affect your metabolism, such as diabetes
- conditions that affect your hormones, such as hypothyroidism
- inflammation linked to diverticular disease or proctitis
- intestinal obstructions, including anorectal blockage and tumors
- anatomic problems of your digestive tract

How Do Doctors Find the Cause of Constipation?

Doctors use your medical and family history, a physical exam, or medical tests to diagnose and find the cause of your constipation.

Medical and Family History

Your doctor will ask you questions about your medical history, such as:

- Whether you have ever had surgery to your digestive tract
- If you have recently lost or gained weight
- If you have a history of anemia

Your doctor also is likely to ask questions about your symptoms, such as:

- How often do you have a bowel movement?
- How long have you had symptoms?
- What do your stools look like?
- Do your stools have red streaks in them?
- Are there streaks of blood on your toilet paper when you wipe?

Your doctor is likely to ask questions about your routines, such as:

- What are your eating habits?
- What is your level of physical activity?
- What medicines, including supplements, and complementary and alternative medicines, do you take?

You may want to track your bowel movements and what your stools look like for several days or weeks before your doctor's visit. Write down or record the information so you can share it with your doctor.

If you've been constipated a long time, your healthcare professional may ask whether anyone in your family has a history of conditions that may cause long-lasting constipation, such as:

- Anatomic problems of the digestive tract
- Intestinal obstruction
- Diverticular disease
- Colon or rectal cancer

Physical Exam

During a physical exam, a healthcare professional may:

- Check your blood pressure, temperature, and heart rate
- Check for dehydration
- Use a stethoscope to listen to sounds in your abdomen
- Check your abdomen for:
  - Swelling
  - Tenderness or pain
  - Masses, or lumps
- Perform a rectal exam

What Medical Tests Do Doctors Use to Find the Cause of Constipation?

Depending on your symptoms and health, your doctor may first try a treatment to improve your symptoms before using tests.

Lab Tests

Your doctor may use one or more of the following lab tests to look for signs of certain diseases and conditions that may be causing your constipation.

- Blood tests can show signs of anemia, hypothyroidism, and celiac disease.

- Stool tests can show the presence of blood and signs of infection and inflammation.

- Urine tests can show signs of diseases such as diabetes.

Endoscopy

Your doctor may perform an endoscopy to look inside your anus, rectum, and colon for signs of problems in your lower digestive tract. Endoscopies for constipation include:

- Colonoscopy

- Flexible sigmoidoscopy

During these two tests, your doctor may also perform a biopsy. A biopsy is a procedure that involves taking small pieces of tissue and examining them under a microscope. A doctor can use a biopsy to look for signs of cancer or other problems.

Colorectal Transit Studies

Your doctor may use bowel function tests called colorectal transit studies to see how well your stool moves through your colon.

- Radiopaque markers—an X-ray that tracks radioactive markers while they pass through your digestive system. You swallow capsules with the markers, which take about 3–7 days to come out with a bowel movement.

- Scintigraphy—a test that involves eating a meal with a small dose of a radioactive substance. Your doctor tracks the substance using special computers and cameras as the substance passes through your intestines.

Other Bowel Function Tests

Your doctor may also use one or more of the following tests to look for signs of certain diseases and conditions that may be causing your constipation:

- Defecography—an X-ray of the area around the anus and rectum to see how well you can hold and release stool

- Anorectal manometry—a test to check how sensitive your rectum is, how well it works, and how well the anal sphincters work

- Balloon expulsion test—a test that involves pushing a small water balloon from your rectum to see if you have a problem pushing out stool

Imaging Tests

To look for other problems that may be causing your constipation, your doctor may perform an imaging test such as:

- Lower gastrointestinal (GI) series

- Magnetic resonance imaging (MRI)

- Computed tomography (CT) scan

How Can I Treat My Constipation?

You can most often treat your constipation at home by doing the following:

Change What You Eat and Drink

Changing what you eat and drink may make your stools softer and easier to pass. To help relieve your symptoms:

- eat more high-fiber foods

- drink plenty of water and other liquids if you eat more fiber or take a fiber supplement

Read about what you should eat and drink to help relieve constipation. Depending on your age and sex, adults should get 25–31 grams of fiber a day.

Get Regular Physical Activity

Getting regular physical activity may help relieve your symptoms.

Try Bowel Training

Your doctor may suggest that you try to train yourself to have a bowel movement at the same time each day to help you become more regular. For example, trying to have a bowel movement 15–45 minutes after breakfast may help, because eating helps your colon move stool. Make sure you give yourself enough time to have a bowel movement, and use the bathroom as soon as you feel the need to go. Try to relax your muscles or put your feet on a footstool to make yourself more comfortable.

Stop Taking Certain Medicines or Dietary Supplements

If you think certain medicines or dietary supplements are causing your constipation, talk with your doctor. He or she may change the dose or suggest a different medicine that does not cause constipation. Don't change or stop any medicine or supplement without talking with a healthcare professional.

Take Over-the-Counter (OTC) Medicines

Your healthcare professional may recommend using a laxative for a short time. He or she will tell you what type of laxative is best for you:

- Bulk-forming agents (Citrucel, FiberCon)
- Osmotic agents (Milk of Magnesia, Miralax)
- Stool softeners (Colace, Docusate)
- Lubricants, such as mineral oil (Fleet)
- Stimulants (Correctol, Dulcolax)

You should only use stimulants if your constipation is severe or other treatments have not worked. If you've been taking laxatives for a long time and can't have a bowel movement without taking a laxative, talk with your doctor about how you can slowly stop using them. If you stop taking laxatives, over time, your colon should start moving stool normally.

How Do Doctors Treat Constipation?

If self-care treatments don't work, your doctor may prescribe a medicine to treat your constipation. If you're taking an over-the-counter (OTC) or prescription medicine or supplement that can cause constipation, your doctor may suggest you stop taking it, change the dose, or switch to a different one. Talk with your doctor before changing or stopping any medicines.

Prescription Medicines

Your doctor may prescribe one of the following medicines for constipation:

- Lubiprostone—a medicine prescribed to increase fluid in your digestive tract, which can help reduce pain in your abdomen, make your stool softer, and increase how often you have bowel movements

- Linaclotide or plecanatide—medicines that help make your bowel movements regular if you have irritable bowel syndrome with constipation or long-lasting constipation without a known cause

Biofeedback Therapy

If you have problems with the muscles that control bowel movements, your doctor may recommend biofeedback therapy to retrain your muscles. By using biofeedback therapy, you can change how you make your muscles work.

Surgery

Your doctor may recommend surgery to treat an anorectal blockage caused by rectal prolapse if other treatments don't work. Your doctor may perform surgery to remove your colon if your colon muscles don't work correctly. If your doctor recommends surgery, ask about the benefits and risks.

How Can I Prevent Constipation?

You can help prevent constipation by doing some of the same things that treat constipation:

- Get enough fiber in your diet.

- Drink plenty of water and other liquids.

- Get regular physical activity.

- Try to have a bowel movement at the same time every day.

What Should I Eat and Drink If I'm Constipated?

Eat enough fiber. Drink plenty of liquids to help the fiber work better.

Fiber

Depending on your age and sex, adults should get 25–31 grams of fiber a day. Older adults sometimes don't get enough fiber because they may lose interest in food.

Talk with a healthcare professional, such as a dietitian, to plan meals with the right amount of fiber for you. Be sure to add fiber to your diet a little at a time so your body gets used to the change.

Good sources of fiber are:

- Whole grains, such as whole wheat bread and pasta, oatmeal, and bran flake cereals

- Legumes, such as lentils, black beans, kidney beans, soybeans, and chickpeas

- Fruits, such as berries, apples with the skin on, oranges, and pears

- Vegetables, such as carrots, broccoli, green peas, and collard greens

- Nuts, such as almonds, peanuts, and pecans

Plenty of Water

You should drink water and other liquids, such as naturally sweetened fruit and vegetable juices and clear soups, to help the fiber work better. This change should make your stools softer and easier to pass. Drinking enough water and other liquids is also a good way to avoid dehydration. Staying hydrated is good for your overall health and can help you avoid getting constipated. Ask a healthcare professional how much liquid you should drink each day based on your size, health, activity level, and where you live.

What Should I Avoid Eating or Drinking If I'm Constipated?

To help prevent or relieve constipation, avoid foods with little to no fiber, such as:

- Chips

- Fast food

- Meat

- Prepared foods, such as some frozen meals and snack foods

- Processed foods, such as hot dogs or some microwavable dinners

Section 3.6

Fecal Incontinence

This section includes text excerpted from "Bowel Control Problems (Fecal Incontinence)," National Institute of Diabetes and Digestive and Kidney Diseases (NIDDK), July 2017.

What Is Fecal Incontinence?

Fecal incontinence, also called accidental bowel leakage, is the accidental passing of bowel movements—including solid stools, liquid stools, or mucus—from your anus. The most common type of fecal incontinence is called urge incontinence. When you have urge incontinence, you feel a strong urge to have a bowel movement but cannot stop it before reaching a toilet. If you have urge incontinence, your pelvic floor muscles may be too weak to hold back a bowel movement due to muscle injury or nerve damage.

Another type of fecal incontinence is called passive incontinence. When you have passive incontinence, leakage occurs without you knowing it. If you have passive incontinence, your body may not be able to sense when your rectum is full. Fecal incontinence can be upsetting and embarrassing. Some people may feel ashamed and try to hide the problem. You may be afraid or embarrassed to talk about

47

fecal incontinence with your doctor. However, talking openly and honestly with your doctor is important in diagnosing and treating your fecal incontinence.

Fecal incontinence is also called:

- Accidental bowel leakage

- Bowel incontinence

- Encopresis—a term used mostly for fecal incontinence in children

How Common Is Fecal Incontinence?

Medical experts consider fecal incontinence a common problem, affecting about one in three people who see a primary healthcare provider.

- Fecal incontinence is more common in older adults.

- Among adults who are not in hospitals or nursing homes, between 7 and 15 out of 100 have fecal incontinence.

- Among adults who are in hospitals, between 18 and 33 out of 100 have fecal incontinence.

- Among adults who are in nursing homes, between 50 and 70 out of 100 have fecal incontinence.

Fecal incontinence occurs in about 2 out of 100 children.

Who Is More Likely to Have Fecal Incontinence?

You may be more likely to have fecal incontinence if you:

- are older than age 65

- are not physically active

- have certain chronic diseases, medical conditions, or health problems

- have had your gallbladder removed

- are a current smoker

Children who were born with certain birth defects of the spinal cord, anus, or rectum are more likely to have fecal incontinence. Children who are constipated are also more likely to have fecal incontinence.

What Other Health Problems Do People with Fecal Incontinence Have?

If you have fecal incontinence, you may also have other health problems, including:

- Diarrhea
- Poor overall health
- Chronic diseases and disorders such as:
  - Irritable bowel syndrome (IBS)
  - Type 2 diabetes
  - Diseases that affect the nerves of your anus, pelvic floor, or rectum
  - Inflammatory bowel disease (IBD)
- Damage to or weakness of the muscles of your anus, pelvic floor, or rectum
- Damage to the nerves in your anus, pelvic floor, or rectum
- Urinary incontinence
- Proctitis

What Problems May Fecal Incontinence Cause?

The problems that fecal incontinence may cause include:

- Discomfort or irritation of the skin around the anus
- Emotional and social distress, such as fear, embarrassment, social isolation, loss of self-esteem, anger, or depression
- Quality of life (QOL) issues, such as not being able to exercise, work, attend school, or go to social gatherings

What Are the Symptoms of Fecal Incontinence?

The symptoms of fecal incontinence depend on the type.

- If you have urge fecal incontinence, you will know when you need to pass stool but not be able to control passing stool before reaching a toilet.
- If you have passive fecal incontinence, you will pass stool or mucus from your anus without knowing it.

Some medical experts include streaks or stains of stool or mucus on your underwear—called soiling—as a symptom of fecal incontinence.

When Should I See a Doctor for Fecal Incontinence?

You should see a doctor if your fecal incontinence is frequent or severe. Although some people are able to manage mild or infrequent fecal incontinence on their own, you should see a doctor if your fecal incontinence is affecting your QOL or causing emotional or social distress.

What Causes Fecal Incontinence

Fecal incontinence has many causes, including digestive tract disorders and chronic diseases. Some causes of fecal incontinence, such as childbirth by vaginal delivery, happen only in women.

Diarrhea

Loose, watery stools from diarrhea fill your rectum quickly and are harder to hold in than solid stools. Diarrhea is the most common risk factor for fecal incontinence for people not staying in hospitals, nursing homes, or other similar institutions. Diarrhea may be caused by digestive tract problems such as:

- Inflammatory bowel disease (IBD)
- Irritable bowel syndrome (IBS)
- Proctitis

Constipation

Constipation can lead to large, hard stools that are difficult to pass. The hard stools stretch and, over time, weaken the muscles in your rectum. The weakened muscles let watery stools that build up behind the hard stool leak out.

Muscle Injury or Weakness

If the muscles in your anus, pelvic floor, or rectum are injured or weakened, they may not be able to keep your anus closed, letting stool leak out. These muscles can be injured or weakened by:

- Surgery to:
  - Remove cancer in the anus or rectum

50

- Remove hemorrhoids
- Treat anal abscesses and fistulas
- Trauma

Nerve Damage

If the nerves that control your anus, pelvic floor, and rectum are damaged, the muscles can't work the way they should. Damage to the nerves that tell you when there is stool in your rectum makes it hard to know when you need to look for a toilet. Nerves can be damaged by:

- A long-term habit of straining to pass stool
- Brain injury
- Spinal cord injury (SCI)

Neurologic Diseases

Neurologic diseases that affect the nerves of the anus, pelvic floor, or rectum can cause fecal incontinence. These diseases include:

- Dementia
- Multiple sclerosis (MS)
- Parkinson disease (PD)
- Stroke
- Type 2 diabetes

Loss of Stretch in the Rectum

If your rectum is scarred or inflamed, it becomes stiff and can't stretch as much to hold stool. Your rectum can get full quickly, and stool can leak out. Rectal surgery, radiation therapy in the pelvic area, and inflammatory bowel disease can cause scarring and inflammation in your rectum.

Hemorrhoids

Hemorrhoids can keep the muscles around your anus from closing completely, which lets small amounts of stool or mucus to leak out.

Rectal Prolapse

Rectal prolapse—a condition that causes your rectum to drop down through your anus—can also keep the muscles around your anus from closing completely, which lets small amounts of stool or mucus leak out.

Physical Inactivity

If you are not physically active, especially if you spend many hours a day sitting or lying down, you may be holding a lot of stool in your rectum. Liquid stool can then leak around the more solid stool. Frail, older adults are most likely to develop constipation-related fecal incontinence for this reason.

Childbirth by Vaginal Delivery

Childbirth sometimes causes injuries to the anal sphincters, which can cause fecal incontinence. The chances are greater if:

- Your baby was large

- Forceps were used to help deliver your baby

- You had a vacuum-assisted delivery

- The doctor made a cut, called an episiotomy, in your vaginal area to prevent the baby's head from tearing your vagina during birth

Rectocele

Rectocele is a condition that causes your rectum to bulge out through your vagina. Rectocele can happen when the thin layer of muscles separating your rectum from your vagina becomes weak. Stool may stay in your rectum because the rectocele makes it harder to push stool out.

What Causes Fecal Incontinence in Children

For children older than four, the most common cause of fecal incontinence is constipation with a large amount of stool in the rectum. When this happens, a child may not be able to sense when a new stool is coming into the rectum. The child may not know that he or she needs to have a bowel movement. A large amount of stool in the rectum can cause the internal anal sphincters to become chronically relaxed, which lets soft stool seep around hard stool in the rectum and leak out.

Birth defects of the anus, rectum, or colon, such as Hirschsprung disease, can cause fecal incontinence in children. These birth defects may weaken pelvic floor muscles or damage nerves in the anus or rectum. Injuries to the nerves in the anus and rectum can also cause fecal incontinence, as can spinal cord injuries and birth defects of the spinal cord.

How Do Doctors Diagnose Fecal Incontinence?

Doctors use your medical history, a physical exam, and medical tests to diagnose fecal incontinence and its causes.

Medical History

In addition to reviewing your general medical history, your doctor may ask the following questions:

- When did your fecal incontinence start?
- Did your fecal incontinence start after:
  - The birth of your child?
  - A motor vehicle accident?
  - A fall?
  - The start of another illness?
- How often does your fecal incontinence happen?
- How much stool passes?
- Do you pass liquid or solid stool?
- Do you have a strong urge to have a bowel movement before your fecal incontinence happens?
- Do you know when you need to have a bowel movement before it happens?
- Does your fecal incontinence happen without you knowing?
- Do you leak liquid stool or mucus?
- Do you have fecal incontinence when you have diarrhea or constipation?
- Is your fecal incontinence worse after eating?
- Do certain foods seem to make your fecal incontinence worse?
- How does fecal incontinence affect your daily life?

Your doctor may ask you to keep a stool diary to help answer these questions. A stool diary is a chart for recording details of your daily bowel movements. Your doctor may give you a stool diary form that he or she has created. Or, you can create your own stool diary form or record your bowel movement details in a notebook.

You may feel embarrassed or shy about answering your doctor's questions. However, your doctor will not be shocked or surprised. The more details and examples you can give about your problem, the better your doctor will be able to help you. You can play an active role in your diagnosis by talking openly and honestly with your doctor.

Physical Exam

Your doctor will perform a physical exam, including:

- Digital rectal exam

- Pelvic exam—an exam to check if internal female reproductive organs are normal by feeling their shape and size

What Medical Tests Do Doctors Use to Diagnose Fecal Incontinence?

Lab Tests

Your doctor may use one or more of the following lab tests to look for signs of certain diseases and conditions that may be causing your fecal incontinence.

- Blood tests can show signs of anemia, inflammation, and infection.

- Stool tests can show the presence of blood and signs of infection and inflammation.

- Urine tests can show signs of diseases such as type 2 diabetes.

Bowel Function Tests

Your doctor may perform one or more of the following tests to see how well the muscles and nerves in your anus, pelvic floor, and rectum are working:

- Anorectal manometry—a test that checks how sensitive your rectum is, how well it works, and how well the anal sphincters work

- Defecography—an X-ray of the area around the anus and rectum to see how well you can hold and release stool

- Electromyography—a test that checks how well the muscles and nerves of your anus and pelvic floor are working

Endoscopy

Your doctor may perform an endoscopy to look inside your anus, rectum, and colon for signs of inflammation and digestive tract problems that may be causing your fecal incontinence. Endoscopies for fecal incontinence include:

- Anoscopy

- Colonoscopy

- Flexible sigmoidoscopy

- Rectoscopy—a procedure similar to an anoscopy to look inside your rectum

Imaging Tests

To look for problems in the anus, pelvic floor, or rectum that may be causing your fecal incontinence, your doctor may perform an imaging test such as:

- Lower GI series

- Magnetic resonance imaging (MRI)

- Ultrasound

Treatment of Fecal Incontinence

The first step in treating your fecal incontinence is to see a doctor. Your doctor will talk to you about the causes of fecal incontinence and how they can be treated. Simple treatments—such as diet changes, medicines, bowel training, and exercises to strengthen your pelvic floor muscles—can improve symptoms by about 60 percent. These treatments can stop fecal incontinence in 1 out of 5 people.

Your doctor can recommend ways you can help manage and treat your fecal incontinence. Your doctor can also recommend ways to relieve anal discomfort and cope with your fecal incontinence.

You can play an active role in your treatment by talking openly and honestly with your doctor about your symptoms and how well your treatments are working.

How Can I Manage and Treat My Fecal Incontinence?

You can help manage and treat your fecal incontinence in the following ways.

Wearing Absorbent Pads

Wearing absorbent pads inside your underwear is the most frequently used treatment for fecal incontinence. For milder forms of fecal incontinence—few bowel leakage accidents, small volumes of stool, or staining of underwear—wearing absorbent pads may make a big difference in your quality of life. Wearing absorbent pads can be combined with other treatments.

Diet Changes

Changing what you eat can help prevent or relieve your fecal incontinence. If diarrhea is the problem, your doctor will recommend avoiding foods and drinks that make your diarrhea worse. To find out which foods and drinks make your fecal incontinence better or worse, your doctor may recommend keeping a food diary to track:

- What you eat each day
- How much of certain foods you eat
- When you eat
- What symptoms you have
- What types of bowel movements you have, such as diarrhea or constipation
- When your fecal incontinence happens
- Which foods or drinks make your fecal incontinence better or worse
- Take your food diary to your doctor to talk about the foods and drinks that affect your fecal incontinence

If constipation or hemorrhoids are causing your fecal incontinence, your doctor may recommend eating more fiber and drinking more liquids. Talk with your doctor or a dietitian about how much fiber and liquids is right for you.

Over-the-Counter (OTC) Medicines

Depending on the cause, OTC medicines can help reduce or relieve your fecal incontinence. If diarrhea is causing your fecal incontinence, your doctor may recommend medicines such as loperamide (Imodium) and bismuth subsalicylate (Pepto-Bismol, Kaopectate). If constipation is causing your fecal incontinence, your doctor may recommend laxatives, stool softeners, or fiber supplements such as psyllium (Metamucil) or methylcellulose (Citrucel).

Bowel Training

Your doctor may recommend that you train yourself to have bowel movements at certain times of the day, such as after meals. Developing regular bowel movements may take weeks to months to improve fecal incontinence.

Pelvic Floor Muscle Exercises

Pelvic floor muscle exercises, also called Kegel exercises, can improve fecal incontinence symptoms. Tightening and relaxing your pelvic floor muscles many times a day can strengthen the muscles in your anus, pelvic floor, and rectum. Your doctor can help make sure you're doing the exercises the right way.

How Do Doctors Treat Fecal Incontinence?

How doctors treat fecal incontinence depends on the cause. Your doctor may recommend one or more of the following treatments:

Biofeedback Therapy

Biofeedback therapy uses devices to help you learn how to do exercises to strengthen your pelvic floor muscles. This therapy can also help you learn how to:

- sense when stool is filling your rectum if you have passive incontinence
- control strong sensations of urgency if you have urge incontinence

Biofeedback therapy can be more effective than learning pelvic floor exercises on your own. Ask your doctor about getting a biofeedback machine or device.

Sacral Nerve Stimulation (SNS)

The sacral nerves control the anal sphincters, colon, and rectum. Doctors use sacral nerve stimulation—a type of electrical stimulation—when the nerves are not working properly. For this treatment, your doctor places thin wires under your skin near the sacral nerves, just above the tailbone. A battery-operated device sends mild electrical pulses through the wires to the sacral nerves.

Electrical stimulation of the sacral nerves helps them work properly. The electrical pulses do not hurt. You can turn the electrical stimulation on or off at any time.

Prescription Medicines

If OTC medicines to treat your fecal incontinence aren't helping your symptoms, your doctor may prescribe prescription medicines that are stronger. These medicines may treat the causes of fecal incontinence, such as irritable bowel syndrome, Crohn disease, and ulcerative colitis.

Vaginal Balloons

For women with fecal incontinence, your doctor may prescribe a device that inflates a balloon inside your vagina. The balloon puts pressure on the wall of your rectum through the vaginal wall. Pressure on the wall of your rectum keeps stool from passing. After your doctor makes sure the device fits right, you can add or remove air from the device as needed to control the passing of stool.

Nonabsorbable Bulking Agents

Nonabsorbable bulking agents are substances injected into the wall of your anus to bulk up the tissue around the anus. The bulkier tissues make the opening of your anus narrower so the sphincters are able to close better.

Surgery

Surgery may be an option for fecal incontinence that fails to improve with other treatments, or for fecal incontinence caused by injuries to the pelvic floor muscles or anal sphincters.

Sphincteroplasty. Sphincteroplasty—the most common fecal incontinence surgery—reconnects the separated ends of an anal sphincter torn by childbirth or another injury.

Artificial anal sphincter. This surgery involves placing a cuff around your anus and implanting a small pump under the skin so that you can inflate or deflate the cuff. Inflating the cuff controls the passage of stool. This surgery is not a common treatment because it may cause side effects.

Colostomy. Colostomy is a surgery in which the colon is brought through an opening in the abdominal wall, and stools are collected in a bag on the outside of the abdomen. Doctors may recommend this surgery as a last resort for the treatment of fecal incontinence. However, this surgery is rarely used to treat fecal incontinence because of the colostomy's effect on quality of life.

Other surgeries. Doctors may perform other surgeries to treat the causes of fecal incontinence, such as:

- Hemorrhoids
- Rectal prolapse
- Rectocele

What Should I Do about Anal Discomfort?

Fecal incontinence can cause anal discomfort such as irritation, pain, or itching. You can help relieve anal discomfort by:

- Washing the anal area after a bowel movement
- Changing soiled underwear as soon as possible
- Keeping the anal area dry
- Using a moisture-barrier cream in the area around your anus
- Using nonmedicated powders
- Using wicking pads or disposable underwear
- Wearing clothes and underwear that let air pass through easily
- Talk with your doctor or a healthcare professional about which moisture-barrier creams and nonmedicated powders are right for you.

How Do I Cope with My Fecal Incontinence?

Doing the following can help you cope with your fecal incontinence:

- Using the toilet before leaving home
- Carrying a bag with cleanup supplies and a change of clothes when leaving the house
- Finding public restrooms before one is needed
- Wearing absorbent pads inside your underwear
- Wearing disposable underwear
- Using fecal deodorants—OTC pills that reduce the smell of stool and gas
- Taking OTC medicines to help prevent diarrhea before eating in restaurants or at social gatherings

As part of coping with your fecal incontinence, remember that fecal incontinence:

- Isn't something to be ashamed of—it's simply a medical problem
- Can often be treated—a wide range of successful treatments are available
- Isn't always a normal part of aging
- Won't usually go away on its own—most people need treatment

What Should I Do If My Child Has Fecal Incontinence?

If your child has fecal incontinence and is older than age four and toilet trained, you should see a doctor to find out the cause. How the doctor treats your child's incontinence depends on the cause.

How Can My Diet Help Prevent or Relieve Fecal Incontinence?

Depending on the cause, changing what you eat and drink can help prevent or relieve your fecal incontinence.

What Should I Eat If I Have Fecal Incontinence?

You should eat a healthy, well-balanced diet. Your doctor or a dietitian can recommend a healthy eating plan that is right for you. If your fecal incontinence is caused by constipation or hemorrhoids, eating more fiber and drinking more liquids can improve your symptoms. Talk with your doctor or a dietitian about how much fiber and liquids are right for you.

What Should I Avoid Eating If I Have Fecal Incontinence?

If your fecal incontinence is caused by diarrhea, you should avoid foods that make your symptoms worse, such as:

- Alcoholic beverages
- Drinks and foods containing caffeine
- Dairy products such as milk, cheese, and ice cream
- Fatty and greasy foods
- Drinks and foods containing fructose
- Fruits such as apples, peaches, and pears
- Spicy foods
- Products, including candy and gum, with sweeteners ending in "–ol," such as sorbitol, mannitol, xylitol, and maltitol

Keeping a Food Diary

Your doctor or dietitian may recommend keeping a food diary, which can help you find out which foods and drinks make your symptoms better or worse. After a few days, the diary may show a link between certain foods and drinks and your fecal incontinence. Changing the foods and drinks linked to your fecal incontinence may improve your symptoms.

Chapter 4

Cyclic Vomiting Syndrome

What Is Cyclic Vomiting Syndrome?

Cyclic vomiting syndrome, or CVS, is a functional gastrointestinal (GI) disorder that causes sudden, repeated attacks—called episodes—of severe nausea and vomiting. Episodes can last from a few hours to several days. The episodes are separated by periods without nausea or vomiting. The time between episodes can be a few weeks to several months. Episodes can happen regularly or at random. Episodes can be so severe that you may have to stay in bed for days, unable to go to school or work. You may need treatment at an emergency room or a hospital during episodes. Cyclic vomiting syndrome can affect you for years or decades.

CVS is not chronic vomiting that lasts weeks without stopping. CVS is not a condition that has a definite cause, such as chemotherapy.

How Common Is Cyclic Vomiting Syndrome?

Experts don't know how common cyclic vomiting syndrome is in adults. However, experts believe that cyclic vomiting syndrome may be just as common in adults as in children. Doctors diagnose about 3 out of 100,000 children with cyclic vomiting syndrome every year.

This chapter includes text excerpted from "Cyclic Vomiting Syndrome," National Institute of Diabetes and Digestive and Kidney Diseases (NIDDK), December 2017.

Who Is More Likely to Get Cyclic Vomiting Syndrome?

You may be more likely to get cyclic vomiting syndrome if you have:

- Migraines or a family history of migraines
- A history of long-term marijuana use
- A tendency to get motion sickness

Among adults with cyclic vomiting syndrome, about 6 out of 10 are Caucasian.

What Are the Complications of Cyclic Vomiting Syndrome?

The severe vomiting and retching that happen during cyclic vomiting episodes may cause the following complications:

- Dehydration
- Esophagitis
- Mallory-Weiss tears
- Tooth decay or damage to tooth enamel

What Are the Symptoms of Cyclic Vomiting Syndrome?

The main symptoms of cyclic vomiting syndrome are sudden, repeated attacks—called episodes—of severe nausea and vomiting. You may vomit several times an hour. Episodes can last from a few hours to several days. Episodes may make you feel very tired and drowsy.

Each episode of cyclic vomiting syndrome tends to start at the same time of day, last the same length of time, and happen with the same symptoms and intensity as previous episodes. Episodes may begin at any time but often start during the early morning hours.

Other symptoms of cyclic vomiting syndrome may include one or more of the following:

- Retching—trying to vomit but having nothing come out of your mouth, also called dry vomiting
- Pain in the abdomen
- Abnormal drowsiness

- Pale skin

- Headaches

- Lack of appetite

- Not wanting to talk

- Drooling or spitting

- Extreme thirst

- Sensitivity to light or sound

- Dizziness

- Diarrhea

- Fever

What Are the Phases of Cyclic Vomiting Syndrome?

Cyclic vomiting syndrome has four phases:

- Prodrome phase

- Vomiting phase

- Recovery phase

- Well phase

How Do the Symptoms Vary in the Phases of Cyclic Vomiting Syndrome?

The symptoms will vary as you go through the four phases of cyclic vomiting syndrome:

- **Prodrome phase.** During the prodrome phase, you feel an episode coming on. Often marked by intense sweating and nausea—with or without pain in your abdomen—this phase can last from a few minutes to several hours. Your skin may look unusually pale.

- **Vomiting phase.** The main symptoms of this phase are severe nausea, vomiting, and retching. At the peak of this phase, you may vomit several times an hour. You may be:

  - Quiet and able to respond to people around you

  - Unable to move and unable to respond to people around you

- Twisting and moaning with intense pain in your abdomen

Nausea and vomiting can last from a few hours to several days.

- **Recovery phase.** Recovery begins when you stop vomiting and retching and you feel less nauseated. You may feel better gradually or quickly. The recovery phase ends when your nausea stops and your healthy skin color, appetite, and energy return.

- **Well phase.** The well phase happens between episodes. You have no symptoms during this phase.

What Causes Cyclic Vomiting Syndrome

Experts aren't sure what causes cyclic vomiting syndrome. However, some experts believe the following conditions may play a role:

- Problems with nerve signals between the brain and digestive tract

- Problems with the way the brain and endocrine system react to stress

- Mutations in certain genes that are associated with an increased chance of getting CVS

How Do Doctors Diagnose Cyclic Vomiting Syndrome?

Doctors diagnose cyclic vomiting syndrome based on family and medical history, a physical exam, pattern of symptoms, and medical tests. Your doctor may perform medical tests to rule out other diseases and conditions that may cause nausea and vomiting.

Family and Medical History

Your doctor will ask about your family and medical history. He or she may ask for details about your history of health problems such as migraines, irritable bowel syndrome, and gastroparesis. Your doctor may also ask about your history of mental health problems, use of substances such as marijuana, and cigarette smoking.

Physical Exam

During a physical exam, your doctor will:

- Examine your body

- Check your abdomen for unusual sounds, tenderness, or pain
- Check your nerves, muscle strength, reflexes, and balance

Pattern or Cycle of Symptoms in Children

A doctor will often suspect cyclic vomiting syndrome in a child when all of the following are present:

- At least five episodes over any time period, or a minimum of three episodes over a six-month period
- Episodes lasting 1 hour to 10 days and happening at least one week apart
- Episodes similar to previous ones, tending to start at the same time of day, lasting the same length of time, and happening with the same symptoms and intensity
- Vomiting during episodes happening at least four times an hour for at least one hour
- Episodes are separated by weeks to months, usually with no symptoms between episodes
- After appropriate medical evaluation, symptoms cannot be attributed to another medical condition

Pattern or Cycle of Symptoms in Adults

A doctor will often suspect cyclic vomiting syndrome in adults when all of the following are present:

- Three or more separate episodes in the past year and two episodes in the past six months, happening at least one week apart
- Episodes that are usually similar to previous ones, meaning that episodes tend to start at the same time of day and last the same length of time—less than one week
- No nausea or vomiting between episodes, but other milder symptoms can be present between episodes
- No metabolic, gastrointestinal, central nervous system, structural, or biochemical disorders

A personal or family history of migraines supports the doctor's diagnosis of cyclic vomiting syndrome. Your doctor may diagnose cyclic vomiting syndrome even if your pattern of symptoms or your child's pattern of symptoms do not fit the patterns described here. Talk to your doctor if your symptoms or your child's symptoms are like the symptoms of cyclic vomiting syndrome.

What Medical Tests Do Doctors Use to Diagnose Cyclic Vomiting Syndrome?

Doctors use lab tests, upper GI endoscopy, and imaging tests to rule out other diseases and conditions that cause nausea and vomiting. Once other diseases and conditions have been ruled out, a doctor will diagnose cyclic vomiting syndrome based on the pattern or cycle of symptoms.

Lab Tests

Your doctor may use the following lab tests:

- Blood tests can show signs of anemia, dehydration, inflammation, infection, and liver problems.
- Urine tests can show signs of dehydration, infection, and kidney problems.

Blood and urine tests can also show signs of mitochondrial diseases.

Upper GI Endoscopy

Your doctor may perform an upper GI endoscopy to look for problems in your upper digestive tract that may be causing nausea and vomiting.

Imaging Tests

A doctor may perform one or more of the following imaging tests:

- Ultrasound of the abdomen
- Gastric emptying test is also called gastric emptying scintigraphy. This test involves eating a bland meal, such as eggs or an egg substitute, that contains a small amount of radioactive material. An external camera scans the abdomen to show where the radioactive material is located. A radiologist can then measure how quickly the stomach empties after the meal. Healthcare professionals perform gastric emptying tests only between episodes.

- Upper GI series
- Magnetic resonance imaging (MRI) scan or computed tomography (CT) scan of the brain

How Do Doctors Treat Cyclic Vomiting Syndrome?

How doctors treat cyclic vomiting syndrome depends on the phase. Your doctor may:

- Prescribe medicines
- Treat health problems that may trigger the disorder
- Recommend
  - Staying away from triggers
  - Ways to manage triggers
  - Getting plenty of sleep and rest

Prodrome Phase

Taking medicines early in this phase can sometimes help stop an episode from happening. Your doctor may recommend over-the-counter (OTC) medicines or prescribe medicines such as:

- Ondansetron (Zofran) or promethazine (Phenergan) for nausea
- Sumatriptan (Imitrex) for migraines
- Lorazepam (Ativan) for anxiety
- Ibuprofen for pain

Your doctor may recommend OTC medicines to reduce the amount of acid your stomach makes, such as:

- Famotidine (Pepcid)
- Ranitidine (Zantac)
- Omeprazole (Prilosec)
- Esomeprazole (Nexium)

Vomiting Phase

During this phase, you should stay in bed and sleep in a dark, quiet room. You may have to go to a hospital if your nausea and vomiting are severe or if you become severely dehydrated. Your doctor may recommend or prescribe the following for children and adults:

- Medicines for:
  - Nausea
  - Migraines
  - Anxiety
  - Pain
- Medicines that reduce the amount of acid your stomach makes

If you go to a hospital, your doctor may treat you with:

- Intravenous (IV) fluids for dehydration
- Medicines for symptoms
- IV nutrition if an episode continues for several days

Recovery Phase

During the recovery phase, you may need IV fluids for a while. Your doctor may recommend that you drink plenty of water and liquids that contain glucose and electrolytes, such as:

- Broths
- Caffeine-free soft drinks
- Fruit juices
- Sports drinks
- Oral rehydration solutions, such as Pedialyte

If you've lost your appetite, start drinking clear liquids and then move slowly to other liquids and solid foods. Your doctor may prescribe medicines to help prevent future episodes.

Well Phase

During the well phase, your doctor may prescribe medicines to help prevent episodes and how often and how severe they are, such as:

- Amitriptyline (Elavil)
- Cyproheptadine (Periactin)

- Propranolol (Inderal)
- Topiramate (Topamax)
- Zonisamide (Zonegran)

Your doctor may also recommend coenzyme Q_{10}, levocarnitine (L-carnitine), or riboflavin as dietary supplements to help prevent episodes.

How Can I Prevent Cyclic Vomiting Syndrome?

Knowing and managing your triggers can help prevent cyclic vomiting syndrome, especially during the well phase. You should also:

- Get enough sleep and rest
- Treat infections and allergies
- Learn how to reduce or manage stress and anxiety
- Avoid foods and food additives that trigger episodes

How Do Doctors Treat the Complications of Cyclic Vomiting Syndrome?

Doctors treat the complications of cyclic vomiting syndrome as follows:

- Dehydration—plenty of liquids with glucose and electrolytes, or IV fluids and hospitalization for severe dehydration
- Esophagitis—medicines to reduce the amount of acid your stomach makes
- Mallory-Weiss tears—medicines or medical procedures to stop bleeding if the tears don't heal on their own, which they generally do
- Tooth decay or damage to tooth enamel—dental fillings, fluoride toothpaste, or mouth rinses

How Can My Diet Help Prevent or Relieve Cyclic Vomiting Syndrome?

Your diet will not help prevent or relieve episodes, but will help you recover and keep you healthy. Your doctor may recommend coenzyme

Q_{10}, levocarnitine (L-carnitine), or riboflavin as dietary supplements to help prevent episodes.

What Should I Eat and Drink If I Have Cyclic Vomiting Syndrome?

When your nausea and vomiting stop, you can generally go back to your regular diet right away. In some cases, you may want to start with clear liquids and go slowly back to your regular diet. You should eat well-balanced and nutritious meals between your episodes. Your doctors will recommend that you not skip meals in between episodes. If you are dehydrated, drink plenty of liquids that contain glucose and electrolytes, such as:

• Broths

• Caffeine-free soft drinks

• Fruit juices

• Sports drinks

• Oral rehydration solutions, such as Pedialyte

What Should I Avoid Eating If I Have Cyclic Vomiting Syndrome?

In between episodes, you should avoid eating foods that may have triggered past episodes. Eating certain foods such as chocolate, cheese, and foods with monosodium glutamate (MSG) may trigger an episode in some people. Adults should avoid drinking alcohol.

Chapter 5

Smoking and Your Digestive System

Smoking affects the entire body, increasing the risk of many life-threatening diseases—including lung cancer, emphysema, and heart disease. Smoking also contributes to many cancers and diseases of the digestive system. Estimates show that about one-fifth of all adults smoke, and each year at least 443,000 Americans die from diseases caused by cigarette smoking.

What Is the Digestive System?

The digestive system is made up of the gastrointestinal (GI) tract—also called the digestive tract—and the liver, pancreas, and gallbladder. The GI tract is a series of hollow organs joined in a long, twisting tube from the mouth to the anus. The hollow organs that make up the GI tract are the mouth, esophagus, stomach, small intestine, large intestine—which includes the colon and rectum—and anus. Food enters the mouth and passes to the anus through the hollow organs of the GI tract. The liver, pancreas, and gallbladder are the solid organs of the digestive system. The digestive system helps the body digest food, which includes breaking food down into nutrients the body needs.

This chapter includes text excerpted from "Smoking and the Digestive System," National Institute of Diabetes and Digestive and Kidney Diseases (NIDDK), September 2013. Reviewed September 2018.

Nutrients are substances the body uses for energy, growth, and cell repair.

Does Smoking Increase the Risk of Cancers of the Digestive System?

Smoking has been found to increase the risk of cancers of the:

- Mouth
- Esophagus
- Stomach
- Pancreas

Research suggests that smoking may also increase the risk of cancers of the:

- Liver
- Colon
- Rectum

What Are the Other Harmful Effects of Smoking on the Digestive System?

Smoking contributes to many common disorders of the digestive system, such as heartburn and gastroesophageal reflux disease (GERD), peptic ulcers, and some liver diseases. Smoking increases the risk of Crohn disease, colon polyps, and pancreatitis, and it may increase the risk of gallstones.

How Does Smoking Affect Heartburn and Gastroesophageal Reflux Disease (GERD)?

Smoking increases the risk of heartburn and GERD. Heartburn is a painful, burning feeling in the chest caused by reflux, or stomach contents flowing back into the esophagus—the organ that connects the mouth to the stomach. Smoking weakens the lower esophageal sphincter (LES), the muscle between the esophagus and stomach that keeps stomach contents from flowing back into the esophagus. The stomach is naturally protected from the acids it makes to help break down food. However, the esophagus is not protected from the acids. When the lower esophageal sphincter weakens, stomach contents may reflux into the esophagus, causing heartburn and possibly damaging the lining of the esophagus.

GERD is persistent reflux that occurs more than twice a week. Chronic, or long lasting, GERD can lead to serious health problems such as bleeding ulcers in the esophagus, narrowing of the esophagus that causes food to get stuck, and changes in esophageal cells that can lead to cancer.

How Does Smoking Affect Peptic Ulcers?

Smoking increases the risk of peptic ulcers. Peptic ulcers are sores on the inside lining of the stomach or duodenum, the first part of the small intestine. The two most common causes of peptic ulcers are infection with a bacterium called *Helicobacter pylori* (*H. pylori*) and long-term use of nonsteroidal anti-inflammatory drugs (NSAIDs) such as aspirin and ibuprofen.

Researchers are studying how smoking contributes to peptic ulcers. Studies suggest that smoking increases the risk of *H. pylori* infection, slows the healing of peptic ulcers, and increases the likelihood that peptic ulcers will recur. The stomach and duodenum contain acids, enzymes, and other substances that help digest food. However, these substances may also harm the lining of these organs. Smoking has not been shown to increase acid production. However, smoking does increase the production of other substances that may harm the lining, such as pepsin, an enzyme made in the stomach that breaks down proteins.

Smoking also decreases factors that protect or heal the lining, including:

- Blood flow to the lining

- Secretion of mucus, a clear liquid that protects the lining from acid

- Production of sodium bicarbonate—a salt like substance that neutralizes acid—by the pancreas

The increase in substances that may harm the lining and decrease in factors that protect or heal the lining may lead to peptic ulcers.

How Does Smoking Affect Liver Disease?

Smoking may worsen some liver diseases, including:

- Primary biliary cirrhosis, a chronic liver disease that slowly destroys the bile ducts in the liver

75

- Nonalcoholic fatty liver disease (NAFLD), a condition in which fat builds up in the liver

Researchers are still studying how smoking affects primary biliary cirrhosis, NAFLD, and other liver diseases. Liver diseases may progress to cirrhosis, a condition in which the liver slowly deteriorates and malfunctions due to chronic injury. Scar tissue then replaces healthy liver tissue, partially blocking the flow of blood through the liver and impairing liver functions.

The liver is the largest organ in the digestive system. The liver carries out many functions, such as making important blood proteins and bile, changing food into energy, and filtering alcohol and poisons from the blood. Research has shown that smoking harms the liver's ability to process medications, alcohol, and other toxins and remove them from the body. In some cases, smoking may affect the dose of medication needed to treat an illness.

How Does Smoking Affect Crohn Disease?

Current and former smokers have a higher risk of developing Crohn disease than people who have never smoked. Crohn disease is an inflammatory bowel disease that causes irritation in the GI tract. The disease, which typically causes pain and diarrhea, most often affects the lower part of the small intestine; however, it can occur anywhere in the GI tract. The severity of symptoms varies from person to person, and the symptoms come and go. Crohn disease may lead to complications such as blockages of the intestine and ulcers that tunnel through the affected area into surrounding tissues. Medications may control symptoms. However, many people with Crohn disease require surgery to remove the affected portion of the intestine.

Among people with Crohn disease, people who smoke are more likely to:

- Have more severe symptoms, more frequent symptoms, and more complications

- Need more medications to control their symptoms

- Require surgery

- Have symptoms recur after surgery

The effects of smoking are more pronounced in women with Crohn disease than in men with the disease. Researchers are studying why smoking increases the risk of Crohn disease and makes the disease worse. Some researchers believe smoking might lower the intestines' defenses, decrease blood flow to the intestines, or cause immune system changes that result in inflammation. In people who inherit genes that make them susceptible to developing Crohn disease, smoking may affect how some of these genes work.

How Does Smoking Affect Colon Polyps?

People who smoke are more likely to develop colon polyps. Colon polyps are growths on the inside surface of the colon or rectum. Some polyps are benign, or noncancerous, while some are cancerous or may become cancerous. Among people who develop colon polyps, those who smoke have polyps that are larger, more numerous, and more likely to recur.

How Does Smoking Affect Pancreatitis?

Smoking increases the risk of developing pancreatitis. Pancreatitis is inflammation of the pancreas, which is located behind the stomach and close to the duodenum. The pancreas secretes digestive enzymes that usually do not become active until they reach the small intestine. When the pancreas is inflamed, the digestive enzymes attack the tissues of the pancreas.

How Does Smoking Affect Gallstones?

Some studies have shown that smoking may increase the risk of developing gallstones. However, research results are not consistent and more study is needed. Gallstones are small, hard particles that develop in the gallbladder, the organ that stores bile made by the liver. Gallstones can move into the ducts that carry digestive enzymes from the gallbladder, liver, and pancreas to the duodenum, causing inflammation, infection, and abdominal pain.

Can the Damage to the Digestive System from Smoking Be Reversed?

Quitting smoking can reverse some of the effects of smoking on the digestive system. For example, the balance between factors that harm and protect the stomach and duodenum lining returns to normal within a few hours of a person quitting smoking. The effects of smoking on how the liver handles medications also disappear when a person stops smoking. However, people who stop smoking continue to have a higher risk of some digestive diseases, such as colon polyps and pancreatitis, than people who have never smoked. Quitting smoking can improve the symptoms of some digestive diseases or keep them from getting worse. For example, people with Crohn disease who quit smoking have less severe symptoms than smokers with the disease.

Eating, Diet, and Nutrition

Eating, diet, and nutrition can play a role in causing, preventing, and treating some of the diseases and disorders of the digestive system that are affected by smoking, including heartburn and GERD, liver diseases, Crohn disease, colon polyps, pancreatitis, and gallstones.

Chapter 6

Effects of Common Medicines on the Gastrointestinal Tract

Medications taken for certain illnesses may sometimes affect the digestive system and cause gastrointestinal (GI) disorders. Both prescribed and over-the-counter (OTC) medicines can be responsible for such harmful side effects. At times, combinations of medicines, when taken together, may interact with each other and cause adverse effects on the gastrointestinal tract. Hence, it is important to be aware of the medication-induced gastrointestinal disorders. Some of the common medication-induced gastrointestinal disorders are as follows.

Stomach Ache

Nonsteroidal anti-inflammatory drugs (NSAIDs) are widely known to cause stomach irritation or stomach ache. NSAIDs are generally used as painkillers as they suppress the secretion of prostaglandins, which are responsible for inflammation and pain. On the other hand, prostaglandins are also responsible for the creation of mucosa that forms a lining on the stomach wall and protects it from digestive juices.

By suppressing prostaglandins, NSAIDs tend to affect the stomach lining and cause ulcers, bleeding, and stomach ache.

Prevention of Stomach Irritation

- Take only prescribed amount of NSAIDs.
- Discuss with your healthcare provider and take coated tablets.
- Drink water and milk while taking NSAIDs.
- Do not drink alcohol while taking NSAIDs.

Esophagitis

If the ingested tablet or pill stays in the esophagus for a relatively long period of time, it may release chemicals that can rupture the layers of the esophagus and cause ulcers. This condition is called "pill-induced esophagitis." Various risk factors can contribute to the prolonged presence of pills in the esophagus: the increased age of the patient; increased size of the pill; strictures (narrowing of esophagus); and scleroderma (hardening of the skin). The severity of the injury depends upon the chemical composition of the pill. The medicines that are commonly known to cause esophagitis are aspirin, iron supplements, NSAIDs, potassium chloride, and tetracyclines.

Prevention of Esophagitis

- Always take tablets or pills with water.
- Sit or stand erect while swallowing tablets or pills.
- Stay upright for at least 30 minutes after swallowing tablets or pills.
- Consult with your healthcare provider and take an alternative drug that is less likely to cause esophagitis.

Gastroesophageal Reflux Disease (GERD)

A sphincter muscle lies between the esophagus and the stomach and enables the smooth passage of food particles. Some medicines affect the functioning of this muscle and can result in gastroesophageal reflux. This condition allows excessive stomach acids to enter the esophagus and cause gastric disorders. A few common medicines that can cause this disease are anticholinergics, birth-control pills, calcium channel blockers, dopamine, methylxanthines, nitrates, NSAIDs, and progesterone.

Prevention of Esophagitis

- Avoid food items that are more likely to worsen reflux such as fatty foods, acidic foods, and spicy foods.

- Avoid smoking and alcohol drinking.

- Do not lie down soon after eating.

- Elevate the head of your bed so that the entry of gastric acids into the esophagus can be prevented by gravity.

Diarrhea

Antibiotics frequently cause diarrhea. The antibiotics sometimes kill the good bacteria that are normally present in the intestine. This, in turn, disturbs the intestinal bacteria content and leads to the overgrowth of pathogenic bacteria called *Clostridium difficile (C. difficile)*. The habitation of *C. difficile* causes colitis, resulting in loose and watery stools. *C. difficile*-induced diarrhea can be life threatening at times. The most common antibiotics known to cause this type of diarrhea are cephalosporins, clindamycin, and penicillin. *C. difficile*-induced diarrhea is treated with another antibiotic that acts against *C. difficile*. Other medicines such as colchicine and magnesium-containing antacids can also cause diarrhea by altering the fluid content in the colon without involving *C. difficile*.

Prevention of Diarrhea

- Avoid unhygienic food.

- Avoid uncooked meat.

- Drink more water.

Take antibiotics if diarrhea is caused by a bacterial infection.

Constipation

Chemicals in certain medicines intervene with the nerve and muscle activity of the colon that are responsible for emptying the stomach. This can bind the intestinal fluids and make the stool harder, which results in delayed gastric emptying, or constipation. Opioid pain relievers such as oxycodone and hydrocodone are known to cause constipation, along with belly cramps and bloating. Opioid-induced constipation can be so severe that doctors usually prescribe laxatives whenever long-term use of opioid is anticipated. Other common medications that can cause constipation are antacids containing aluminum hydroxide, antihypertensives, anticholinergics, cholestyramine, frusemide, iron supplements, levothyroxine, and verapamil.

Prevention of Constipation

- Stay active.

- Eat more fiber-rich food.

- Drink water frequently and stay hydrated.

- Consult with your doctor and take suitable laxatives.

References

1. "Medicines and the Digestive System," University of Rochester Medical Center (URMC), February 1, 2002.

2. "Drug-Induced Gastrointestinal Disorders," National Center for Biotechnology Information (NCBI), January 2014.

3. Tresca, Amber J. "Effects of Medications on the Stomach," Verywell Health, August 20, 2018.

4. "Which Medicines Can Cause Stomach Pain?" WebMD, May 22, 2017.

Part Two

Diagnostic and Surgical Procedures Used for Gastrointestinal Disorders

Chapter 7

Endoscopic Procedures and Related Concerns

Chapter Contents

Section 7.1

Colonoscopy

This section includes text excerpted from "Colonoscopy,"
National Institute of Diabetes and Digestive and Kidney
Diseases (NIDDK), July 2017.

What Is Colonoscopy?

Colonoscopy is a procedure in which a doctor uses a colonoscope
or scope, to look inside your rectum and colon. Colonoscopy can show
irritated and swollen tissue, ulcers, polyps, and cancer.

Why Do Doctors Use Colonoscopy?

A colonoscopy can help a doctor find the cause of symptoms, such as:

- Bleeding from your anus
- Changes in your bowel activity, such as diarrhea
- Pain in your abdomen
- Unexplained weight loss

Doctors also use colonoscopy as a screening tool for colon polyps and
cancer. Screening is testing for diseases when you have no symptoms.
Screening may find diseases at an early stage, when a doctor has a
better chance of curing the disease.

Screening for Colon and Rectal Cancer

Your doctor will recommend screening for colon and rectal cancer—also called colorectal cancer—starting at age 50 if you don't have
health problems or risk factors that make you more likely to develop
colon cancer.

You have risk factors for colorectal cancer if you:

- are male
- are African American
- or someone in your family has had polyps or colorectal cancer
- have a personal history of inflammatory bowel disease (IBD),
  such as ulcerative colitis (UC) and Crohn disease

- have Lynch syndrome (LS), or another genetic disorder that increases the risk of colorectal cancer

- have other factors, such as that you weigh too much or smoke cigarettes

If you are more likely to develop colorectal cancer, your doctor may recommend screening at a younger age, and more often. If you are older than age 75, talk with your doctor about whether you should be screened. Government health insurance plans, such as Medicare, and private insurance plans sometimes change whether and how often they pay for cancer screening tests. Check with your insurance plan to find out how often your plan will cover a screening colonoscopy.

How Do I Prepare for a Colonoscopy?

To prepare for a colonoscopy, you will need to talk with your doctor, change your diet for a few days, clean out your bowel, and arrange for a ride home after the procedure.

Talk with Your Doctor

You should talk with your doctor about any health problems you have and all prescribed and over-the-counter (OTC) medicines, vitamins, and supplements you take, including:

- Arthritis medicines

- Aspirin or medicines that contain aspirin

- Blood thinners

- Diabetes medicines

- Nonsteroidal anti-inflammatory drugs (NSAIDs) such as ibuprofen or naproxen

- Vitamins that contain iron or iron supplements

Change Your Diet and Clean out Your Bowel

A healthcare professional will give you written bowel prep instructions to follow at home before the procedure so that little or no stool remains in your intestine. A complete bowel prep lets you pass stool that is clear and liquid. Stool inside your intestine can prevent your doctor from clearly seeing the lining.

You may need to follow a clear liquid diet for one to three days before the procedure. You should avoid red and purple-colored drinks or gelatin. The instructions will include details about when to start and stop the clear liquid diet. In most cases, you may drink or eat the following:

- Fat-free bouillon or broth

- Gelatin in flavors such as lemon, lime, or orange

- Plain coffee or tea, without cream or milk

- Sports drinks in flavors such as lemon, lime, or orange

- Strained fruit juice, such as apple or white grape—avoid orange juice

- Water

Different bowel preps may contain different combinations of laxatives—pills that you swallow or powders that you dissolve in water or clear liquids. Some people will need to drink a large amount, often a gallon, of liquid laxative over a scheduled amount of time—most often the night before and the morning of the procedure. Your doctor may also prescribe an enema.

The bowel prep will cause diarrhea, so you should stay close to a bathroom. You may find this part of the bowel prep hard; however, finishing the prep is very important. Call a healthcare professional if you have side effects that keep you from finishing the prep. Your doctor will tell you how long before the procedure you should have nothing by mouth.

Arrange for a Ride Home

For safety reasons, you can't drive for 24 hours after the procedure, as the sedatives or anesthesia need time to wear off. You will need to make plans for getting a ride home after the procedure.

How Do Doctors Perform a Colonoscopy?

A doctor performs a colonoscopy in a hospital or an outpatient center. A colonoscopy usually takes 30–60 minutes. A healthcare professional will place an intravenous (IV) needle in a vein in your arm or hand to give you sedatives, anesthesia, or pain medicine, so you won't be aware or feel pain during the procedure. The healthcare staff will check your vital signs and keep you as comfortable as possible.

For the procedure, you'll lie on a table while the doctor inserts a colonoscope through your anus and into your rectum and colon. The scope inflates your large intestine with air for a better view. The camera sends a video image to a monitor, allowing the doctor to examine your large intestine.

The doctor may move you several times on the table to adjust the scope for better viewing. Once the scope reaches the opening to your small intestine, the doctor slowly removes the scope and examines the lining of your large intestine again.

During the procedure, the doctor may remove polyps and will send them to a lab for testing. You will not feel the polyp removal. Colon polyps are common in adults and are harmless in most cases. However, most colon cancer begins as a polyp, so removing polyps early helps to prevent cancer. If your doctor finds an abnormal tissue, he or she may perform a biopsy. You won't feel the biopsy.

What Should I Expect after a Colonoscopy?

After a colonoscopy, you can expect the following:

- The anesthesia takes time to wear off completely. You'll stay at the hospital or outpatient center for one to two hours after the procedure.

- You may feel cramping in your abdomen or bloating during the first hour after the procedure.

- After the procedure, you—or a friend or family member— will receive instructions on how to care for yourself after the procedure. You should follow all instructions.

- You'll need your prearranged ride home, since you won't be able to drive after the procedure.

- You should expect a full recovery and return to your normal diet by the next day.

After the sedatives or anesthesia wear off, your doctor may share what was found during the procedure with you or, if you choose, with a friend or family member.

If the doctor removed polyps or performed a biopsy, you may have light bleeding from your anus. This bleeding is normal. A pathologist will examine the biopsy tissue, and results take a few days or longer to come back. A healthcare professional will call you or schedule an appointment to go over the results.

What Are the Risks of Colonoscopy?

The risks of colonoscopy include:

- Bleeding

- Perforation of the colon

- Reaction to the sedative, including breathing or heart problems

- Severe pain in your abdomen

- Death, although this risk is rare

A study of screening colonoscopies found roughly 4–8 serious complications for every 10,000 procedures. Bleeding and perforation are the most common complications from colonoscopy. Most cases of bleeding occur in patients who have polyps removed. The doctor can treat bleeding that happens during the colonoscopy right away.

You may have delayed bleeding up to two weeks after the procedure. The doctor can diagnose and treat delayed bleeding with a repeat colonoscopy. The doctor may need to treat perforation with surgery.

Seek Care Right Away

If you have any of the following symptoms after a colonoscopy, seek medical care right away:

- Severe pain in your abdomen

- Fever

- Bloody bowel movements that do not get better

- Bleeding from the anus that does not stop

- Dizziness

- Weakness

Section 7.2

Virtual Colonoscopy

This section includes text excerpted from "Virtual Colonoscopy," National Institute of Diabetes and Digestive and Kidney Diseases (NIDDK), August 2016.

What Is Virtual Colonoscopy?

Virtual colonoscopy is a procedure in which a radiologist uses X-rays and a computer to create images of your rectum and colon from outside the body. Virtual colonoscopy can show ulcers, polyps, and cancer. Virtual colonoscopy is also called computerized tomography (CT) colonography.

How Is Virtual Colonoscopy Different from Colonoscopy?

Colonoscopy and virtual colonoscopy are different in several ways. Colonoscopy is a procedure in which a trained specialist uses a long, flexible, narrow tube with a light and tiny camera on one end, called a colonoscope or scope, to look inside your rectum and colon. Virtual colonoscopy is an X-ray test, takes less time, and does not require a doctor to insert a scope into the entire length of your colon. Unlike colonoscopy, virtual colonoscopy does not require sedation or anesthesia.

However, virtual colonoscopy may not be as effective as colonoscopy at finding certain polyps. Also, doctors cannot remove polyps or treat certain other problems during virtual colonoscopy, as they can during colonoscopy. Your health insurance coverage for virtual colonoscopy and colonoscopy also may be different.

Why Do Doctors Use Virtual Colonoscopy?

Doctors mainly use virtual colonoscopy to screen for polyps or cancer. Screening may find diseases at an early stage, when a doctor has a better chance of curing the disease. Occasionally, doctors may use virtual colonoscopy when colonoscopy is incomplete or not possible due to other medical reasons.

Screening for Colon and Rectal Cancer

Your doctor will recommend screening for colon and rectal cancer at age 50 if you don't have health problems or other factors that make you more likely to develop colon cancer.

Factors that make you more likely to develop colorectal cancer include:

- Someone in your family has had polyps or cancer of the colon or rectum

- A personal history of inflammatory bowel disease, such as ulcerative colitis or Crohn disease

- Other factors, such as if you weigh too much or smoke cigarettes

If you are more likely to develop colorectal cancer, your doctor may recommend screening at a younger age, and you may need to be tested more often.

If you are older than age 75, talk with your doctor about whether you should be screened. Government health insurance plans, such as Medicare, and private health insurance plans sometimes change whether and how often they pay for cancer screening tests. Check with your insurance plan to find out if and how often your insurance will cover a screening virtual colonoscopy.

How Do I Prepare for a Virtual Colonoscopy?

To prepare for a virtual colonoscopy, you will need to talk with your doctor, change your diet, clean out your bowel, and drink a special liquid called contrast medium. The contrast medium makes your rectum and colon easier to see in the X-rays.

Talk with Your Doctor

You should talk with your doctor about any medical conditions you have and all prescribed and over-the-counter (OTC) medicines, vitamins, and supplements you take, including:

- Arthritis medicines
- Aspirin or medicines that contain aspirin
- Blood thinners
- Diabetes medicines

- Nonsteroidal anti-inflammatory drugs (NSAIDs), such as ibuprofen or naproxen

- Vitamins that contain iron or iron supplements

X-rays may interfere with personal medical devices. Tell your doctor if you have any implanted medical devices, such as a pacemaker. Doctors don't recommend X-rays for pregnant women because X-rays may harm the fetus. Tell your doctor if you are, or may be, pregnant. Your doctor may suggest a different procedure, such as a colonoscopy.

Change Your Diet and Clean out Your Bowel

As in colonoscopy, a healthcare professional will give you written bowel prep instructions to follow at home before the procedure. A healthcare professional orders a bowel prep so that little or no stool is present in your intestine. A complete bowel prep lets you pass stool that is clear and liquid. Stool inside your colon can prevent the X-ray machine from taking clear images of the lining of your intestine.

You may need to follow a clear liquid diet the day before the procedure. The instructions will provide specific direction about when to start and stop the clear liquid diet. In most cases, you may drink or eat the following:

- Fat-free bouillon or broth

- Gelatin in flavors such as lemon, lime, or orange

- Plain coffee or tea, without cream or milk

- Sports drinks in such flavors as lemon, lime, or orange

- Strained fruit juice, such as apple or white grape—doctors recommend avoiding orange juice and red or purple beverages

- Water

Your doctor will tell you how long before the procedure you should have nothing by mouth. A healthcare professional will ask you to follow the directions for a bowel prep before the procedure. The bowel prep will cause diarrhea, so you should stay close to a bathroom. Different bowel preps may contain different combinations of laxatives—pills that you swallow or powders that you dissolve in water and other clear liquids, and enemas. Some people will need to drink a large amount, often a gallon, of liquid laxative over a scheduled amount of time—most often the night before the procedure. You may find this part of the bowel prep difficult; however, completing the prep is very important. The images will not be clear if the prep is incomplete.

Drink Contrast Medium

The night before the procedure, you will drink a contrast medium. Contrast medium is visible on X-rays and can help your doctor tell the difference between stool and polyps.

How Do Healthcare Professionals Perform a Virtual Colonoscopy?

A specially trained X-ray technician performs a virtual colonoscopy at an outpatient center or a hospital. You do not need anesthesia. For the procedure, you will lie on a table while the technician inserts a thin tube through your anus and into your rectum. The tube inflates your large intestine with air for a better view. The table slides into a tunnel-shaped device where the technician takes the X-ray images. The technician may ask you to hold your breath several times during the procedure to steady the images. The technician will ask you to turn over on your side or stomach so he or she can take different images of the large intestine. The procedure lasts about 10–15 minutes.

What Should I Expect after a Virtual Colonoscopy?

After a virtual colonoscopy, you can expect to:

- feel cramping or bloating during the first hour after the test
- resume your regular activities right after the test
- return to a normal diet

After the test, a radiologist looks at the images to find any problems and sends a report to your doctor. If the radiologist finds problems, your doctor may perform a colonoscopy the same day or at a later time.

What Are the Risks of a Virtual Colonoscopy?

Inflating the colon with air has a small risk of perforating the lining of the large intestine. The doctor may need to treat perforation with surgery.

Section 7.3

Upper GI Endoscopy

This section includes text excerpted from "Diagnostic
Tests—Upper GI Endoscopy," National Institute of Diabetes
and Digestive and Kidney Diseases (NIDDK), July 2017.

What Is Upper Gastrointestinal (GI) Endoscopy?

Upper gastrointestinal (GI) endoscopy is a procedure in which a
doctor uses an endoscope—a flexible tube with a camera—to see the
lining of your upper GI tract. A gastroenterologist, surgeon, or other
trained healthcare professional performs the procedure, most often
while you receive light sedation to help you relax. Healthcare professionals may also call the procedure endoscopy, upper endoscopy, EGD
or esophagogastroduodenoscopy.

Why Do Doctors Use Upper GI Endoscopy?

Doctors use upper GI endoscopy to help diagnose and treat symptoms and conditions that affect the esophagus, stomach, and upper
intestine or duodenum.

Upper GI endoscopy can help find the cause of unexplained symptoms, such as:

- Persistent heartburn
- Bleeding
- Nausea and vomiting
- Pain
- Problems swallowing
- Unexplained weight loss

Upper GI endoscopy can be used to identify many different diseases:

- Gastroesophageal reflux disease
- Ulcers
- Cancer
- Inflammation or swelling
- Precancerous abnormalities such as Barrett esophagus

- Celiac disease

- Strictures or narrowing of the esophagus

- Blockages

Upper GI endoscopy can check for damage after a person eats or drinks harmful chemicals.

During upper GI endoscopy, a doctor obtains biopsies by passing an instrument through the endoscope to obtain a small piece of tissue for testing. Biopsies are needed to diagnose conditions such as:

- Cancer

- Celiac disease

- Gastritis

Doctors also use upper GI endoscopy to:

- treat conditions such as bleeding from ulcers, esophageal varices, or other conditions

- dilate or open up strictures with a small balloon passed through the endoscope

- remove objects, including food, that may be stuck in the upper GI tract

- remove polyps or other growths

- place feeding tubes or drainage tubes

Doctors are also starting to use upper GI endoscopy to perform weight loss procedures for some people with obesity.

How Do I Prepare for an Upper GI Endoscopy?
Talk with Your Doctor

You should talk with your doctor about your medical history, including medical conditions and symptoms you have, allergies, and all prescribed and over-the-counter (OTC) medicines, vitamins, and supplements you take, including:

- Aspirin or medicines that contain aspirin

- Arthritis medicines

- Blood thinners

- Blood pressure medicines

- Diabetes medicines

- Nonsteroidal anti-inflammatory drugs (NSAIDs) such as ibuprofen and naproxen

You can take most medicines as usual, but you may need to adjust or stop some medicines for a short time before your upper GI endoscopy. Your doctor will tell you about any necessary changes to your medicines before the procedure.

Arrange for a Ride Home

For safety reasons, you can't drive for 24 hours after the procedure, as the sedatives used during the procedure need time to wear off. You will need to make plans for getting a ride home after the procedure.

Do Not Eat or Drink before the Procedure

To see your upper GI tract clearly, your doctor will most likely ask you not to eat or drink up to eight hours before the procedure.

How Do Doctors Perform an Upper GI Endoscopy?

A doctor performs an upper GI endoscopy in a hospital or an outpatient center. Before the procedure, you will likely get a sedative or a medicine to help you stay relaxed and comfortable during the procedure. The sedative will be given to you through an intravenous (IV) needle in your arm. In some cases, the procedure can be done without getting a sedative. You may also be given a liquid medicine to gargle or a spray to numb your throat and help prevent you from gagging during the procedure. The healthcare staff will monitor your vital signs and keep you as comfortable as possible.

You'll be asked to lie on your side on an exam table. The doctor will carefully pass the endoscope down your esophagus and into your stomach and duodenum. A small camera mounted on the endoscope will send a video image to a monitor, allowing close examination of the lining of your upper GI tract. The endoscope pumps air into your stomach and duodenum, making them easier to see.

During the upper GI endoscopy, the doctor may:

- take small samples of tissue, cells, or fluid in your upper GI tract for testing

- stop any bleeding

- perform other procedures, such as opening up strictures

The upper GI endoscopy most often takes between 15 and 30 minutes. The endoscope does not interfere with your breathing, and many people fall asleep during the procedure.

What Should I Expect after an Upper GI Endoscopy?

After an upper GI endoscopy, you can expect the following:

- To stay at the hospital or outpatient center for one to two hours after the procedure so the sedative can wear off

- To rest at home for the rest of the day

- Bloating or nausea for a short time after the procedure

- A sore throat for one to two days

- To go back to your normal diet once your swallowing returns to normal

After the procedure, you—or a friend or family member who is with you if you're still groggy—will receive instructions on how to care for yourself when you are home. You should follow all instructions. Some results from an upper GI endoscopy are available right away. Your doctor will share these results with you or, if you choose, with your friend or family member. A pathologist will examine the samples of tissue, cells, or fluid that were taken to help make a diagnosis. Biopsy results take a few days or longer to come back. The pathologist will send a report to your healthcare professional to discuss with you.

What Are the Risks of an Upper GI Endoscopy?

Upper GI endoscopy is considered a safe procedure. The risks of complications from an upper GI endoscopy are low, but may include:

- Bleeding from the site where the doctor took the tissue samples or removed a polyp

- Perforation in the lining of your upper GI tract

- An abnormal reaction to the sedative, including breathing or heart problems

Bleeding caused by the procedure often is minor and stops without treatment. Serious complications such as perforation are uncommon. Your doctor may need to perform surgery to treat some complications. Your doctor can also treat an abnormal reaction to a sedative with medicines or IV fluids during or after the procedure.

Seek Care Right Away

If you have any of the following symptoms after an upper GI endoscopy, seek medical care right away:

- Chest pain

- Problems breathing

- Problems swallowing or throat pain that gets worse

- Vomiting—particularly if your vomit is bloody or looks like coffee grounds

- Pain in your abdomen that gets worse

- Bloody or black, tar-colored stool

- Fever

Section 7.4

Endoscopic Ultrasound

This section includes text excerpted from "Endoscopic Ultrasound," U.S. Department of Veterans Affairs (VA), May 26, 2017.

New technology has allowed for the development of a specialized endoscope that has ultrasound capabilities. This enables the physician to visualize the internal layers of the wall of the esophagus, stomach, first part of the small intestine, liver, and pancreas. Being able to see an ultrasound image of the structures beyond the wall of the esophagus, stomach, and small intestine, allows the doctor to pass a small needle through the scope to take biopsy samples of pancreatic tumors, lymph nodes, and other types of abnormalities. This technology can also be used in the staging of cancerous tumors of the esophagus, stomach, pancreas, and liver providing valuable information to the physicians for planning their patients care and treatment.

Preparing for Endoscopic Ultrasound

Follow these and any other instructions you are given before your endoscopic ultrasound. If you don't follow the doctor's instructions carefully, the test may need to be rescheduled.

- Tell your healthcare provider before the exam if you are taking any medications or have any medical problems.

- Do not eat or drink anything after midnight the night before your exam.

- If your exam is in the afternoon, drink only clear liquids in the morning, and do not eat or drink anything for six hours before the exam.

- On the morning of the procedure, take all important medications (for heart, high blood pressure, or seizure disorders) as prescribed with a small amount of water.

- Female patients under the age of 55 who have not had a hysterectomy will be required to provide a urine specimen upon arrival.

- Bring your X-rays and any other test results you have.

- Bring a responsible adult (over 18 years old) to your appointment. The doctor will ask them to wait in the lobby and take you home after the procedure. If you arrive without a responsible adult, even if you complete the prep, your procedure may need to be rescheduled, or you may need to spend the night in the hospital. Please call your Patient Aligned Care Team (PACT) to discuss options in advance if you do not have someone to come with you to the appointment.

The Procedure

- You lie on the endoscopy table.

- You are given sedating (relaxing) medication through an intravenous (IV) line.

- You swallow the ultrasound scope. This is thinner than most pieces of food that you swallow. It will not affect your breathing. The medication helps keep you from gagging.

- Air is inserted to expand your gastrointestinal (GI) tract. It can make you burp.

- The ultrasound scope carries images of your upper GI tract to a video screen.

After the Test

- You may discuss the preliminary results with your doctor at your visit. If tissue is removed, a letter with biopsy results will be mailed to your home address within two weeks.

- After the procedure is done, plan to rest for the remainder of the day.

- You will be able to eat after you leave the procedure area, unless your doctor advises otherwise.

- You may feel a little bloating or have a sore throat for the first day.

Risks and Possible Complications

- Bleeding
- A puncture or tear in the GI tract
- Risks of anesthesia or sedating medications

Section 7.5

Flexible Sigmoidoscopy

This section includes text excerpted from "Flexible Sigmoidoscopy," National Institute of Diabetes and Digestive and Kidney Diseases (NIDDK), July 2016.

What Is Flexible Sigmoidoscopy?

Flexible sigmoidoscopy is a procedure in which a trained medical professional uses a flexible, narrow tube with a light and tiny camera on one end, called a sigmoidoscope or scope, to look inside your rectum and lower colon, also called the sigmoid colon and descending colon. Flexible sigmoidoscopy can show irritated or swollen tissue, ulcers, polyps, and cancer.

Why Do Doctors Use Flexible Sigmoidoscopy?

A flexible sigmoidoscopy can help a doctor find the cause of unexplained symptoms, such as:

- Bleeding from your anus
- Changes in your bowel activity such as diarrhea
- Pain in your abdomen
- Unexplained weight loss

Doctors also use flexible sigmoidoscopy as a screening tool for colon polyps and colon and rectal cancer. Screening may find diseases at an early stage, when a doctor has a better chance of curing the disease.

Screening for Colon and Rectal Cancer

Your doctor will recommend screening for colon and rectal cancer at age 50 if you don't have health problems or other factors that make you more likely to develop colon cancer.

Factors that make you more likely to develop colorectal cancer include:

- Someone in your family has had polyps or cancer of the colon or rectum
- A personal history of inflammatory bowel disease (IBD), such as ulcerative colitis or Crohn disease

- Other factors, such as if you weigh too much or smoke cigarettes

If you are more likely to develop colorectal cancer, your doctor may recommend screening at a younger age, and you may need to be tested more often. If you are older than age 75, talk with your doctor about whether you should be screened.

Most doctors recommend colonoscopy to screen for colon cancer because colonoscopy shows the entire colon and can remove colon polyps. However, preparing for and performing a flexible sigmoidoscopy may take less time and you may not need anesthesia. Healthcare providers may combine flexible sigmoidoscopy with other tests.

If your doctor finds an abnormal tissue or one or more polyps during a flexible sigmoidoscopy, you should have a colonoscopy to examine the rest of your colon.

Government health insurance plans, such as Medicare, and private health insurance plans sometimes change whether and how often they pay for cancer screening tests. Check with your insurance plan to find out how often your insurance will cover a screening flexible sigmoidoscopy.

How Do I Prepare for a Flexible Sigmoidoscopy?

To prepare for a flexible sigmoidoscopy, you will need to talk with your doctor, change your diet, and clean out your bowel.

Talk with Your Doctor

You should talk with your doctor about any medical conditions you have and all prescribed and over-the-counter (OTC) medicines, vitamins, and supplements you take, including:

- Arthritis medicines

- Aspirin or medicines that contain aspirin

- Blood thinners

- Diabetes medicines

- Nonsteroidal anti-inflammatory drugs (NSAIDs), such as ibuprofen or naproxen

- Vitamins that contain iron or iron supplements

Change Your Diet and Clean out Your Bowel

A healthcare professional will give you written bowel prep instructions to follow at home before the procedure. A healthcare professional orders a bowel prep so that little or no stool is present in your intestine. A complete bowel prep lets you pass stool that is clear and liquid. Stool inside your colon can prevent your doctor from clearly seeing the lining of your intestine.

You may need to follow a clear liquid diet the day before the procedure. The instructions will provide specific direction about when to start and stop the clear liquid diet. In most cases, you may drink or eat the following:

- Fat-free bouillon or broth

- Gelatin in flavors such as lemon, lime, or orange

- Plain coffee or tea, without cream or milk

- Sports drinks in flavors such as lemon, lime, or orange

- Strained fruit juice, such as apple or white grape—doctors recommend avoiding orange juice and red or purple liquids

- Water

Your doctor will tell you how long before the procedure you should have nothing by mouth. A healthcare professional will ask you to follow the directions for a bowel prep before the procedure. The bowel prep will cause diarrhea, so you should stay close to a bathroom.

Different bowel preps may contain different combinations of laxatives—pills that you swallow or powders that you dissolve in water and other clear liquids—and enemas. Some people will need to drink a large amount, often a gallon, of liquid laxative over a scheduled amount of time—most often the night before the procedure.

You may find this part of the bowel prep difficult; however, completing the prep is very important. Your doctor will not be able to see your sigmoid colon clearly if the prep is incomplete. Call a healthcare professional if you have side effects that prevent you from finishing the prep.

How Do Doctors Perform a Flexible Sigmoidoscopy?

A trained medical professional performs a flexible sigmoidoscopy during an office visit or at a hospital or an outpatient center. You typically do not need sedatives or anesthesia, and the procedure takes about 20 minutes.

For the procedure, you'll be asked to lie on a table while the doctor inserts a sigmoidoscope into your anus and slowly guides it through your rectum and into your sigmoid colon. The scope pumps air into your large intestine to give the doctor a better view. The camera sends a video image of your intestinal lining to a monitor, allowing the doctor to examine the tissues lining your sigmoid colon and rectum. The doctor may ask you to move several times on the table to adjust the scope for better viewing. Once the scope has reached your transverse colon, the doctor slowly withdraws it and examines the lining of your sigmoid colon again.

During the procedure, your doctor may remove polyps and send them to a lab for testing. Colon polyps are common in adults and are harmless in most cases. However, most colon cancer begins as a polyp, so removing polyps early is an effective way to prevent cancer.

If your doctor finds an abnormal tissue, he or she may perform a biopsy. You won't feel the biopsy. If your doctor found polyps or other abnormal tissue during a flexible sigmoidoscopy, your doctor may suggest you return for a colonoscopy.

What Should I Expect after a Flexible Sigmoidoscopy?

After a flexible sigmoidoscopy, you can expect the following:

- You may have cramping in your abdomen or bloating during the first hour after the procedure.

- You can resume regular activities right away after the procedure.

- You can return to a normal diet.

A healthcare professional will give you written instructions on how to take care of yourself after the procedure and will review them with you. You should follow all instructions.

If the doctor removed polyps or performed a biopsy, you may have light bleeding from your anus. This bleeding is normal. Some results from a flexible sigmoidoscopy are available right after the procedure, and your doctor will share these results with you. A pathologist will examine the biopsy tissue. Biopsy results take a few days or longer to come back.

What Are the Risks of a Flexible Sigmoidoscopy?

The risks of a flexible sigmoidoscopy include:

- Bleeding

- Perforation of the colon

- Severe pain in your abdomen

- Death, although this risk is rare

Bleeding and perforation are the most common complications from flexible sigmoidoscopy. Most cases of bleeding occur in patients who have polyps removed. The doctor can treat bleeding that occurs during the flexible sigmoidoscopy right away. However, you may have delayed bleeding up to two weeks after the procedure. The doctor diagnoses and treats delayed bleeding with a colonoscopy or repeat flexible sigmoidoscopy. The doctor may need to treat perforation with surgery.

Section 7.6

Endoscopic Retrograde Cholangiopancreatography

This section includes text excerpted from "Endoscopic Retrograde Cholangiopancreatography (ERCP)," National Institute of Diabetes and Digestive and Kidney Diseases (NIDDK), June 2016.

What Is Endoscopic Retrograde Cholangiopancreatography?

Endoscopic retrograde cholangiopancreatography (ERCP) is a procedure that combines upper gastrointestinal (GI) endoscopy and X-rays to treat problems of the bile and pancreatic ducts.

What Are the Bile and Pancreatic Ducts?

Your bile ducts are tubes that carry bile from your liver to your gallbladder and duodenum. Your pancreatic ducts are tubes that carry pancreatic juice from your pancreas to your duodenum. Small pancreatic ducts empty into the main pancreatic duct. Your common bile duct and main pancreatic duct join before emptying into your duodenum.

Why Do Doctors Use Endoscopic Retrograde Cholangiopancreatography?

Doctors use ERCP to treat problems of the bile and pancreatic ducts. Doctors also use ERCP to diagnose problems of the bile and pancreatic ducts if they expect to treat problems during the procedure. For diagnosis alone, doctors may use noninvasive tests—tests that do not physically enter the body—instead of ERCP. Noninvasive tests such as magnetic resonance cholangiopancreatography (MRCP)—a type of magnetic resonance imaging (MRI)—are safer and can also diagnose many problems of the bile and pancreatic ducts.

Doctors perform ERCP when your bile or pancreatic ducts have become narrowed or blocked because of:

- Gallstones that form in your gallbladder and become stuck in your common bile duct
- Infection
- Acute pancreatitis
- Chronic pancreatitis
- Trauma or surgical complications in your bile or pancreatic ducts
- Pancreatic pseudocysts
- Tumors or cancers of the bile ducts
- Tumors or cancers of the pancreas

How Do I Prepare for Endoscopic Retrograde Cholangiopancreatography?

To prepare for ERCP, talk with your doctor, arrange for a ride home, and follow your doctor's instructions.

Talk with Your Doctor

You should talk with your doctor about any allergies and medical conditions you have and all prescribed and over-the-counter (OTC) medicines, vitamins, and supplements you take, including:

- Arthritis medicines

- Aspirin or medicines that contain aspirin

- Blood thinners

- Blood pressure medicines

- Diabetes medicines

- Nonsteroidal anti-inflammatory drugs (NSAIDs) such as ibuprofen and naproxen

Your doctor may ask you to temporarily stop taking medicines that affect blood clotting or interact with sedatives. You typically receive sedatives during ERCP to help you relax and stay comfortable.

Tell your doctor if you are, or may be, pregnant. If you are pregnant and need ERCP to treat a problem, the doctor performing the procedure may make changes to protect the fetus from X-rays. Research has found that ERCP is generally safe during pregnancy.

Arrange for a Ride Home

For safety reasons, you can't drive for 24 hours after ERCP, as the sedatives or anesthesia used during the procedure needs time to wear off. You will need to make plans for getting a ride home after ERCP.

Don't Eat, Drink, Smoke, or Chew Gum

To see your upper GI tract clearly, your doctor will most likely ask you not to eat, drink, smoke, or chew gum during the eight hours before ERCP.

How Do Doctors Perform Endoscopic Retrograde Cholangiopancreatography?

Doctors who have specialized training in ERCP perform this procedure at a hospital or an outpatient center. An intravenous (IV) needle will be placed in your arm to provide a sedative. Sedatives help you stay relaxed and comfortable during the procedure. A healthcare professional will give you a liquid anesthetic to gargle or will spray anesthetic on the back of your throat. The anesthetic numbs your throat and helps prevent gagging during the procedure. The healthcare staff will monitor your vital signs and keep you as comfortable as possible. In some cases, you may receive general anesthesia.

You'll be asked to lie on an examination table. The doctor will carefully feed the endoscope down your esophagus, through your stomach, and into your duodenum. A small camera mounted on the endoscope will send a video image to a monitor. The endoscope pumps air into your stomach and duodenum, making them easier to see.

During ERCP, the doctor:

- locates the opening where the bile and pancreatic ducts empty into the duodenum

- slides a thin, flexible tube called a catheter through the endoscope and into the ducts

- injects a special dye, also called contrast medium, into the ducts through the catheter to make the ducts more visible on X-rays

- uses a type of X-ray imaging, called fluoroscopy, to examine the ducts and look for narrowed areas or blockages

The doctor may pass tiny tools through the endoscope to:

- open blocked or narrowed ducts

- break up or remove stones

- perform a biopsy or remove tumors in the ducts

- insert stents—tiny tubes that a doctor leaves in narrowed ducts to hold them open. A doctor may also insert temporary stents to stop bile leaks that can occur after gallbladder surgery

The procedure most often takes between one and two hours.

What Should I Expect after Endoscopic Retrograde Cholangiopancreatography?

After ERCP, you can expect the following:

- You will most often stay at the hospital or outpatient center for one to two hours after the procedure so the sedation or anesthesia can wear off. In some cases, you may need to stay overnight in the hospital after ERCP.

- You may have bloating or nausea for a short time after the procedure.

- You may have a sore throat for one to two days.

- You can go back to a normal diet once your swallowing has returned to normal.

- You should rest at home for the remainder of the day.

Following the procedure, you—or a friend or family member who is with you if you're still groggy—will receive instructions on how to care for yourself after the procedure. You should follow all instructions.

Some results from ERCP are available right away after the procedure. After the sedative has worn off, the doctor will share results with you or, if you choose, with your friend or family member.

If the doctor performed a biopsy, a pathologist will examine the biopsy tissue. Biopsy results take a few days or longer to come back.

What Are the Risks of Endoscopic Retrograde Cholangiopancreatography?

The risks of ERCP include complications such as the following:

- Pancreatitis

- Infection of the bile ducts or gallbladder

- Excessive bleeding, called hemorrhage

- An abnormal reaction to the sedative, including respiratory or cardiac problems

- Perforation in the bile or pancreatic ducts, or in the duodenum near the opening where the bile and pancreatic ducts empty into it

- Tissue damage from X-ray exposure

- Death, although this complication is rare

Research has found that these complications occur in about 5–10 percent of ERCP procedures. People with complications often need treatment at a hospital.

Chapter 8

Upper and Lower GI Series

Chapter Contents

Section 8.1

Upper GI Series

This section includes text excerpted from "Upper GI Series,"
National Institute of Diabetes and Digestive and Kidney
Diseases (NIDDK), August 2016.

What Is an Upper Gastrointestinal (GI) Series?

An upper gastrointestinal (GI) series is a procedure in which a doctor uses X-rays, fluoroscopy, and a chalky liquid called barium to view your upper GI tract. The barium will make your upper GI tract more visible on an X-ray.

The two types of upper GI series are:

1. A standard barium upper GI series, which uses only barium

2. A double-contrast upper GI series, which uses both air and barium for a clearer view of your stomach lining

Why Do Doctors Use Upper GI Series?

An upper GI series can help a doctor find the cause of:

- Nausea and vomiting
- Pain in the abdomen
- Problems swallowing
- Unexplained weight loss

An upper GI series can also show:

- Abnormal growths such as cancer
- Esophageal varices
- Gastroesophageal reflux (GER)
- A hiatal hernia
- Scars or strictures
- Ulcers

How Do I Prepare for an Upper GI Series?

To prepare for an upper GI series, don't eat, drink, smoke, or chew gum. You also will need to talk with your doctor.

Don't Eat, Drink, Smoke, or Chew Gum

In order to see your upper GI tract clearly, your doctor will most likely ask you not to eat, drink, smoke, or chew gum during the eight hours before the upper GI series.

Talk with Your Doctor

You should talk with your doctor about any medical conditions you have and all prescribed and over-the-counter (OTC) medicines, vitamins, and supplements you take.

Doctors don't recommend X-rays for pregnant women because X-rays may harm the fetus. Tell your doctor if you are, or may be, pregnant. Your doctor may suggest a different procedure. A doctor may recommend an upper GI series for your child when the benefits of the procedure outweigh the relatively small risk of X-rays. Talk with your child's doctor about safety measures used to lower your child's exposure to X-rays during the procedure.

How Do Doctors Perform an Upper GI Series?

An X-ray technician and a radiologist perform an upper GI series at a hospital or an outpatient center. You do not need anesthesia. The procedure usually takes about two hours. The procedure can take up to five hours if the barium moves slowly through your small intestine. For the procedure, you'll be asked to stand or sit in front of an X-ray machine and drink barium, which coats the lining of your upper GI tract. You will then lie on the X-ray table, and the radiologist will watch the barium move through your GI tract on the X-ray and fluoroscopy. The technician may press on your abdomen or ask you to change position several times to evenly coat your upper GI tract with the barium. If you are having a double-contrast study, you will swallow gas-forming crystals that mix with the barium coating your stomach. Gas forms when the crystals and barium mix. The gas expands your stomach, which lets the radiologist see more details of your upper GI tract lining. The technician will then take additional X-rays.

What Should I Expect after an Upper GI Series?

After an upper GI series, you can expect the following:

- You may have cramping in your abdomen and bloating during the first hour after the procedure.

- You may resume most normal activities after leaving the hospital or outpatient center.

- For several days, your stools may be white or light colored from the barium in your GI tract.

- A healthcare professional will give you instructions on how to care for yourself after the procedure. The instructions will explain how to flush the remaining barium from your GI tract. You should follow all instructions.

- A specialist will read the X-rays and send a report of the findings to your doctor.

What Are the Risks of an Upper GI Series?

The risks of an upper GI series include:

- Constipation from the barium—the most common complication of an upper GI series

- An allergic reaction to the barium or flavoring in the barium

- Intestinal obstruction

Section 8.2

Lower GI Series (Barium Enema)

This section includes text excerpted from "Lower GI Series,"
National Institute of Diabetes and Digestive and Kidney
Diseases (NIDDK), June 2016.

What Is Lower Gastrointestinal (GI) Series?

A lower gastrointestinal (GI) series is a procedure in which a doctor uses X-rays and a chalky liquid called barium to view your large intestine. The barium will make your large intestine more visible on an X-ray.

The two types of lower GI series are:

1. A single-contrast lower GI series, which uses only barium

2. A double-contrast or air-contrast lower GI series, which uses both barium and air for a clearer view of your large intestine

Lower GI series is also called a barium enema.

Why Do Doctors Use Lower GI Series?

A lower GI series can help a doctor find the cause of:

*   Bleeding from your anus
*   Changes in your bowel activity
*   Chronic diarrhea
*   Pain in your abdomen
*   Unexplained weight loss

A lower GI series can also show:

*   Cancerous growths
*   Diverticula
*   A fistula
*   Polyps
*   Ulcers

How Do I Prepare for a Lower GI Series?

To prepare for a lower GI series, you will need to talk with your doctor, change your diet, and clean out your bowel.

Talk with Your Doctor

You should talk with your doctor about any medical conditions you have and all prescribed and over-the-counter (OTC) medicines, vitamins, and supplements you take.

Also, tell your doctor whether you've had a colonoscopy with a biopsy or polyp removal in the last four weeks. Doctors don't recommend X-rays for pregnant women because X-rays may harm the fetus. Tell your doctor if you are, or may be, pregnant. Your doctor may suggest a different procedure.

Change Your Diet and Clean out Your Bowel

A healthcare professional will give you written bowel prep instructions to follow at home before the procedure. A healthcare professional orders a bowel prep so that little to no stool is present in your intestine. A complete bowel prep lets you pass stool that is clear and liquid. Stool inside your colon can prevent the X-ray machine from taking clear images of your intestine.

You may need to follow a clear liquid diet for one to three days before the procedure. The instructions will provide specific direction about when to start and stop the clear liquid diet. In most cases, you may drink or eat the following:

- Fat-free bouillon or broth

- Gelatin in flavors such as lemon, lime, or orange

- Plain coffee or tea, without cream or milk

- Sports drinks in flavors such as lemon, lime, or orange

- Strained fruit juice, such as apple or white grape—doctors recommend avoiding orange juice

- Water

Your doctor will tell you how long before the procedure you should have nothing by mouth.

A healthcare professional will ask you to follow the directions for a bowel prep before the procedure. The bowel prep will cause diarrhea, so you should stay close to a bathroom.

Different bowel preps may contain different combinations of laxatives—pills that you swallow or powders that you dissolve in water and other clear liquids—and enemas. Some people will need to drink a large amount, often a gallon, of liquid laxative during a scheduled amount of time—most often the night before the procedure.

You may find this part of the bowel prep difficult; however, completing the prep is very important. Your doctor will not be able to see your large intestine clearly if the prep is incomplete. Call a healthcare professional if you have side effects that prevent you from finishing the prep.

How Do Doctors Perform a Lower GI Series?

An X-ray technician and a radiologist perform a lower GI series at a hospital or an outpatient center. You do not need anesthesia. The procedure usually takes 30–60 minutes.

For the procedure, you'll be asked to lie on a table while the radiologist inserts a flexible tube into your anus and fills your large intestine with barium. The radiologist prevents barium from leaking from your anus by inflating a balloon on the end of the tube. You may be asked to change position several times to evenly coat the large intestine with the barium. If you are having a double-contrast lower GI series, the radiologist will inject air through the tube to inflate the large intestine.

During the procedure, you may have some discomfort and feel the urge to have a bowel movement. You will need to hold still in various positions while the radiologist and technician take X-ray images and possibly an X-ray video, called fluoroscopy.

The radiologist or technician will deflate the balloon on the tube when the imaging is complete. Most of the barium will drain through the tube. You will push out the remaining barium into a bedpan or nearby toilet. A healthcare professional may give you an enema to flush out the rest of the barium.

What Should I Expect after a Lower GI Series?

After a lower GI series, you can expect the following:

- You may have cramping in your abdomen and bloating during the first hour after the procedure.

- You may resume most normal activities after leaving the hospital or outpatient center.

- For several days, your stools may be white or light colored from the barium in your large intestine.

- A healthcare professional will give you instructions on how to care for yourself after the procedure. The instructions will explain how to flush the remaining barium from your large intestine. You should follow all instructions.

The radiologist will read the X-rays and send a report of the findings to your doctor.

What Are the Risks of a Lower GI Series?

The risks of a lower GI series include:

- Constipation from the barium enema—the most common complication of a lower GI series

117

- An allergic reaction to the barium

- Intestinal obstruction

- Leakage of barium into your abdomen through a tear or hole in the lining of the large intestine

Chapter 9

Diagnostic Liver Tests

Chapter Contents

Section 9.1

Tests for Liver Damage

This section includes text excerpted from "Viral Hepatitis—
Tests of the Liver," U.S. Department of Veterans Affairs (VA),
February 14, 2018.

Most people with chronic liver disease will have no ongoing symptoms, and the damage will be detected only by blood tests. The tests (called a "liver panel") measure:

- Your level of liver enzymes

- Your level of bilirubin, which rises when the liver is not working well

- A protein called albumin, whose levels go down when the liver is damaged

Doctors can run more blood tests if they need to in order to find out what is causing the damage to your liver. Ultrasound, computed tomography (CT) scans, and magnetic resonance imaging (MRI) are the three main methods of taking pictures of the liver. They can often show if the liver injury has become serious. A liver biopsy, in which a needle is used to take a sample of the liver itself, can tell even more about the liver's health.

Some people with liver problems can have a swollen liver. Others may have severe scarring or a shrunken liver. During an examination, a doctor can feel the liver to find out if it is shrunken, hard, or swollen.

There's a handful of liver tests and it is helpful to know what each of them means. Here, common liver blood tests and how to understand your results are explained:

Liver Panel

A "liver panel" usually refers to several lab tests performed as a group. Depending on the physician or the laboratory, a liver panel usually includes tests for aspartate aminotransferase (AST), alanine aminotransferase (ALT), bilirubin, and alkaline phosphatase.

Liver Enzymes

Usually, the term "liver enzymes" refers to the AST and the ALT.

Liver Function Tests (LFTs)

The phrase "liver function tests" or "LFTs" is commonly used by patients and physicians. Many patients and physicians use the term to describe the aspartate aminotransferase (AST) and alanine amino-transferase (ALT). However, this is not correct—the AST and ALT do not measure the function of the liver.

The true function of the liver is actually best measured by the prothrombin time (PT), international normalized ratio (INR), and albumin. Therefore, if you are getting a PT, INR or albumin, these tests can determine how the liver is "functioning."

Alanine Aminotransferase (ALT)

ALT, or alanine aminotransferase, is one of the two "liver enzymes." It is sometimes known as serum glutamic-pyruvic transaminase, or SGPT. It is a protein made only by liver cells. When liver cells are damaged, ALT leaks out into the bloodstream and the level of ALT in the blood is higher than normal.

Explanation of Test Results

A high ALT level often means there is some liver damage, but it may not be related to hepatitis C. It is important to realize the ALT level goes up and down in most patients with hepatitis C. The ALT level does not tell you exactly how much liver damage there is, and small changes should be expected. Changes in the ALT level do not mean the liver is doing any better or any worse. The ALT level does not tell you how much scarring (fibrosis) is in the liver and it does not predict how much liver damage will develop.

Other Things to Know

- Many patients with hepatitis C will have a normal ALT level.

- Patients can have very severe liver disease and cirrhosis and still have a normal ALT level.

- When a patient takes treatment for hepatitis C, it is helpful to see if the ALT level goes down.

Aspartate Aminotransferase (AST)

AST, or aspartate aminotransferase, is one of the two "liver enzymes." It is also known as serum glutamic-oxaloacetic

121

transaminase, or SGOT. AST is a protein made by liver cells. When liver cells are damaged, AST leaks out into the bloodstream and the level of AST in the blood becomes higher than normal. AST is different from ALT because AST is found in parts of the body other than the liver—including the heart, kidneys, muscles, and brain. When cells in any of those parts of the body are damaged, AST can be elevated.

Explanation of Test Results

A high AST level often means there is some liver damage, but it is not necessarily caused by hepatitis C. A high AST with a normal ALT may mean that the AST is coming from a different part of the body. It is important to realize that the AST level in most patients with hepatitis C goes up and down. The exact AST level does not tell you how much liver damage there is, or whether the liver is getting better or worse, and small changes should be expected. However, for patients receiving treatment for hepatitis C, it is helpful to see if the AST level goes down.

Other Things to Know

- The AST level is not as helpful as the ALT level for checking the liver.
- Many patients with hepatitis C will have a normal AST level.
- Patients can have very severe liver disease or cirrhosis and still have a normal AST level.

Bilirubin

Bilirubin is a yellowish substance that is created by the breakdown (destruction) of hemoglobin, a major component of red blood cells (RBCs).

Explanation of Test Results

As red blood cells age, they are broken down naturally in the body. Bilirubin is released from the destroyed red blood cells and passed on to the liver. The liver excretes the bilirubin in fluid called bile. If the liver is not functioning correctly, the bilirubin will not be properly excreted. Therefore, if the bilirubin level is higher than normal, it may mean that the liver is not functioning correctly.

Other Things to Know

- Levels of bilirubin in the blood go up and down in patients with hepatitis C.

- When bilirubin levels remain high for prolonged periods, it usually means there is severe liver disease and possibly cirrhosis.

- High levels of bilirubin can cause jaundice (yellowing of the skin and eyes, darker urine, and lighter-colored bowel movements).

- Elevated bilirubin levels can be caused by reasons other than liver disease.

- Total bilirubin is made up of two components: direct bilirubin and indirect bilirubin.

- Direct bilirubin + indirect bilirubin = total bilirubin.

Albumin

Albumin is a protein made by the liver. Albumin prevents fluid from leaking out of blood vessels into tissues.

Explanation of Test Results

A low albumin level in patients with hepatitis C can be a sign of cirrhosis (advanced liver disease). Albumin levels can go up and down slightly. Very low albumin levels can cause symptoms of edema, or fluid accumulation, in the abdomen (called ascites) or in the leg.

Other Things to Know

- A low albumin level can also come from kidney disease or malnutrition or acute illness.

- A low albumin level causing fluid overload is often treated with diuretic medications, or "water pills."

Prothrombin Time (PT)

Prothrombin is a protein made by the liver. Prothrombin helps blood to make normal clots. The "prothrombin time" (PT) is one way of measuring how long it takes blood to form a clot, and it is measured in seconds (such as 13.2 seconds). A normal PT indicates that a normal amount of blood-clotting protein is available.

Explanation of Test Results

When the PT is high, it takes longer for the blood to clot (17 seconds, for example). This usually happens because the liver is not making the right amount of blood clotting proteins, so the clotting process takes longer. A high PT usually means that there is serious liver damage or cirrhosis.

Other Things to Know

- Some patients take a drug called Coumadin (warfarin), which elevates the PT for the purpose of "thinning" the blood. This is not related to having liver disease because it is the Coumadin causing the PT to be high.

- The test called INR measures the same factors as PT and is used instead of PT by many doctors.

Alkaline Phosphatase (ALP)

Alkaline phosphatase (ALP) (often shortened to alk phos) is an enzyme made in liver cells and bile ducts. The alk phos level is a common test that is usually included when liver tests are performed as a group.

Explanation of Test Results

A high alk phos level does not reflect liver damage or inflammation. A high alk phos level occurs when there is a blockage of flow in the biliary tract or a buildup of pressure in the liver—often caused by a gallstone or scarring in the bile ducts.

Other Things to Know

- Many patients with hepatitis C have normal alk phos levels.
- Hepatitis C treatment usually does not affect alk phos levels.
- Alk phos is produced in other organs besides the liver—it is also found in the bones and the kidneys.
- If your alk phos level is high, your doctor will probably order additional tests to determine why.

International Normalized Ratio (INR)

International normalized ratio (INR) is a blood-clotting test. It is a test used to measure how quickly your blood forms a clot, compared with normal clotting time.

Explanation of Test Results

A normal INR is 1.0. Each increase of 0.1 means the blood is slightly thinner (it takes longer to clot). INR is related to the prothrombin time (PT). If there is serious liver disease and cirrhosis, the liver may not produce the normal amount of proteins and then the blood is not able to clot normally. When your doctor is evaluating the function of your liver, a high INR usually means that the liver is not working as well as it could because it is not making the blood clot normally.

Other Things to Know

- Some patients take a drug called Coumadin (warfarin), which elevates the INR, for the purpose of "thinning" the blood.

- The INR is another way of measuring the blood-clotting time and it is easier to determine than the PT.

Platelets

Platelets are cells that help the blood to form clots. The platelet number or "platelet count" in the blood is measured as part of the complete blood count (CBC).

Explanation of Test Results

Platelet counts in a patient who has cirrhosis are often low. But low platelet counts can also come from other causes, including certain medications. Interferon treatment can reduce platelet counts. When the platelet count is extremely reduced, this condition is known as "thrombocytopenia." If a platelet count is too low, the patient cannot make normal clots and may bruise more easily.

Other Things to Know

- If the platelet count drops too low (below 50,000, for example) when a patient is receiving interferon, doctors may recommend that the interferon dosage be reduced.

Total Protein

Total protein level is a measure of a number of different proteins in the blood. Total protein can be divided into the albumin and globulin fractions.

Explanation of Test Results

Low levels of total protein in the blood can occur because of impaired function of the liver.

Section 9.2

Liver Biopsy

This section includes text excerpted from "Liver Biopsy," National Institute of Diabetes and Digestive and Kidney Diseases (NIDDK), May 2014. Reviewed September 2018.

What Is a Liver Biopsy?

A liver biopsy is a procedure that involves taking a small piece of liver tissue for examination with a microscope for signs of damage or disease. The three types of liver biopsy are the following:

1. Percutaneous biopsy—the most common type of liver biopsy—involves inserting a hollow needle through the abdomen into the liver. The abdomen is the area between the chest and hips.

2. Transvenous biopsy involves making a small incision in the neck and inserting a needle through a hollow tube called a sheath through the jugular vein to the liver.

3. Laparoscopic biopsy involves inserting a laparoscope, a thin tube with a tiny video camera attached, through a small incision to look inside the body to view the surface of organs. The healthcare provider will insert a needle through a plastic, tube-like instrument called a cannula to remove the liver tissue sample.

What Is the Liver and What Does It Do?

The liver is the body's largest internal organ. The liver is called the body's metabolic factory because of the important role it plays in metabolism—the way cells change food into energy after food is digested and absorbed into the blood. The liver has many functions, including:

- Taking up, storing, and processing nutrients from food— including fat, sugar, and protein—and delivering them to the rest of the body when needed

- Making new proteins, such as clotting factors and immune factors

- Producing bile, which helps the body absorb fats, cholesterol, and fat-soluble vitamins

- Removing waste products the kidneys cannot remove, such as fats, cholesterol, toxins, and medications

A healthy liver is necessary for survival. The liver can regenerate most of its own cells when they become damaged.

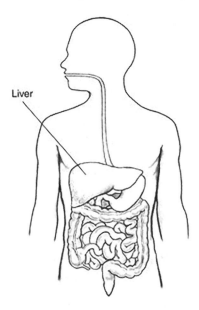

Liver

Figure 9.1. *Liver*

The liver, the body's largest internal organ, has many important functions.

Why Is a Liver Biopsy Performed?

A healthcare provider will perform a liver biopsy to:

- diagnose liver diseases that cannot be diagnosed with blood or imaging tests

- estimate the degree of liver damage, a process called staging
- help determine the best treatment for liver damage or disease

How Does a Person Prepare for a Liver Biopsy?

A person prepares for a liver biopsy by:

- talking with a healthcare provider
- having blood tests
- arranging for a ride home
- fasting before the procedure

Talking with a healthcare provider. People should talk with their healthcare provider about medical conditions they have and all prescribed and over-the-counter (OTC) medications, vitamins, and supplements they take, including:

- Antibiotics
- Antidepressants
- Aspirin
- Asthma medications
- Blood pressure medications
- Blood thinners
- Diabetes medications
- Dietary supplements
- Nonsteroidal anti-inflammatory drugs (NSAIDs) such as ibuprofen and naproxen

The healthcare provider may tell the person to stop taking medications temporarily that affect blood clotting or interact with anesthesia, which people sometimes receive during a liver biopsy.

Having blood tests. A person will have a test to show how well his or her blood clots. A person will have a test to show how well his or her blood clots. A technician or nurse draws a blood sample during an office visit or at a commercial facility and sends the sample to a lab for analysis. People with severe liver disease often have blood-clotting problems that can increase their chance of bleeding after the biopsy.

A healthcare provider may give the person a medication called clotting factor concentrates just before a liver biopsy to reduce the chance of bleeding.

Arranging for a ride home after the procedure. For safety reasons, most people cannot drive home after the procedure. A healthcare provider will ask a person to make advance arrangements for getting home after the procedure.

Fasting before the procedure. A healthcare provider will ask a person not to eat or drink for eight hours before the procedure if the provider anticipates using anesthesia or sedation.

How Is a Liver Biopsy Performed?

A healthcare provider performs the liver biopsy at a hospital or an outpatient center and determines which type of biopsy is best for the person.

Percutaneous Liver Biopsy

A person lies face up on a table and rests the right hand above the head. A healthcare provider gives the person a local anesthetic on the area where he or she will insert the biopsy needle. If needed, the healthcare provider will give the person sedatives and pain medication.

The healthcare provider either taps on the abdomen to locate the liver or uses one of the following imaging techniques:

- Ultrasound
- Computerized tomography (CT) scan

Research has shown fewer complications after biopsy when healthcare providers use ultrasound to locate the liver compared with tapping on the abdomen. Healthcare providers may select ultrasound over a CT scan because it is quicker and less expensive, and can show the biopsy needle in real time.

The healthcare provider will:

- make a small incision in the right side of the person's abdomen, either toward the bottom of or just below the rib cage
- insert the biopsy needle
- ask the person to exhale and hold his or her breath while the healthcare provider inserts the needle and quickly removes a sample of liver tissue

- insert and remove the needle several times if multiple samples are needed

- place a bandage over the incision

After the biopsy, the person must lie on his or her right side for up to two hours to reduce the chance of bleeding. Medical staff monitors the person for signs of bleeding for two to four more hours.

Transvenous Liver Biopsy

When a person's blood clots slowly or the person has ascites—a buildup of fluid in the abdomen—the healthcare provider may perform a transvenous liver biopsy.

For this procedure, the person lies face up on an X-ray table, and a healthcare provider applies local anesthetic to one side of the neck. The healthcare provider will give sedatives and pain medication if the person needs them.

The healthcare provider will:

- make a small incision in the neck

- insert a sheath into the jugular vein and thread the sheath down the jugular vein, along the side of the heart, and into one of the veins in the liver

- inject contrast medium into the sheath and take an X-ray. The contrast medium makes the blood vessels and the location of the sheath clearly visible on the X-ray images.

- thread a biopsy needle through the sheath and into the liver and quickly remove a liver tissue sample

- insert and remove the biopsy needle several times if multiple samples are needed

- carefully withdraw the sheath and close the incision with a bandage

Medical staff monitors the person for four to six hours afterward for signs of bleeding.

Laparoscopic Liver Biopsy

Healthcare providers use this type of biopsy to obtain a tissue sample from a specific area or from multiple areas of the liver, or when the risk of spreading cancer or infection exists. A healthcare provider may take a liver tissue sample during laparoscopic surgery performed for other reasons, including liver surgery.

The person lies on his or her back on an operating table. A nurse or technician will insert an intravenous (IV) needle into the person's arm to give anesthesia. The healthcare provider will:

- make a small incision in the abdomen, just below the rib cage

- insert a thin tube into the incision and fill the abdomen with gas to provide space to work inside the abdominal cavity and to see the liver

- insert a biopsy needle through the cannula and into the liver and quickly remove a liver tissue sample

- insert and remove the biopsy needle several times if multiple samples are needed

- remove the thin tube and close the incisions with dissolvable stitches

The healthcare provider can easily spot any bleeding from the procedure with the camera on the laparoscope and treat it using an electric probe. The person stays at the hospital or an outpatient center for a few hours while the anesthesia wears off.

What Can a Person Expect after a Liver Biopsy?

After a liver biopsy, a person can expect:

- Full recovery in one to two days

- To avoid intense activity, exercise, or heavy lifting for up to one week

- Soreness around the biopsy or incision site for about a week. Acetaminophen (Tylenol) or other pain medications that do not interfere with blood clotting may help. People should check with their healthcare provider before taking any pain medications.

- A member of the healthcare team to review the discharge instructions with the person—or with an accompanying friend or family member if the person is still groggy—and provide a written copy. The person should follow all instructions given.

Liver biopsy results take a few days to come back. The liver sample goes to a pathology lab where a technician stains the tissue. Staining highlights important details within the liver tissue and helps identify any signs of liver disease. The pathologist—a doctor who specializes in diagnosing diseases—looks at the tissue with a microscope and sends a report to the person's healthcare provider.

What Are the Risks of Liver Biopsy?

The risks of a liver biopsy include:

- Pain and bruising at the biopsy or incision site—the most common complication after a liver biopsy. Most people experience mild pain that does not require medication; however, some people need medications to relieve the pain.

- Prolonged bleeding from the biopsy or incision site or internal bleeding. A person may require hospitalization, transfusions, and sometimes surgery or another procedure to stop the bleeding.

- Infection of the biopsy site or incision site that may cause sepsis. Sepsis is an illness in which the body has a severe response to bacteria or a virus.

- Pneumothorax also called collapsed lung occurs when air or gas builds up in the pleural space. The pleural space is thin layers of tissue that wrap around the outside of the lungs and line the inside of the chest cavity. Pneumothorax may happen when the biopsy needle punctures the pleural space.

- Hemothorax, or the buildup of blood in the pleural space

- Puncture of other organs

Chapter 10

Other Diagnostic Tests of the Gastrointestinal Tract

Chapter Contents

Section 10.1

Esophageal Manometry Testing

This section includes text excerpted from "Esophageal Manometry,"
U.S. Department of Veterans Affairs (VA), March 27, 2017.

Esophageal manometry is a test to measure the strength and function of the esophagus (the "food pipe"). Results can help identify causes of heartburn, swallowing problems, or chest pain. The test can also help plan surgery and determine the success of previous surgery.

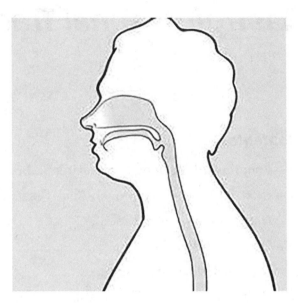

Figure 10.1. *Esophagus* (Source: "Where's the Feeding Tube?" Agency for Healthcare Research and Quality (AHRQ), U.S. Department of Health and Human Services (HHS).)

Preparing for the Test

Be sure to talk to your doctor about any medications you take. Some medications can affect the test results. Also ask any questions you have about the risks of the test. These include irritation to the nose and throat. Be sure not to smoke, eat, or drink for up to 12 hours before the test. Morning of the procedure take all important medications (for heart, high blood pressure, or seizure disorders) as prescribed with a small amount of water.

During the Test

Manometry takes about an hour. Usually, you lie down during the test. Your nose and throat are numbed. Then a soft, thin tube is placed through the nose and down the esophagus. At first, you may notice a gagging feeling. You will be asked to swallow several times. Holes along the tube measure the pressure while you swallow. Measurements are printed out as tracings, much like a heart test tracing. After the test, another catheter may be left in the esophagus for up to 24 hours to measure acid (pH) levels.

After Esophageal Manometry

You'll probably discuss the results of the test with your doctor at another appointment. This is because time is needed to review the tracings. You may have a mild sore throat for a short time. As soon as the numbness in your throat is gone, you can return to eating and your normal activities.

Section 10.2

Gastric Analysis (Stomach Acid Test)

This section includes text excerpted from "Gastric Analysis," Clinical Center, National Institutes of Health (NIH), March 1, 2016.

You are scheduled for gastric analysis. This test measures how much acid your stomach makes. For this test, the contents of your stomach will be collected through a tube inserted through your nose called a nasogastric tube.

Preparation

- Do not eat or drink after midnight on the day of the test, until the test is over.

- Your doctor will decide which medications you should stop taking before the test.

- For your comfort during the test, empty your bladder beforehand.

- Tell your doctor if you have a deviated septum or have ever broken your nose.

Procedure

- The test will be done in your room or in the endoscopy suite.

- A small tube will be inserted through your nose into your stomach. To help with this process, you will be asked to take small sips of water. You may feel pressure at the back of your nose for about five minutes.

- You will be asked to lie on your back or on your left side.

- A nurse will collect the contents of your stomach through the tube and place it in a container.

- You may be given medications during the test by injection. You may also have an IV (intravenous) line inserted. Blood samples may also be taken.

- The procedure usually starts early in the morning and lasts two hours or longer, depending on the type of test your doctor ordered.

After the Procedure

- After the test, the nasogastric tube will be removed.

- If you have questions about the procedure, your nurse and doctor will gladly answer your questions and are ready to assist you at all times.

Section 10.3

Helicobacter pylori *Test*

This section contains text excerpted from the following sources: Text in this section begins with excerpts from *"Helicobacter pylori* Infections," MedlinePlus, National Institutes of Health (NIH), April 23, 2018; Text under the heading "Lab Tests" is excerpted from "Diagnosis of Peptic Ulcers (Stomach Ulcers)," National Institute of Diabetes and Digestive and Kidney Diseases (NIDDK), November 2014. Reviewed September 2018.

Helicobacter pylori (H. pylori) is a type of bacteria that causes infection in the stomach. It is the main cause of peptic ulcers, and it can also cause gastritis and stomach cancer. About 30–40 percent of people in the United States get an *H. pylori* infection. Most people get it as a child. *H. pylori* usually does not cause symptoms. But it can break down the inner protective coating in some people's stomachs and cause inflammation. This can lead to gastritis or a peptic ulcer.

Researchers aren't sure how *H. pylori* spreads. They think that it may spread by unclean food and water, or through contact with an infected person's saliva and other body fluids. A peptic ulcer causes a dull or burning pain in your stomach, especially when you have an empty stomach. It lasts for minutes to hours, and it may come and go for several days or weeks. It may also cause other symptoms, such as bloating, nausea, and weight loss. If you have the symptoms of a peptic ulcer, your healthcare provider will check to see whether you have *H. pylori*. There are blood, breath, and stool tests to check for *H. pylori*. In some cases, you may need an upper endoscopy, often with a biopsy.

Lab Tests

To see if you have a *H. pylori* infection, your doctor will order these tests:

- **Blood test.** A blood test involves drawing a sample of your blood at your doctor's office or a commercial facility. A healthcare professional tests the blood sample to see if the results fall within the normal range for different disorders or infections.

- **Urea breath test.** For a urea breath test, you will drink a special liquid that contains urea, a waste product that your body makes as it breaks down protein. If *H. pylori* are present, the bacteria will change this waste product into carbon dioxide (CO_2)—a harmless gas. Carbon dioxide normally appears in your breath when you exhale.

A healthcare professional will take a sample of your breath by having you breathe into a bag at your doctor's office or at a lab. He or she then sends your breath sample to a lab for testing. If your breath sample has higher levels of carbon dioxide than normal, you have *H. pylori* in your stomach or small intestine.

- **Stool test.** Doctors use a stool test to study a sample of your stool. A doctor will give you a container for catching and storing your stool at home. You return the sample to the doctor or a commercial facility, who then sends it to a lab for analysis. Stool tests can show the presence of *H. pylori*.

Section 10.4

Celiac Disease Tests

This section includes text excerpted from "Celiac Disease Testing (For Healthcare Professionals)," National Institute of Diabetes and Digestive and Kidney Diseases (NIDDK), September 2013. Reviewed September 2018.

Serologic tests for celiac disease provide an effective first step in identifying candidates for intestinal biopsy. If serologic or genetic tests indicate the possibility of celiac disease, a biopsy should be done promptly and before initiating any dietary changes. Genetic tests that confirm the presence or absence of specific genes associated with celiac disease may be beneficial in some cases.

Serologic Tests

Serologic tests look for three antibodies common in celiac disease:

- Anti-tissue transglutaminase (tTG) antibodies
- Endomysial antibodies (EMA)

- Deamidated gliadin peptide (DGP) antibodies

The most sensitive antibody tests are of the immunoglobulin A (IgA) class; however, immunoglobulin G (IgG) tests may be used in people with IgA deficiency. Panels are often used because no one serologic test is ideal. However, the tests included in a celiac panel vary by lab, and one or more may be unwarranted. Some reference labs—labs used for specialized tests—have developed cascades of tests in an attempt to minimize the use of less accurate tests whose automatic inclusion in a panel would add little or no sensitivity and/or detract from specificity. For accurate diagnostic test results, patients must be on a gluten-containing diet.

Tissue Transglutaminase (tTG)

The tTG-IgA test is an enzyme-linked immunosorbent assay (ELISA) test. The tTG-IgA test is the preferred screening method and has a sensitivity of 93 percent, yielding few false negative results. The tTG test also has a specificity of more than 98 percent. The performance of the tTG-IgA test may depend on the degree of intestinal damage, making the test less sensitive among people with milder celiac disease. In addition to screening, the tTG test may be used to assess initiation and maintenance of a gluten-free diet. Point-of-care tTG tests have been developed commercially; however, because of lower sensitivity and specificity, assay results may differ from those in the lab. The tTG-IgG test is only useful in those subjects who have IgA deficiency, which is 1/400 of the general population or 2–3 percent of people with celiac disease.

Endomysial Antibodies (EMA)

The test for EMA-IgA is highly specific for celiac disease, with 99 percent accuracy. The reason the test has a variable sensitivity of 70–100 percent may be due in part to the high technical difficulty in performing this test. EMA are measured by indirect immunofluorescent assay, a more expensive and time-consuming process than ELISA testing. In addition, the EMA test is qualitative, making the results more subjective than those for tTG. EMA is often used as an adjunctive test to the routine tTG-IgA test when EMA make celiac disease more certain. A jejunal biopsy may help diagnose patients who are EMA or tTG negative and suspected of having celiac disease.

Deamidated Gliadin Peptide (DGP)

A new generation of tests that use DGP antibodies has sensitivity and specificity that is substantially better than the older gliadin tests. However, based on a meta-analysis of 11 studies, insufficient evidence exists to support the use of DGP over tTG or EMA tests. The tTG test is less expensive than the DGP test and offers better diagnostic performance.

Immunoglobulin A (IgA) Deficiency

If tTG-IgA or EMA-IgA is negative and celiac disease is still suspected, total IgA should be measured to identify selective IgA deficiency. In cases of IgA deficiency, tTG-IgG or DGP-IgG should be measured. DGP-IgG may be sensitive for celiac disease, and it is preferable to tTG-IgG if used in a cascade. DGP-IgG has reasonable sensitivity for celiac disease in IgA-sufficient as well as IgA-deficient patients.

Genetic Screening Tests

Most people with celiac disease have gene pairs that encode for at least one of the human leukocyte antigen (HLA) gene variants, or alleles, designated *HLA-DQ2*—found in 95 percent of people with the disease—and *HLA-DQ8*. However, these alleles are found in about 30–35 percent of Caucasians, and most people with the variants do not develop celiac disease. Negative findings for *HLA-DQ2* and *HLA-DQ8* make current or future celiac disease very unlikely in patients for whom other tests, including biopsy, do not provide a clear diagnostic result. An increased risk of developing celiac disease has recently been described in individuals who carry a new *HLA-G I* allele in addition to *HLA-DQ2*.

Section 10.5

Diagnostic Laparoscopy

"Diagnostic Laparoscopy," © 2018 Omnigraphics.
Reviewed September 2018.

Diagnostic laparoscopy is a minimally invasive exploratory method that uses a fiber optic instrument to visually examine the abdominal and pelvic organs. The laparoscope, a long fiber optic cable system, is introduced into the abdomen through a small incision in the abdominal wall, which allows medical personnel to obtain visuals of the affected area. A high-intensity light source and high-resolution monitor are connected to the laparoscope to enable medical personnel to directly view the peritoneal cavity. Diagnostic laparoscopy, also called "exploratory laparoscopy," is usually recommended when other imaging techniques such as X-ray, computed tomography (CT) scan, magnetic resonance imaging (MRI) scan, or ultrasound fail to provide insight into the nature of the problem or medical condition.

This diagnostic procedure is also a valuable tool for obtaining tissue samples for biopsy (a laboratory test used to determine the underlying pathology of a disease). In addition to diagnostic use, laparoscopy is also widely used for therapeutic interventions instead of conventional open surgeries, which are associated with larger incisions, greater risk of hemorrhaging, more pain, and a relatively longer recovery period.

Indications for Diagnostic Laparoscopy

A laparoscopy is recommended when abdominal organs—which include the stomach, small and large intestines, liver, pancreas, spleen, gallbladder, and the appendix—are to be examined. An exploratory laparoscopy procedure can also be a preparation to laparoscopic surgery of the underlying pathology. Acute or chronic abdominal pain is one of the most common indications for laparoscopic investigation. Abdominal pain can have a number of potential causes, including trauma, appendicitis, inflammation of the abdominal organs, intra-abdominal scar tissue from a previous surgery, intestinal obstruction, abdominal aortic aneurysm, and diverticulitis, among others.

Diagnostic laparoscopy is also used to:

- establish a definitive diagnosis of an abdominal mass or tumor that has been revealed by palpation or X-ray study

- assess the cause of ascites (fluid accumulation in the abdominal cavity) of an unknown origin

- obtain tissue samples for investigative study of liver disease

- serve as a second-look procedure to determine the outcome of a particular treatment, such as a previous surgery or radiation therapy for cancer

Preparation and Procedure

Standard blood and urine analysis and other imaging studies may be needed before an exploratory laparoscopy is performed. Medications such as blood thinners, if routinely taken, may need to be discontinued prior to the procedure. Most procedures are performed in an outpatient setting under general anesthesia, but in some cases, local anesthesia may be used.

The abdominal cavity is inflated with carbon dioxide (CO_2) gas to elevate the abdominal wall above the internal organs for visual clarity. A trocar is introduced through an incision in the abdomen that is usually in, or close to, the umbilicus (belly button). This primary port facilitates intraperitoneal access for entry of the laparoscope. Other trocars introduced through additional incisions serve as ancillary ports for introducing cameras and other laparoscopic instruments such as scissors, graspers, retractors, and so on. The locations of the secondary ports vary depending upon diagnostic or surgical procedure requirements. The doctor examines the organs and removes tissue samples if necessary. After the examination, the carbon dioxide gas used to distend the abdomen is removed. The instruments and trocars are then withdrawn and the abdominal incisions are closed with surgical tape or sutures.

Perioperative Care

Prophylactic measures may be used to reduce postoperative nausea and vomiting. Antibiotics are generally administered to prevent infection at the surgical site. The doctor may prescribe pain medication to relieve soreness around the incision site, which should normally subside on its own within a few days. Most patients can return to normal activities within seven days. Temporary leaks may occur at the operative sites.

Patients should notify their doctors immediately if one or more of the following complications develop:

- Pain, fever, or chills
- Continued nausea or vomiting
- Abdominal swelling or discharge from the operative site
- Chest pain or shortness of breath
- Difficulty urinating

A follow-up appointment is usually scheduled within two weeks of the procedure.

Medical Complications of Laparoscopy

Brief investigative procedures involving laparoscopy are associated with minimal risks and patients are discharged on the same day following the procedure. However, as with any surgical procedure, diagnostic laparoscopy may be associated with a risk of minor complications such as pain, infection, or adverse outcomes from anesthesia. A less serious complication may also arise from incomplete evacuation of carbon dioxide gas from the abdomen following the procedure. Pockets of gas may push against the diaphragm—the muscular partition that separates the abdominal and thoracic cavities—and exert pressure on the phrenic nerve, innervating the diaphragm. This can sometimes lead to shoulder pain. Intra-abdominal trocar insertions can sometimes cause a puncture wound in an underlying organ, which could result in peritonitis or trauma to large blood vessels and hemorrhaging. Minor perforation wounds, if detected early, can be immediately managed by suturing or stapling; major visceral injuries are mostly managed by open surgical repair.

Diagnostic Laparoscopy Disadvantages

Diagnostic laparoscopy has become a quick and effective tool for achieving a conclusive diagnosis in chronic abdominal conditions with uncertain diagnosis, thereby reducing patient distress; but it still is an invasive procedure and may not replace other noninvasive modalities, such as imaging studies. Furthermore, it cannot be performed in all patients. For instance, the procedure is contraindicated in critically ill patients with poor chances of survival. It is also contraindicated in patients with abdominal-wall infections and those who cannot tolerate insufflation of carbon dioxide in the abdominal cavity (pneumoperitoneum). The procedure is also considered less advantageous than an open procedure since small openings reduce the surgeon's range of motion. Limitations resulting from the absence of tactile sensations also pose a major disadvantage for the surgeon as palpation of tissue is an important tool in terms of both diagnosis and execution of delicate surgical procedures.

References

1. "Diagnostic Laparoscopy," Society of American Gastrointestinal and Endoscopic Surgeons (SAGES), n.d.

2. "The Efficacy of Laparoscopy in the Diagnosis and Management of Chronic Abdominal Pain," National Center for Biotechnology Information (NCBI), July 1, 2010.

Section 10.6

Fecal Occult Blood Tests

This section includes text excerpted from "Fecal Occult Blood Test (FOBT)," MedlinePlus, National Institutes of Health (NIH), September 22, 2017.

What Is a Fecal Occult Blood Test?

A fecal occult blood test (FOBT) looks at a sample of your stool (feces) to check for blood. Occult blood means that you can't see it with the naked eye. Blood in the stool means there is likely some kind of bleeding in the digestive tract. It may be caused by a variety of conditions, including:

- Polyps

- Hemorrhoids

- Diverticulosis

- Ulcers

- Colitis, a type of inflammatory bowel disease

Blood in the stool may also be a sign of colorectal cancer, a type of cancer that starts in the colon or rectum. Colorectal cancer is the second leading cause of cancer-related deaths in the United States and the third most common cancer in men and in women. A fecal occult blood test is a screening test that may help find colorectal cancer early, when treatment is most effective.

Other names: FOBT, stool occult blood, occult blood test, Hemoccult test, guaiac smear test, gFOBT, immunochemical FOBT, iFOBT; fecal immunochemical test (FIT)

What Is a Fecal Occult Blood Test Used For?

A fecal occult blood test is used as an early screening test for colorectal cancer. It may also be used to diagnose other conditions that cause bleeding in the digestive tract.

Why Do I Need a Fecal Occult Blood Test?

The National Cancer Institute (NCI) recommends that people get regular screenings for colorectal cancer starting at age 50. The screening may be a fecal occult test, a colonoscopy, or another test. Talk with your healthcare provider about which test is right for you. If you choose a fecal occult blood test, you need to get it every year. If you have a colonoscopy, you only need it every ten years. But it is a more invasive procedure. You may need screening more often if you have certain risk factors. These include:

- A family history of colorectal cancer
- Cigarette smoking
- Obesity
- Excessive alcohol use

What Happens during a Fecal Occult Blood Test?

A fecal occult blood test is a noninvasive test that you can perform at home at your convenience. Your healthcare provider will give you a kit that includes instructions on how to do the test. There are two main types of fecal occult blood tests: the guaiac smear method (gFOBT) and the immunochemical method (iFOBT or FIT). Below are typical instructions for each test. Your instructions may vary slightly depending on the manufacturer of the test kit.

For a guaiac smear test (gFOBT), you will most likely need to:

- collect samples from three separate bowel movements

- for each sample, collect the stool and store in a clean container. Make sure the sample does not mix in with urine or water from the toilet.

- use the applicator from your test kit to smear some of the stool on the test card or slide, also included in your kit

- label and seal all your samples as directed

- mail the samples to your healthcare provider or lab

For a fecal immunochemical test (FIT), you will most likely need to:

- collect samples from two or three bowel movements

- collect the sample from the toilet using the special brush or other device that was included in your kit

- for each sample, use the brush or device to take the sample from the surface of the stool

- brush the sample onto a test card

- label and seal all your samples as directed

- mail the samples to your healthcare provider or lab

Be sure to follow all the instructions provided in your kit, and talk to your healthcare provider if you have any questions.

Will I Need to Do Anything to Prepare for the Test?

Certain foods and drugs may affect the results of a guaiac smear method (gFOBT) test. Your healthcare provider may ask you to avoid the following:

- Nonsteroidal anti-inflammatory drugs (NSAIDs) such as ibuprofen, naproxen, or aspirin for seven days prior to your test. If you take aspirin for heart problems, talk to your healthcare provider before stopping your medicine. Acetaminophen may be safe to use during this time, but check with your healthcare provider before taking it.

- More than 250 mg of vitamin C daily from supplements, fruit juices, or fruit for seven days prior to your test. Vitamin C can affect the chemicals in the test and cause a negative result even if there is blood present.

- Red meat, such as beef, lamb, and pork, for three days prior to the test. Traces of blood in these meats may cause a false-positive result.

There are no special preparations or dietary restrictions for a fecal immunochemical test (FIT).

Are There Any Risks to the Test?

There is no known risk to having a fecal occult blood test.

What Do the Results Mean?

If your results are positive for either type of fecal occult blood test, it means you likely have bleeding somewhere in your digestive tract. But it does not necessarily mean you have cancer. Other conditions that may produce a positive result on a fecal occult blood test include ulcers, hemorrhoids, polyps, and benign tumors. If your test results are positive for blood, your healthcare provider will likely recommend additional testing, such as a colonoscopy, to figure out the exact location and cause of your bleeding. If you have questions about your results, talk to your healthcare provider.

Is There Anything Else I Need to Know about a Fecal Occult Blood Test?

Regular colorectal cancer screenings, such as the fecal occult blood test, are an important tool in the fight against cancer. Studies show that screening tests can help find cancer early, and may reduce deaths from the disease.

Chapter 11

Common Gastrointestinal Surgical Procedures

Chapter Contents

Section 11.1

Ostomy Surgery

This section includes text excerpted from "Ostomy Surgery of the Bowel," National Institute of Diabetes and Digestive and Kidney Diseases (NIDDK), August 2014. Reviewed September 2018.

What Is Ostomy Surgery of the Bowel?

Ostomy surgery of the bowel, also known as bowel diversion, refers to surgical procedures that reroute the normal movement of intestinal contents out of the body when part of the bowel is diseased or removed. Creating an ostomy means bringing part of the intestine through the abdominal wall so that waste exits through the abdominal wall instead of passing through the anus.

Ostomy surgery of the bowel may be temporary or permanent, depending on the reason for the surgery. A surgeon specially trained in intestinal surgery performs the procedure in a hospital. During the surgery, the person receives general anesthesia.

Ostomy surgeries of the bowel include:

- Ileostomy
- Colostomy
- Ileoanal reservoir
- Continent ileostomy

What Is the Bowel?

The bowel is another word for the small and large intestines. The bowel forms the largest part of the gastrointestinal (GI) tract—a series of hollow organs joined in a long, twisting tube from the mouth to the anus. The anus is a one-inch-long opening through which stool leaves the body. Organs that make up the GI tract include the mouth, esophagus, stomach, small intestine, large intestine, and anus. The small intestine measures about 20 feet long in adults and includes:

- The duodenum—the first part of the small intestine nearest the stomach
- The jejunum—the middle section of the small intestine between the duodenum and ileum
- The ileum—the lower end of the small intestine

Peristalsis—a wavelike movement of muscles in the GI tract—moves food and liquid through the GI tract. Peristalsis, along with the release of hormones and enzymes, helps food digest. The small intestine absorbs nutrients from foods and liquids passed from the stomach. Most food digestion and nutrient absorption take place in the small intestine.

The large intestine consists of the cecum, colon, and rectum. The cecum connects to the last part of the ileum and contains the appendix. The large intestine measures about five feet in adults and absorbs water and any remaining nutrients from partially digested food passed from the small intestine. The large intestine then changes waste from liquid to semisolid or solid feces or stool. Stool passes from the colon to the rectum. The rectum measures six to eight inches in adults and is located between the last part of the colon and the anus. The rectum stores stool prior to a bowel movement. During a bowel movement, stool moves from the rectum, through the anus, and out of the body.

Why Does a Person Need Ostomy Surgery of the Bowel?

A person may need ostomy surgery of the bowel if he or she has:

- Cancer of the colon or rectum

- An injury to the small or large intestine

- Inflammatory bowel disease (IBD)—longlasting disorders, such as Crohn disease and ulcerative colitis (UC), that cause irritation or sores in the GI tract

- Obstruction—a blockage in the bowel that prevents the flow of fluids or solids

- Diverticulitis—a condition that occurs when small pouches in the colon called diverticula become inflamed, or irritated and swollen, and infected

What Is a Stoma?

During ostomy surgery of the bowel, a surgeon creates a stoma by bringing the end of the intestine through an opening in the abdomen and attaching it to the skin to create an opening outside the body. A stoma may be three-fourths of an inch to a little less than two inches wide. The stoma is usually located in the lower part of the abdomen, just below the beltline. However, sometimes the stoma is located in the upper abdomen. The surgeon and a wound, ostomy, and continence (WOC) nurse or an enterostomal therapist will work together to select the best location for the stoma. A removable external collection pouch, called an ostomy pouch or ostomy appliance, is attached to the stoma and worn outside the body to collect intestinal contents or stool. Intestinal contents or stool passes through the stoma instead of passing through the anus. The stoma has no muscle, so it cannot control the flow of stool, and the flow occurs whenever other digestive muscles contract. Ileostomy and colostomy are the two main types of ostomy surgery of the bowel during which a surgeon creates a stoma.

What Is an Ileostomy?

An ileostomy is a stoma created from a part of the ileum. For this surgery, the surgeon brings the ileum through the abdominal wall to make a stoma. An ileostomy may be permanent or temporary. An ileostomy is permanent when the surgeon removes or bypasses the entire colon, rectum, and anus. A surgeon may perform a temporary ileostomy for a damaged or an inflamed colon or rectum that only needs time to rest or heal from injury or surgery. After the colon or rectum heals, the surgeon repairs the opening in the abdominal wall and reconnects the ileum so stool will pass into the colon normally. An ileostomy is the most common temporary bowel diversion. A surgeon performs an ileostomy most often to treat inflammatory bowel disease (IBD) or rectal cancer.

What Is a Colostomy?

A colostomy is a stoma created from a part of the colon. For this surgery, the surgeon brings the colon through the abdominal wall and makes a stoma. A colostomy may be temporary or permanent. The colostomy is permanent when the surgeon removes or bypasses the lower end of the colon or rectum. A surgeon may perform a temporary colostomy for a damaged or an inflamed lower part of the colon or rectum that only needs time to rest or heal from injury or surgery. Once the colon or rectum heals, the surgeon repairs the opening in the abdominal wall and reconnects the colon so stool will pass normally. A surgeon performs a colostomy most often to treat rectal cancer, diverticulitis, or fecal incontinence—the accidental loss of stool.

What Is an Ileoanal Reservoir?

An ileoanal reservoir is an internal pouch made from the ileum. This surgery is a common alternative to an ileostomy and does not have a permanent stoma. Also known as a J-pouch or pelvic pouch, the ileoanal reservoir connects to the anus after a surgeon removes the colon and rectum. Stool collects in the ileoanal reservoir and then exits the body through the anus during a bowel movement. An ileoanal reservoir is an option after removal of the entire large intestine when the anus remains intact and disease-free. The surgeon often makes a temporary ileostomy before or at the time of making an ileoanal reservoir. Once the ileoanal reservoir heals from surgery, the surgeon reconnects the ileum to the ileoanal pouch and closes the temporary ileostomy. A person does not need a permanent external ostomy pouch for an ileoanal reservoir.

A surgeon creates an ileoanal reservoir most often to treat ulcerative colitis or familial adenomatous polyposis. Familial adenomatous polyposis is an inherited disease characterized by the presence of 100 or more polyps in the colon. The polyps may lead to colorectal cancer if not treated. People with Crohn disease usually are not candidates for this procedure.

What Is a Continent Ileostomy?

A continent ileostomy is an internal pouch, sometimes called a Kock pouch, fashioned from the end of the ileum just before it exits the abdominal wall as an ileostomy. The surgeon makes a valve inside the pouch so that intestinal contents do not flow out. The person drains the pouch each day by inserting a thin, flexible tube, called a catheter, through the stoma. The person covers the stoma with a simple patch or dressing. A continent ileostomy is an option for people who are not good candidates for an ileoanal reservoir because of damage to the rectum or anus and who do not want to wear an ostomy pouch.

Creating the Kock pouch is a delicate surgical procedure that requires a healthy bowel for proper healing. Therefore, a surgeon usually does not perform Kock pouch surgery during an acute attack of bowel disease. A continent ileostomy is now uncommon, and most hospitals do not have a specialist who knows how to perform this type of surgery. As with ileoanal reservoir surgery, the surgeon usually removes the colon and rectum to treat the original bowel disease, such as ulcerative colitis or familial adenomatous polyposis. People with Crohn disease are not usually candidates for this procedure.

What Are the Complications of Ostomy Surgery of the Bowel?

Complications of ostomy surgery of the bowel may include:

- Skin irritation
- Stoma problems
- Blockage
- Diarrhea
- Bleeding
- Electrolyte imbalance
- Infection
- Irritation of the internal pouch, or pouchitis
- Vitamin B12 deficiency
- Phantom rectum
- Short bowel syndrome
- Rectal discharge

Section 11.2

Colectomy

What Is a Colectomy?

A colectomy is the surgical removal of all or a part of the colon, or large intestine, from the digestive system. The esophagus, stomach, small intestine, and large intestine (colon) are part of the human digestive system. Digestion involves processing vitamins, minerals, carbohydrates, fats, proteins, and water from food and removing waste from the body. When a colectomy is performed, the severed portions of the colon may be reattached to facilitate bowel movement. Otherwise, a surgical procedure known as a colostomy becomes necessary. In this procedure, an opening known as a stoma is made on the outside of the body to excrete stool.

When Is a Colectomy Recommended?

A colectomy is recommended for conditions like bowel obstruction, colon cancer, diverticulitis, inflammatory disease, such as Crohn disease and ulcerative colitis, infection, and bleeding.

What Is the Surgical Procedure Used in a Colectomy?

Surgeons use one of two methods to perform a colectomy:

1. **Open surgery.** The colon is accessed by making a long vertical incision on the abdomen and the surgeon operates on the infected/damaged part. This is termed an "open colectomy."

2. **Laparoscopic surgery.** The surgeon makes a few small incisions using specialized surgical tools. A video camera is then inserted into one of the incisions so that the surgeon can operate by looking at a screen. This is termed a "laparoscopic-assisted colectomy" and is the procedure of choice for certain types of cancerous conditions. There is less pain and blood loss and recovery is usually faster than after an open surgery.

What Are the Categories of Colectomy?

Depending on whether all or part of the colon is removed, a colectomy is categorized into the following types:

- **Total colectomy.** The entire colon is surgically removed.

- **Segmental resection.** Removal is confined to only the affected part of the colon.

- **Partial colectomy.** Part of the colon is removed. This is also known as a subtotal colectomy.

- **Sigmoidectomy.** The lower section of the colon is removed in this procedure.

- **Hemicolectomy.** Only the right or left quadrant of the colon is removed.

- **Total proctocolectomy.** The entire colon and the rectum are removed and the small intestine is attached to the anus for excretion of stool.

- **Abdominal perineal resection.** This involves the removal of the sigmoid colon, rectum, and anus and replaced with a permanent colostomy.

- **Low anterior resection.** The top section of the rectum is removed.

How Do I Prepare before Surgery?

A few days before surgery you need to take care of a few things as listed below:

- Follow the diet advised by the surgeon.

- Stay hydrated with at least eight glasses of water daily.

- Cleanse your colon by following the instructions given by your surgeon. This could include laxatives, enemas, and special liquid preparations and diets.

- Take medicines as prescribed by your surgeon.

- Shower with an antibacterial soap the night before the procedure.

- Make arrangements for help at home and have someone drive you to hospital.

- Wear comfortable clothing.

- Stop taking regular medication as instructed by your surgeon.

What Happens in a Colectomy?

During a laparoscopic colectomy, the surgeon makes an incision that is less than half an inch long in the abdomen and inserts a tube-like instrument known as a cannula or port into the abdomen. Carbon dioxide (CO_2) gas is pumped into the abdomen through the cannula to create enough space to carry out the procedure. A laparoscope is then inserted through the cannula. The laparoscope is a device with a camera and light source on it. It illuminates the surgical site and relays images of it to a high-definition monitor for the surgeon to view.

Up to four ports are used to insert specialized surgical instruments for the surgeon to perform the surgery. One of the incisions is made slightly bigger than the others and the portion of the colon targeted for removal is pulled out of the abdomen through it. Depending on the type of surgery, the ends of the intestines are then joined together and inserted back into the abdomen.

An open surgery happens more or less the same way, except that the surgeon uses handheld instruments through a large incision made in the abdomen.

If most of the colon is removed, reattachment may not be possible and an ileostomy or a colostomy may be required. A stoma, or opening, is made in the abdominal wall and the open end of the intestine is attached to it. This allows waste to exit from the stoma. The patient will need to wear an ostomy bag which collects the waste material. Depending on the patient, the stoma could be temporary or permanent. People are able to lead healthy and active lives even with a permanent stoma.

What Are the Complications and Side Effects Associated with a Colectomy?

A colectomy is a generally safe procedure. But as with any operation, there are risks. If you are concerned, discuss them with your healthcare provider.

Some of the risks include:

- Bleeding

- Difficulty breathing

- Heart attack

- Injury to nearby organs during surgery

- Blood clots in the legs and lungs

- Obstruction caused by scar tissue after surgery

- Infection

- Tearing of sutures

- Anastomotic leaks in the colon because of failure of sutures

- Hematoma (accumulation of blood in the wound)

What Happens after the Procedure?

You may need to spend up to a week in the hospital after surgery to recover. You will be administered pain medication and put on a limited liquid diet. After a few days, solid food may be advised. Your surgeon, as well as other doctors (such as your oncologist or general practitioner), will schedule a series of follow-up appointments. Make sure you attend all of them. You will also be given instructions on specific things to watch out for in order to spot complications that may arise when you are at home. Make sure you remain alert to them. You will also be given information on how to take care of the stoma.

How Should I Take Care of Myself at Home after Surgery?

Keep the following things in mind for a normal recovery and to identify complications at home:

- Watch for problems such as swelling, redness, bleeding, or discharge at the site of surgery. Contact your healthcare provider immediately if you find something.

- If you experience pain, chills, or fever, contact your healthcare provider immediately.

- Do not lift heavy weights and do not engage in demanding activities at home for up to six weeks.

- Seek help at home for your daily activities until you can take care of yourself again.

- Follow a diet as per instructions from your healthcare provider.

- Do not expose the surgical site to water.

- Drink plenty of water to stay hydrated.

- Do not drive while on narcotic medication for pain.

- Follow instructions on showering, sexual activity, and taking care of your stoma.

- Use a thermometer to check for fever.

- Wear loose-fitting clothes.

- Remain on medication as directed for pain, infection, and constipation. Call your healthcare provider if in doubt.

- Engage in deep breathing and relaxation techniques if you find yourself getting anxious.

What Is the Outcome of a Colectomy?

The outcome of a colectomy depends on why exactly you needed the procedure. For cancerous conditions, if the diseased section has been removed entirely, the possibility of a good outcome is greater. For precancerous conditions, such as polyps and ulcerative colitis, the outcome is similar. Most people go on to lead a healthy and productive lives postsurgery.

References

1. "Frequently Asked Questions about Colectomy (Colon Resection)," The University of Chicago Medical Center, n.d.

2. Tresca, Amber J. "Types of Colectomy Surgery," VeryWell, January 4, 2017.

3. "Surgical Procedures: Colectomy," Trustees of the University of Pennsylvania, September 19, 2016.

4. "Colectomy," EBSCO Publishing, n.d.

5. "Colectomy," The Regents of the University of California, n.d.

6. "Colectomy," The Johns Hopkins University, The Johns Hopkins Hospital, and Johns Hopkins Health System, n.d.

7. Mayo Clinic Staff, "Colectomy," Mayo Foundation for Medical Education and Research (MFMER), November 17, 2015.

Section 11.3

Bariatric Surgery

This section includes text excerpted from "Bariatric Surgery," National Institute of Diabetes and Digestive and Kidney Diseases (NIDDK), July 2016.

What Is Obesity?

Obesity is defined as having a body mass index (BMI) of 30 or more. BMI is a measure of your weight in relation to your height. Class 1 obesity means a BMI of 30–35, Class 2 obesity is a BMI of 35–40, and Class 3 obesity is a BMI of 40 or more. Classes 2 and 3, also known as severe obesity, are often hard to treat with diet and exercise alone.

What Is Bariatric Surgery?

Bariatric surgery is an operation that helps you lose weight by making changes to your digestive system. Some types of bariatric surgeries make your stomach smaller, allowing you to eat and drink less at one time and making you feel full sooner. Other bariatric surgeries also change your small intestine—the part of your body that absorbs calories and nutrients from foods and beverages.

Bariatric surgery may be an option if you have severe obesity and have not been able to lose weight or keep from gaining back any weight you lost using other methods such as lifestyle treatment or medications. Bariatric surgery also may be an option if you have serious health problems, such as type 2 diabetes or sleep apnea, related to obesity. Bariatric surgery can improve many of the medical conditions linked to obesity, especially type 2 diabetes.

Does Bariatric Surgery Always Work?

Studies show that many people who have bariatric surgery lose about 15–30 percent of their starting weight on average, depending on the type of surgery they have. However, no method, including surgery, is sure to produce and maintain weight loss. Some people who have bariatric surgery may not lose as much as they hoped. Over time, some people regain a portion of the weight they lost. The amount of weight people regain may vary. Factors that affect weight regain may include a person's level of obesity and the type of surgery he or she had.

Bariatric surgery does not replace healthy habits, but may make it easier for you to consume fewer calories and be more physically active. Choosing healthy foods and beverages before and after the surgery may help you lose more weight and keep it off long term. Regular physical activity after surgery also helps keep the weight off. To improve your health, you must commit to a lifetime of healthy lifestyle habits and following the advice of your healthcare providers.

Types of Bariatric Surgery

The type of surgery that may be best to help a person lose weight depends on a number of factors. You should discuss with your doctor what kind of surgery might be best for you or your teen.

What Is the Difference between Open and Laparoscopic Surgery?

In open bariatric surgery, surgeons make a single, large cut in the abdomen. More often, surgeons now use laparoscopic surgery, in which they make several small cuts and insert thin surgical tools through the cuts. Surgeons also insert a small scope attached to a camera that projects images onto a video monitor. Laparoscopic surgery has fewer risks than open surgery and may cause less pain and scarring than open surgery. Laparoscopic surgery also may lead to a faster recovery.

Open surgery may be a better option for certain people. If you have a high level of obesity, have had stomach surgery before, or have other complex medical problems, you may need open surgery.

What Are the Surgical Options?

In the United States, surgeons use three types of operations most often:

1. Laparoscopic adjustable gastric band

2. Gastric sleeve surgery, also called sleeve gastrectomy

3. Gastric bypass

Surgeons use a fourth operation, biliopancreatic diversion with duodenal switch, less often.

Laparoscopic Adjustable Gastric Band

In this type of surgery, the surgeon places a ring with an inner inflatable band around the top of your stomach to create a small pouch. This makes you feel full after eating a small amount of food. The band has a circular balloon inside that is filled with salt solution. The surgeon can adjust the size of the opening from the pouch to the rest of your stomach by injecting or removing the solution through a small device called a port placed under your skin.

After surgery, you will need several follow-up visits to adjust the size of the band opening. If the band causes problems or is not helping you lose enough weight, the surgeon may remove it.

The U.S. Food and Drug Administration (FDA) has approved use of the gastric band for people with a BMI of 30 or more who also have at least one health problem linked to obesity, such as heart disease or diabetes.

Gastric Sleeve

In gastric sleeve surgery, also called vertical sleeve gastrectomy, a surgeon removes most of your stomach, leaving only a banana-shaped section that is closed with staples. Like gastric band surgery, this surgery reduces the amount of food that can fit in your stomach, making you feel full sooner. Taking out part of your stomach may also affect gut hormones or other factors such as gut bacteria that may affect appetite and metabolism. This type of surgery cannot be reversed because some of the stomach is permanently removed.

Gastric Bypass

Gastric bypass surgery, also called Roux-en-Y gastric bypass, has two parts. First, the surgeon staples your stomach, creating a small pouch in the upper section. The staples make your stomach much smaller, so you eat less and feel full sooner.

Next, the surgeon cuts your small intestine and attaches the lower part of it directly to the small stomach pouch. Food then bypasses most of the stomach and the upper part of your small intestine so your body absorbs fewer calories. The surgeon connects the bypassed section farther down to the lower part of the small intestine. This bypassed section is still attached to the main part of your stomach, so digestive juices can move from your stomach and the first part of your small intestine into the lower part of your small intestine. The bypass also changes gut hormones, gut bacteria, and other factors that may affect appetite and metabolism. Gastric bypass is difficult to reverse, although a surgeon may do it if medically necessary.

Duodenal Switch

This surgery, also called biliopancreatic diversion with duodenal switch, is more complex than the others. The duodenal switch involves two separate surgeries. The first is similar to gastric sleeve surgery. The second surgery redirects food to bypass most of your small intestine. The surgeon also reattaches the bypassed section to the last part of the small intestine, allowing digestive juices to mix with food.

This type of surgery allows you to lose more weight than the other three. However, this surgery is also the most likely to cause surgery-related problems and a shortage of vitamins, minerals, and protein in your body. For these reasons, surgeons do not perform this surgery as often.

What Should I Expect before Surgery?

Before surgery, you will meet with several healthcare providers, such as a dietitian, a psychiatrist or psychologist, an internist, and a bariatric surgeon.

- The doctor will ask about your medical history, do a thorough physical exam, and order blood tests. If you are a smoker, he or she will likely ask you to stop smoking at least six weeks before your surgery.

- The surgeon will tell you more about the surgery, including how to prepare for it and what type of follow-up you will need.

- The dietitian will explain what and how much you will be able to eat and drink after surgery and help you to prepare for how your life will change after surgery.

- The psychiatrist or psychologist may do an assessment to see if bariatric surgery is an option for you.

These healthcare providers also will advise you to become more active and adopt a healthy eating plan before and after surgery. In some cases, losing weight and bringing your blood sugar levels closer to normal before surgery may lower your chances of having surgery-related problems.

Some bariatric surgery programs have groups you can attend before and after surgery that can help answer questions about the surgery and offer support.

What Should I Expect after Surgery?

After surgery, you will need to rest and recover. Although the type of follow-up varies by type of surgery, you will need to take supplements that your doctor prescribes to make sure you are getting enough vitamins and minerals. Walking and moving around the house may help you recover more quickly. Start slowly and follow your doctor's advice about the type of physical activity you can do safely. As you feel more comfortable, add more physical activity. After surgery, most people move from a liquid diet to a soft diet such as cottage cheese, yogurt, or soup, and then to solid foods over several weeks. Your doctor, nurse, or dietitian will tell you which foods and beverages you may have and which ones you should avoid. You will need to eat small meals and chew your food well.

How Much Weight Can I Expect to Lose?

The amount of weight people lose after bariatric surgery depends on the individual and on the type of surgery he or she had. A study following people for 3 years after surgery found that those who had gastric band surgery lost an average of about 45 pounds. People who had gastric bypass lost an average of 90 pounds. Most people regained some weight over time, but weight regain was usually small compared to their initial weight loss.

Researchers know less about the long-term results of gastric sleeve surgery, but the amount of weight loss seems to be similar to or slightly less than gastric bypass.

Your weight loss could be different. Remember, reaching your goal depends not just on the surgery but also on sticking with healthy lifestyle habits throughout your life.

Weight-Loss Devices

The FDA has approved several new weight-loss devices that do not permanently change your stomach or small intestine. These devices cause less weight loss than bariatric surgery, and some are only temporary. The devices may have risks, so talk with your doctor if you're thinking about any of these options. Researchers haven't studied any of them over a long period of time and don't know the long-term risks and benefits.

- The electrical stimulation system uses a device implanted in your abdomen, by way of laparoscopic surgery, that blocks nerve activity between your stomach and brain. The device works on the vagus nerve, which helps signal the brain that the stomach feels full or empty.

- The gastric balloon system consists of one or two balloons placed in your stomach through a tube inserted through your mouth. Your doctor or nurse will give you a sedative before the procedure. Once the balloons are in your stomach, doctors inflate them with salt water so they take up space in your stomach and help you feel fuller. You will need to have the balloons removed after six months or a year.

- A new device uses a pump to drain part of the food in your stomach after a meal. The device includes a tube that goes from the inside of your stomach to a port on the outside of your abdomen. The port is a small valve that fits over the opening in your abdomen. About 20–30 minutes after eating, you attach tubing from the port to the pump and open the valve. The pump drains your stomach contents through a tube into the toilet, so that your body doesn't absorb about 30 percent of calories you ate. You can have the device removed at any time.

What Are the Benefits of Bariatric Surgery?

Bariatric surgery can help you lose weight and improve many health problems related to obesity. These health problems include:

- Type 2 diabetes
- High blood pressure
- Unhealthy cholesterol levels
- Sleep apnea
- Urinary incontinence
- Body pain
- Knee and hip pain

You may be better able to move around and be physically active after surgery. You might also notice your mood improve and feel like your quality of life (QOL) is better.

What Are the Side Effects of Bariatric Surgery?

Side effects may include:

- Bleeding

- Infection

- Leaking from the site where the sections of the stomach or small intestine, or both, are stapled or sewn together

- Diarrhea

- Blood clots in the legs that can move to the lungs and heart

Rarely, surgery-related problems can lead to death. Other side effects may occur later. Your body may not absorb nutrients well, especially if you don't take your prescribed vitamins and minerals. Not getting enough nutrients can cause health problems, such as anemia and osteoporosis. Gallstones can occur after rapid weight loss. Some doctors prescribe medicine for about 6 months after surgery to help prevent gallstones. Gastric bands can erode into the stomach wall and need to be removed.

Other problems that could occur later include strictures and hernias. Strictures—narrowing of the new stomach or connection between the stomach and small intestine—make it hard to eat solid food and can cause nausea, vomiting, and trouble swallowing. Doctors treat strictures with special instruments to expand the narrowing. Two kinds of hernias may occur after bariatric surgery—at the incision site or in the abdomen. Doctors repair hernias with surgery.

Some research suggests that bariatric surgery, especially gastric bypass, may change the way your body absorbs and breaks down alcohol, and may lead to more alcohol-related problems after surgery.

Part Three

Disorders of the Upper Gastrointestinal Tract

Chapter 12

Dyspepsia

What Is Indigestion?

Indigestion, also called dyspepsia or upset stomach, is a general term that describes a group of gastrointestinal (GI) symptoms that occur together. These symptoms most often include:

- Pain, a burning feeling, or discomfort in your upper abdomen

- Feeling full too soon while eating a meal

- Feeling uncomfortably full after eating a meal

Indigestion may be:

- Occasional—happening once in a while

- Chronic—happening regularly for a few weeks or months

- Functional—having chronic symptoms without a specific cause

Indigestion is not a disease. However, indigestion may be a sign of certain digestive tract diseases or conditions. Indigestion is not always related to eating. Sometimes digestive tract diseases such as peptic ulcer disease, gastritis, and stomach cancer cause chronic indigestion. However, most often doctors do not know what causes

This chapter includes text excerpted from "Indigestion (Dyspepsia)," National Institute of Diabetes and Digestive and Kidney Diseases (NIDDK), November 2016.

chronic indigestion. Chronic indigestion without a health problem or digestive tract disease that could explain symptoms is called functional dyspepsia.

How Common Is Indigestion?

Indigestion is a common condition, affecting about one in four people in the United States each year. Of those people with indigestion who see a doctor, almost three in four are diagnosed with functional dyspepsia.

Who Is More Likely to Get Indigestion?

You are more likely to get indigestion if you:

- Drink
  - too many alcoholic beverages
  - too much coffee or too many drinks containing caffeine
- Eat
  - too fast or too much during a meal
  - spicy, fatty, or greasy foods
  - foods that contain a lot of acid, such as tomatoes, tomato products, and oranges
- Feel stressed
- Have certain health problems or digestive tract diseases
- Smoke
- Take certain medicines

What Are the Complications of Indigestion?

In most cases, indigestion does not have complications, although it may affect your quality of life (QOL).

What Are the Symptoms of Indigestion?

When you have indigestion, you may have one or more of the following symptoms:

- Pain, a burning feeling, or discomfort in your upper abdomen
- Feeling full too soon while eating a meal

- Feeling uncomfortably full after eating a meal
- Bloating
- Burping

Other symptoms may include:

- Burping up food or liquid
- Loud growling or gurgling in your stomach
- Nausea
- Gas

Sometimes when you have indigestion, you may also have heartburn. However, heartburn and indigestion are two separate conditions.

Seek Care Right Away

If you have indigestion and any of the following symptoms, you may have a more serious condition and should see a doctor right away:

- Black, tar-like stools
- Bloody vomit
- Difficulty swallowing or painful swallowing
- Frequent vomiting
- Losing weight without trying
- Pain in your chest, jaw, neck, or arm
- Severe and constant pain in your abdomen
- Shortness of breath
- Sweating
- Yellowing of your eyes or skin

You should also see a doctor if your indigestion lasts longer than two weeks.

What Causes Indigestion

Some of the causes of indigestion include:

- Drinking

- too many alcoholic beverages
- too much coffee or too many drinks containing caffeine
- too many carbonated, or fizzy, drinks
- Eating
  - too fast or too much during a meal
  - spicy, fatty, or greasy foods
  - foods that contain a lot of acid, such as tomatoes, tomato products, and oranges
- Feeling stressed
- Smoking

Some medicines can cause indigestion, such as:

- Certain antibiotics—medicines that kill bacteria
- Nonsteroidal anti-inflammatory drugs (NSAIDs)

Health problems and digestive tract diseases and conditions can cause indigestion, including:

- Acid reflux (Gastroesophageal reflux (GER) and gastroesophageal reflux disease (GERD))
- Anxiety or depression
- Gallbladder inflammation
- Gastritis
- Gastroparesis
- *Helicobacter pylori* (*H. pylori*) infection
- Irritable bowel syndrome (IBS)
- Lactose intolerance
- Peptic ulcer disease (PUD)
- Stomach cancer

Researchers do not know what causes functional dyspepsia. Some research suggests that the following factors may play a role in functional dyspepsia:

- Eating

- Gastroparesis
- Problems in the first part of your small intestine, including inflammation, and being overly sensitive to stomach acids
- Infection by microorganisms such as *H. pylori*, *Salmonella*, *Escherichia coli* (*E. coli*), *Campylobacter*, Giardia, or norovirus
- Psychological problems, especially anxiety
- Genes—a trait passed from parent to child

How Do Doctors Diagnose Indigestion?

Your doctor diagnoses indigestion based on your medical history, a physical exam, upper gastrointestinal (GI) endoscopy, and other tests.

Medical History

Your doctor will review your symptoms and medical history. He or she will ask you about your eating and drinking habits, your use of over-the-counter (OTC), prescription medicines, and whether you smoke.

Physical Exam

During a physical exam, your doctor may:

- Check for bloating
- Listen to sounds in your abdomen using a stethoscope
- Tap on your abdomen to check for tenderness, pain, and lumps
- Look for yellowing of your eyes or skin

Upper GI Endoscopy

Your doctor may perform an upper GI endoscopy to diagnose diseases and conditions that may be causing your indigestion, such as:

- Gastritis
- Peptic ulcer disease
- Stomach cancer

A doctor may recommend an upper GI endoscopy for people with indigestion who are older than 55 or for people with indigestion of any age who have:

- A family history of cancer
- Difficulty swallowing
- Evidence of bleeding in the digestive tract
- Frequent vomiting
- Weight loss

During an upper GI endoscopy, your doctor can use tiny tools passed through the endoscope to take small pieces of tissue from the lining of your stomach and duodenum. This procedure is called an upper GI biopsy. A doctor will examine the tissue samples to look for digestive tract diseases and conditions, including *Helicobacter pylori* (*H. pylori*) infection.

Other Tests

- Imaging tests
- *H. pylori* testing
- Blood test
- Stool test
- Urea breath test

How Do Doctors Treat Indigestion?

Treatment for indigestion depends on the cause and may include:

- Over-the-counter (OTC) and prescription medicines
- Changing what you eat and drink
- Psychological therapies

Over-the-Counter (OTC) and Prescription Medicines

You can buy many medicines to treat indigestion without a prescription, such as antacids, H2 blockers, or proton pump inhibitors (PPIs). However, if your indigestion lasts longer than two weeks, you should see your doctor. Your doctor may prescribe acid-suppressing medicines that are stronger than the ones you can buy, antibiotics, prokinetics, or psychological medicines.

Antacids. Doctors often first recommend antacids—OTC medicines that neutralize acids in your stomach. Antacids include:

- Calcium carbonate (Rolaids, Tums)
- Loperamide (Imodium)
- Simethicone (Maalox, Mylanta)
- Sodium bicarbonate (Alka-Seltzer)

Antibiotics. To treat a *Helicobacter pylori* (*H. pylori*) infection, your doctor will prescribe antibiotics—medicines that kill bacteria. He or she will prescribe at least two of the following:

- Amoxicillin (Amoxil)
- Clarithromycin (Biaxin)
- Metronidazole (Flagyl)
- Tetracycline (Sumycin)
- Tinidazole (Tindamax)

H2 blockers. H2 blockers are medicines that decrease the amount of acid your stomach produces. H2 blockers provide short-term or on-demand relief for many people with indigestion. You can buy an H2 blocker or your doctor can prescribe one. H2 blockers include:

- Cimetidine (Tagamet HB)
- Famotidine (Pepcid AC)
- Nizatidine (Axid AR)
- Ranitidine (Zantac 75)

Proton pump inhibitors (PPIs). PPIs are most effective in treating indigestion if you also have heartburn. You can buy some PPIs or your doctor can prescribe one. PPIs include:

- Esomeprazole (Nexium)
- Lansoprazole (Prevacid)
- Omeprazole (Prilosec, Zegerid)
- Pantoprazole (Protonix)

- Rabeprazole (AcipHex)

Prokinetics. Prokinetics help your stomach empty faster. Prescription prokinetics include:

- Bethanechol (Urecholine)
- Metoclopramide (Reglan)

Changes in What You Eat and Drink

Your doctor may recommend that you avoid certain foods and drinks that may cause indigestion or make your symptoms worse, such as:

- Alcoholic beverages
- Carbonated, or fizzy, drinks
- Foods or drinks that contain caffeine
- Foods that contain a lot of acid, such as tomatoes, tomato products, and oranges
- Spicy, fatty, or greasy foods

Psychological Therapies

Your doctor may recommend a type of psychological therapy called "talk therapy" to help treat anxiety and depression that may be causing your indigestion. If stress is causing your indigestion, your doctor may recommend ways to help you reduce your stress, such as meditation, relaxation exercises, or counseling. Talk therapy can also help you learn how to reduce your stress.

What Can I Do to Help Prevent Indigestion?

In addition to making changes in what you eat and drink, you can help prevent indigestion by making lifestyle changes such as:

- Avoiding exercise right after eating
- Chewing food carefully and completely
- Losing weight
- Not eating late-night snacks
- Not taking a lot of nonsteroidal anti-inflammatory drugs
- Quitting smoking

- Trying to reduce stress in your life

- Waiting two to three hours after eating before you lie down

How Can My Diet Help Prevent Indigestion?

You can help prevent indigestion by changing what you eat and drink. You may need to avoid foods and drinks that cause indigestion.

What Foods and Drinks Should I Avoid If I Have Indigestion?

If you have indigestion, avoid foods and drinks that may make your symptoms worse, such as:

- Alcoholic beverages

- Carbonated, or fizzy, drinks

- Foods and drinks that contain caffeine

- Foods that contain a lot of acid, such as tomatoes, tomato products, and oranges

- Spicy, fatty, or greasy foods

What Can I Eat If I Have Indigestion?

You should eat a healthy, well-balanced diet. A healthy diet can improve your overall health, help manage certain diseases and conditions, and reduce the chance of disease.

Chapter 13

Barrett Esophagus

What Is Barrett Esophagus?

Barrett esophagus is a condition in which tissue that is similar to the lining of your intestine replaces the tissue lining your esophagus. Doctors call this process intestinal metaplasia (IM).

How Common Is Barrett Esophagus?

Experts are not sure how common Barrett esophagus is. Researchers estimate that it affects 1.6–6.8 percent of people.

Who Is More Likely to Develop Barrett Esophagus?

Men develop Barrett esophagus twice as often as women, and Caucasian men develop this condition more often than men of other races. The average age at diagnosis is 55. Barrett esophagus is uncommon in children.

What Are the Symptoms of Barrett Esophagus?

While Barrett esophagus itself doesn't cause symptoms, many people with Barrett esophagus have gastroesophageal reflux disease (GERD), which does cause symptoms.

This chapter includes text excerpted from "Barrett's Esophagus," National Institute of Diabetes and Digestive and Kidney Diseases (NIDDK), March 2017.

What Causes Barrett Esophagus

Experts don't know the exact cause of Barrett esophagus. However, some factors can increase or decrease your chance of developing Barrett esophagus.

What Factors Increase a Person's Chances of Developing Barrett Esophagus?

Having GERD increases your chances of developing Barrett esophagus. GERD is a more serious, chronic form of gastroesophageal reflux, a condition in which stomach contents flow back up into your esophagus. Refluxed stomach acid that touches the lining of your esophagus can cause heartburn and damage the cells in your esophagus. Between 10 and 15 percent of people with GERD develop Barrett esophagus. Obesity—specifically high levels of belly fat—and smoking also increase your chances of developing Barrett esophagus. Some studies suggest that your genetics, or inherited genes, may play a role in whether or not you develop Barrett esophagus.

What Factors Decrease a Person's Chances of Developing Barrett Esophagus?

Having a *Helicobacter pylori* (*H. pylori*) infection may decrease your chances of developing Barrett esophagus. Doctors are not sure how *H. pylori* protects against Barrett esophagus. While the bacteria damage your stomach and the tissue in your duodenum, some researchers believe the bacteria make your stomach contents less damaging to your esophagus if you have GERD. Researchers have found that other factors may decrease the chance of developing Barrett esophagus, including:

- Frequent use of aspirin or other nonsteroidal anti-inflammatory drugs

- A diet high in fruits, vegetables, and certain vitamins

How Do Doctors Diagnose Barrett Esophagus?

Doctors diagnose Barrett esophagus with an upper gastrointestinal (GI) endoscopy and a biopsy. Doctors may diagnose Barrett esophagus while performing tests to find the cause of a patient's gastroesophageal reflux disease (GERD) symptoms.

Medical History

Your doctor will ask you to provide your medical history. Your doctor may recommend testing if you have multiple factors that increase your chances of developing Barrett esophagus.

Upper Gastrointestinal (GI) Endoscopy and Biopsy

In an upper GI endoscopy, a gastroenterologist, surgeon, or other trained healthcare provider uses an endoscope to see inside your upper GI tract, most often while you receive light sedation. The doctor carefully feeds the endoscope down your esophagus and into your stomach and duodenum. The procedure may show changes in the lining of your esophagus. The doctor performs a biopsy with the endoscope by taking a small piece of tissue from the lining of your esophagus. You won't feel the biopsy. A pathologist examines the tissue in a lab to determine whether Barrett esophagus cells are present. A pathologist who has expertise in diagnosing Barrett esophagus may need to confirm the results. Barrett esophagus can be difficult to diagnose because this condition does not affect all the tissue in your esophagus. The doctor takes biopsy samples from at least eight different areas of the lining of your esophagus.

Who Should Be Screened for Barrett Esophagus?

Your doctor may recommend screening for Barrett esophagus if you are a man with chronic—lasting more than five years—and/or frequent—happening weekly or more—symptoms of GERD and two or more risk factors for Barrett esophagus. These risk factors include:

- Being age 50 and older

- Being Caucasian

- Having high levels of belly fat

- Being a smoker or having smoked in the past

- Having a family history of Barrett esophagus or esophageal adenocarcinoma

How Do Doctors Treat Barrett Esophagus?

Your doctor will talk about the best treatment options for you based on your overall health, whether you have dysplasia, and its severity.

Treatment options include medicines for GERD, endoscopic ablative therapies, endoscopic mucosal resection (EMR), and surgery.

Periodic Surveillance Endoscopy

Your doctor may use upper gastrointestinal endoscopy with a biopsy periodically to watch for signs of cancer development. Doctors call this approach surveillance. Experts aren't sure how often doctors should perform surveillance endoscopies. Talk with your doctor about what level of surveillance is best for you. Your doctor may recommend endoscopies more frequently if you have high-grade dysplasia rather than low-grade or no dysplasia.

Medicines

If you have Barrett esophagus and gastroesophageal reflux disease (GERD), your doctor will treat you with acid-suppressing medicines called proton pump inhibitors (PPIs). These medicines can prevent further damage to your esophagus and, in some cases, heal existing damage.

PPIs include:

- Pmeprazole (Prilosec, Zegerid)

- Lansoprazole (Prevacid)

- Pantoprazole (Protonix)

- Rabeprazole (AcipHex)

- Esomeprazole (Nexium)

- Dexlansoprazole (Dexilant)

All of these medicines are available by prescription. Omeprazole and lansoprazole are also available in over-the-counter (OTC) strength. Your doctor may consider anti-reflux surgery if you have GERD symptoms and don't respond to medicines. However, research has not shown that medicines or surgery for GERD and Barrett esophagus lower your chances of developing dysplasia or esophageal adenocarcinoma.

Endoscopic Ablative Therapies

Endoscopic ablative therapies use different techniques to destroy the dysplasia in your esophagus. After the therapies, your body should begin making normal esophageal cells.

A doctor, usually a gastroenterologist or surgeon, performs these procedures at certain hospitals and outpatient centers. You will receive local anesthesia and a sedative. The most common procedures are the following:

- **Photodynamic therapy.** Photodynamic therapy uses a light-activated chemical called porfimer (Photofrin), an endoscope, and a laser to kill precancerous cells in your esophagus. A doctor injects porfimer into a vein in your arm, and you return 24–72 hours later to complete the procedure. Complications of photodynamic therapy may include:

  - Sensitivity of your skin and eyes to light for about six weeks after the procedure

  - Burns, swelling, pain, and scarring in nearby healthy tissue

  - Coughing, trouble swallowing, stomach pain, painful breathing, and shortness of breath

- **Radiofrequency ablation.** Radiofrequency ablation uses radio waves to kill precancerous and cancerous cells in the Barrett tissue. An electrode mounted on a balloon or an endoscope creates heat to destroy the Barrett tissue and precancerous and cancerous cells. Complications of radiation ablation may include:

  - Chest pain

  - Cuts in the lining of your esophagus

  - Strictures

Clinical trials have shown that complications are less common with radiofrequency ablation compared with photodynamic therapy.

Endoscopic Mucosal Resection (EMR)

In endoscopic mucosal resection (EMR), your doctor lifts the Barrett tissue, injects a solution underneath or applies suction to the tissue, and then cuts the tissue off. The doctor then removes the tissue with an endoscope. Gastroenterologists perform this procedure at certain hospitals and outpatient centers. You will receive local anesthesia to numb your throat and a sedative to help you relax and stay comfortable. Before performing an EMR for cancer, your doctor will do an endoscopic ultrasound. Complications can include bleeding or tearing of your esophagus. Doctors sometimes combine EMR with photodynamic therapy.

Surgery

Surgery called esophagectomy is an alternative to endoscopic therapies. Many doctors prefer endoscopic therapies because these procedures have fewer complications. Esophagectomy is the surgical removal of the affected sections of your esophagus. After removing sections of your esophagus, a surgeon rebuilds your esophagus from part of your stomach or large intestine. The surgery is performed at a hospital. You'll receive general anesthesia, and you'll stay in the hospital for 7–14 days after the surgery to recover. Surgery may not be an option if you have other medical problems. Your doctor may consider the less-invasive endoscopic treatments or continued frequent surveillance instead.

How Can Your Diet Help Prevent Barrett Esophagus?

Researchers have not found that diet and nutrition play an important role in causing or preventing Barrett esophagus. If you have gastroesophageal reflux (GER) or gastroesophageal reflux disease (GERD), you can prevent or relieve your symptoms by changing your diet. Dietary changes that can help reduce your symptoms include:

- Decreasing fatty foods
- Eating small, frequent meals instead of three large meals

Avoid eating or drinking the following items that may make GER or GERD worse:

- Chocolate
- Coffee
- Peppermint
- Greasy or spicy foods
- Tomatoes and tomato products
- Alcoholic drinks

Chapter 14

Gastroesophageal Reflux Disease

Chapter Contents

Section 14.1

Gastroesophageal Reflux (GER) and Gastroesophageal Reflux Disease (GERD) in Infants

This section includes text excerpted from "Acid Reflux (GER and GERD) in Infants," National Institute of Diabetes and Digestive and Kidney Diseases (NIDDK), April 2015.

What Is Gastroesophageal Reflux (GER)?

Gastroesophageal reflux (GER) happens when stomach contents come back up into the esophagus. Infants—babies younger than two years—with GER spit up liquid mostly made of saliva and stomach acid. Stomach acid that touches the lining of the infant's esophagus can cause heartburn, also called acid indigestion.

Does GER Have Another Name?

Doctors also refer to GER as:

- Acid indigestion
- Acid reflux
- Acid regurgitation
- Heartburn
- Reflux

How Common Is GER in Infants?

GER is common in infants. About half of all infants spit up or regurgitate, many times a day in the first three months of their lives. In most cases, infants stop spitting up between the ages of 12 and 14 months.

What Is Gastroesophageal Reflux Disease (GERD)?

Gastroesophageal reflux disease (GERD) is a more serious and long-lasting form of GER in which acid reflux irritates the esophagus.

What Is the Difference between GER and GERD?

Infants with symptoms that prevent them from feeding or those with GER that lasts more than 12–14 months may actually have GERD. If you think your infant has GERD, you should take him or her to see a doctor or a pediatrician.

How Common Is GERD in Infants?

GERD is common in infants. Two-thirds of 4-month-olds have symptoms of GERD. By 1 year old, up to 10 percent of infants have symptoms of GERD.

What Are the Symptoms of GERD in Infants?

The main symptom of GERD in infants is spitting up more than they normally do. Infants with GERD can also have some or all of the following recurring symptoms:

- Arching of the back, often during or right after feeding
- Colic—crying that lasts for more than three hours a day with no medical cause
- Coughing
- Gagging or trouble swallowing
- Irritability, particularly after feeding
- Pneumonia—an infection in one or both of the lungs
- Poor feeding or refusal to feed
- Poor growth and malnutrition
- Poor weight gain
- Trouble breathing
- Vomiting
- Weight loss
- Wheezing—a high-pitched whistling sound that happens while breathing

What Causes GER and GERD in Infants

Gastroesophageal reflux (GER) happens when an infant's lower esophageal sphincter is not fully developed, and the muscle lets the stomach contents back up the esophagus. Once the stomach contents move up into the esophagus, the infant will regurgitate, or spit up. Once an infant's sphincter muscle fully develops, he or she should no longer spit up. GERD happens when an infant's lower esophageal sphincter muscle becomes weak or relaxes when it shouldn't. This weakness or relaxation lets the stomach contents come back up into the esophagus.

When Should I Seek a Doctor's Help?

Call a doctor right away if an infant:

- Vomits large amounts
- Has regular projectile, or forceful, vomiting, particularly in infants younger than two months
- Vomits fluid that is:
  - Green or yellow
  - Looks like coffee grounds
  - Contains blood
- Has problems breathing after vomiting or spitting up
- Often refuses feedings, causing weight loss or poor growth
- Cries three or more hours a day and is more irritable than usual
- Shows signs of dehydration, such as having dry diapers or extreme fussiness

How Do Doctors Diagnose GER in Infants?

In most cases, a doctor diagnoses GER by reviewing an infant's symptoms and medical history. If symptoms of GER do not improve with feeding changes and antireflux medicines, he or she may need testing.

How Do Doctors Diagnose GERD in Infants?

The doctor may recommend testing for gastroesophageal reflux disease (GERD) if:

- an infant's symptoms don't improve

- he or she is not gaining weight

- he or she is having lung problems

The doctor may refer the infant to a pediatric gastroenterologist to diagnose and treat GERD.

What Tests Do Doctors Use to Diagnose GERD in Infants?

Several tests can help a doctor diagnose GERD. A doctor may order more than one test to make a diagnosis.

Upper Gastrointestinal (GI) Endoscopy and Biopsy

In an upper gastrointestinal (GI) endoscopy, a gastroenterologist, surgeon, or other trained healthcare professional uses an endoscope to see inside an infant's upper GI tract. This procedure takes place at a hospital or an outpatient center. A healthcare professional will use an upper GI endoscopy especially if an infant has growth or breathing problems.

An intravenous (IV) needle is placed into one of the veins in the infant's arms, hands, or feet to give him or her medicines to keep him or her relaxed during the endoscopy procedure. The infant will receive extra oxygen throughout the procedure. The healthcare professional carefully feeds the endoscope down the infant's esophagus and into the stomach and duodenum. A small camera mounted on the endoscope sends a video image to a monitor, allowing close examination of the lining of the upper GI tract. The endoscope pumps air into the infant's GI tract, making them easier to see.

The doctor may perform a biopsy with the endoscope by taking a small piece of tissue from the lining of the infant's esophagus. He or she won't feel the biopsy. A pathologist examines the tissue in a lab. In most cases, the procedure only diagnoses GERD if the infant has moderate to severe symptoms

Upper GI Series

An upper GI series looks at the shape of an infant's upper GI tract. An X-ray technician performs this procedure at a hospital or an outpatient center. A radiologist reads and reports on the X-ray images. The infant doesn't need anesthesia. If possible, you shouldn't feed the infant before the procedure. Check with the doctor about what to do to prepare the infant for an upper GI series.

During the procedure, a healthcare professional will give the infant liquid contrast (barium) in a bottle or mixed with food to coat the inner lining of the upper GI tract. The X-ray technician takes several X-rays as the contrast moves through the GI tract. The technician or radiologist will often change the position of the infant to get the best view of the GI tract. The barium shows up on the X-ray and can help find problems related to GERD. For several days afterward, the infant may have white or light-colored stools from the barium. A healthcare professional will give you specific instructions about the infant's feeding and drinking after the procedure.

Esophageal pH and Impedance Monitoring

The most accurate procedure to detect acid reflux is esophageal pH and impedance monitoring. Esophageal pH and impedance monitoring measures the amount of acid or liquid in an infant's esophagus while he or she does normal things, such as eating and sleeping.

This procedure takes place at a hospital or outpatient center. A nurse or physician places a thin flexible tube through the infant's nose into the stomach. The tube is then pulled back into the esophagus and is secured in place with tape to the infant's cheek. The end of the tube in the esophagus measures when and how much acid or liquid comes into the esophagus from the stomach. The other end of the tube attaches to a monitor outside his or her body that records the measurements. The placement of the tube is sometimes done while a child is sedated after an upper endoscopy, but can be done while an infant is fully awake.

Most infants will stay overnight in the hospital for 24 hours after the tube is placed. This procedure is most useful to the doctor if you keep a diary of when, what, and how much food the infant eats and his or her GERD symptoms after feeding. The gastroenterologist can see how the symptoms, certain foods, and certain times of day relate to one another. The procedure can also show whether or not reflux triggers any breathing problems.

How Do Doctors Treat GER in Infants?

In most cases, gastroesophageal reflux (GER) in infants goes away before it becomes gastroesophageal reflux disease (GERD), so doctors don't treat GER in infants.

How Do Doctors Treat GERD in Infants?

Treatment for GERD depends on an infant's symptoms and age and may involve feeding changes, medicines, or surgery.

Feeding Changes

A doctor may first recommend treating an infant's GERD by changing the way you feed him or her. The doctor may suggest that you:

- add up to one tablespoon of rice cereal for every two ounces of formula in the infant's bottles. If the mixture is too thick, you can change the nipple size or cut a little "x" in the nipple to make the opening larger. Do not change formulas unless the doctor tells you to.

- add rice cereal to breast milk stored in a bottle for breastfed babies.

- burp infants after they have one to two ounces of formula, or burp breastfed infants after nursing from each breast.

- avoid overfeeding infants. Follow the amount of formula or breast milk recommended.

- hold infants upright for 30 minutes after feedings.

- try putting infants on a hydrolyzed protein formula for two to four weeks if the doctor thinks he or she may be sensitive to milk protein. The protein content of this type of formula is already broken down or "predigested."

Over-the-Counter (OTC) and Prescription Medicines

A doctor may recommend medicines that treat GERD by decreasing the amount of acid in the infant's stomach. The doctor will only prescribe a medicine if the infant still has regular GERD symptoms and if:

- you have tried making feeding changes

- the infant has problems sleeping or feeding

- the infant does not grow properly

The doctor will often prescribe a medicine on a trial basis and will explain any possible complications. You shouldn't give an infant any medicines unless told to do so by a doctor.

H2 blockers. H2 blockers decrease acid production. They provide short-term or on-demand relief for infants with GERD symptoms. They can also help heal the esophagus.

A doctor may prescribe an H2 blocker, such as:

- Cimetidine (Tagamet HB)

- Famotidine (Pepcid AC)

- Nizatidine (Axid AR)

- Ranitidine (Zantac 75)

Proton pump inhibitors (PPIs). PPIs lower the amount of acid the infant's stomach makes. PPIs are better at treating GERD symptoms than H2 blockers. They can heal the esophageal lining in infants. Doctors often prescribe PPIs for long-term GERD treatment. An infant needs to be given these medicines on an empty stomach so that his or her stomach acid can make them work.

Several types of PPIs are available by a doctor's prescription, including:

- Esomeprazole (Nexium)

- Lansoprazole (Prevacid)

- Omeprazole (Prilosec, Zegerid)

- Pantoprazole (Protonix)

- Rabeprazole (AcipHex)

Surgery

A pediatric gastroenterologist will only use surgery to treat GERD in infants in severe cases. Infants must have severe breathing problems or a physical problem that causes GERD symptoms for surgery to be an option.

How Can Diet Prevent or Relieve GER and GERD in Infants?

An infant's doctor will first suggest feeding changes if the infant is not growing well or has malnutrition. If feeding changes don't help an infant's GERD symptoms, the doctor may suggest a higher-calorie formula or tube feedings. For tube feedings, a doctor places a feeding tube through an infant's nose or mouth and into the stomach. An infant feeds from food, liquids, and medicines through the tube.

Section 14.2

Gastroesophageal Reflux (GER) and Gastroesophageal Reflux Disease (GERD) in Children and Teens

This section includes text excerpted from "Acid Reflux
(GER and GERD) in Children and Teens," National
Institute of Diabetes and Digestive and Kidney
Diseases (NIDDK), April 2015.

What Is Gastroesophageal Reflux (GER)?

Gastroesophageal reflux (GER) happens when stomach contents come back up into the esophagus. Stomach acid that touches the lining of the esophagus can cause heartburn, also called acid indigestion.

How Common Is GER in Children and Teens?

Occasional GER is common in children and teens—ages 2 to 19— and doesn't always mean that they have gastroesophageal reflux disease (GERD).

What Is Gastroesophageal Reflux Disease (GERD)?

GERD is a more serious and long-lasting form of GER in which acid reflux irritates the esophagus.

What Is the Difference between GER and GERD?

GER that occurs more than twice a week for a few weeks could be GERD. GERD can lead to more serious health problems over time. If you think your child or teen has GERD, you should take him or her to see a doctor or a pediatrician.

How Common Is GERD in Children and Teens?

Up to 25 percent of children and teens have symptoms of GERD, although GERD is more common in adults.

What Are the Complications of GERD in Children and Teens?

Without treatment, GERD can sometimes cause serious complications over time, such as:

Esophagitis

Esophagitis may lead to ulcerations, a sore in the lining of the esophagus.

Esophageal Stricture

An esophageal stricture happens when a person's esophagus becomes too narrow. Esophageal strictures can lead to problems with swallowing.

Respiratory Problems

A child or teen with GERD might breathe stomach acid into his or her lungs. The stomach acid can then irritate his or her throat and lungs, causing respiratory problems or symptoms, such as:

- Asthma—a long-lasting lung disease that makes a child or teen extra sensitive to things that he or she is allergic to
- Chest congestion, or extra fluid in the lungs
- A dry, long-lasting cough or a sore throat
- Hoarseness—the partial loss of a child or teen's voice
- Laryngitis—the swelling of a child or teen's voice box that can lead to a short-term loss of his or her voice
- Pneumonia—an infection in one or both lungs—that keeps coming back
- Wheezing—a high-pitched whistling sound that happens while breathing

A pediatrician should monitor children and teens with GERD to prevent or treat long-term problems.

What Are the Symptoms of GER and GERD in Children and Teens?

If a child or teen has gastroesophageal reflux (GER), he or she may taste food or stomach acid in the back of the mouth. Symptoms of gastroesophageal reflux disease (GERD) in children and teens can vary depending on their age. The most common symptom of GERD in children 12 years and older is regular heartburn, a painful, burning feeling in the middle of the chest, behind the breastbone, and in the middle of the abdomen. In many cases, children with GERD who are younger than 12 don't have heartburn.

Other common GERD symptoms include:

- Bad breath
- Nausea
- Pain in the chest or the upper part of the abdomen
- Problems swallowing or painful swallowing
- Respiratory problems
- Vomiting
- The wearing away of teeth

What Causes GER and GERD in Children and Teens

GER and GERD happen when a child or teen's lower esophageal sphincter becomes weak or relaxes when it shouldn't, causing stomach contents to rise up into the esophagus. The lower esophageal sphincter becomes weak or relaxes due to certain things, such as:

- Increased pressure on the abdomen from being overweight, obese, or pregnant
- Certain medicines, including:
  - Those used to treat asthma—a long-lasting disease in the lungs that makes a child or teen extra sensitive to things that he or she is allergic to
  - Antihistamines—medicines that treat allergy symptoms
  - Painkillers
  - Sedatives—medicines that help put someone to sleep
  - Antidepressants—medicines that treat depression
- Smoking, which is more likely with teens than younger children, or inhaling secondhand smoke

Other reasons a child or teen develops GERD include:

- Previous esophageal surgery

195

- Having a severe developmental delay or neurological condition, such as cerebral palsy (CP)

When Should I Seek a Doctor's Help?

Call a doctor right away if your child or teen:

- Vomits large amounts
- Has regular projectile, or forceful, vomiting
- Vomits fluid that is:
  - Green or yellow
  - Looks like coffee grounds
  - Contains blood
- Has problems breathing after vomiting
- Has mouth or throat pain when he or she eats
- Has problems swallowing or pain when swallowing
- Refuses food repeatedly, causing weight loss or poor growth
- Shows signs of dehydration, such as no tears when he or she cries

How Do Doctors Diagnose GER in Children and Teens?

In most cases, a doctor diagnoses gastroesophageal reflux (GER) by reviewing a child or teen's symptoms and medical history. If symptoms of GER do not improve with lifestyle changes and antireflux medicines, he or she may need testing.

How Do Doctors Diagnose GERD in Children and Teens?

If a child or teen's GER symptoms do not improve, if they come back frequently, or he or she has trouble swallowing, the doctor may recommend testing for gastroesophageal reflux disease (GERD). The doctor may refer the child or teen to a pediatric gastroenterologist to diagnose and treat GERD.

What Tests Do Doctors Use to Diagnose GERD?

Several tests can help a doctor diagnose GERD. A doctor may order more than one test to make a diagnosis.

Upper Gastrointestinal (GI) Series

An upper gastrointestinal (GI) series looks at the shape of the child or teen's upper GI tract. During the procedure, the child or teen will drink liquid contrast (barium or gastrografin) to coat the lining of the upper GI tract. The X-ray technician takes several X-rays as the contrast moves through the GI tract. The technician or radiologist will often change the position of the child or teen to get the best view of the GI tract. They may press on the child's abdomen during the X-ray procedure.

The upper GI series can't show mild irritation in the esophagus. It can find problems related to GERD, such as esophageal strictures, or problems with the anatomy that may cause symptoms of GERD. Children or teens may have bloating and nausea for a short time after the procedure. For several days afterward, they may have white or light-colored stools from the barium. A healthcare professional will give you specific instructions about the child or teen's eating and drinking after the procedure.

Esophageal pH and Impedance Monitoring

The most accurate procedure to detect acid reflux is esophageal pH and impedance monitoring. Esophageal pH and impedance monitoring measures the amount of acid or liquid in a child or teen's esophagus while he or she does normal things, such as eating and sleeping.

This procedure takes place at a hospital or outpatient center. A nurse or physician places a thin flexible tube through the child or teen's nose into the stomach. The tube is then pulled back into the esophagus and taped to the child or teen's cheek. The end of the tube in the esophagus measures when and how much acid comes up into the esophagus. The other end of the tube attaches to a monitor outside his or her body that records the measurements. The placement of the tube is sometimes done while a child is sedated after an upper endoscopy, but can be done while a child is fully awake.

The child or teen will wear a monitor for the next 24 hours. He or she will return to the hospital or outpatient center to have the tube removed. Children may need to stay in the hospital for the esophageal pH and impedance monitoring.

This procedure is most useful to the doctor if you keep a diary of when, what, and how much food the child or teen eats and his or her GERD symptoms after eating. The gastroenterologist can see how the symptoms, certain foods, and certain times of day relate to one another. The procedure can also help show whether acid reflux triggers any respiratory symptoms the child or teen might have.

Upper GI Endoscopy and Biopsy

In an upper GI endoscopy, a gastroenterologist, surgeon, or other trained healthcare professional uses an endoscope to see inside a child or teen's upper GI tract. This procedure takes place at a hospital or an outpatient center.

An intravenous (IV) needle will be placed in the child or teen's arm to give him or her medicines that keep him or her relaxed and comfortable during the procedure. They may be given a liquid anesthetic to gargle or spray anesthetic on the back of his or her throat. The doctor carefully feeds the endoscope down the child or teen's esophagus then into the stomach and duodenum. A small camera mounted on the endoscope sends a video image to a monitor, allowing close examination of the lining of the upper GI tract. The endoscope pumps air into the child or teen's stomach and duodenum, making them easier to see.

The doctor may perform a biopsy with the endoscope by taking small pieces of tissue from the lining of the child or teen's esophagus, stomach, or duodenum. He or she won't feel the biopsy. A pathologist examines the tissue in a lab. In most cases, the procedure only diagnoses GERD if the child or teen has moderate to severe symptoms.

How Do Doctors Treat GER and GERD in Children and Teens?

You can help control a child or teen's gastroesophageal reflux (GER) or gastroesophageal reflux disease (GERD) by having him or her:

- not eat or drink items that may cause GER, such as greasy or spicy foods

- not overeat

- avoid smoking and secondhand smoke

- lose weight if he or she is overweight or obese

- avoid eating two to three hours before bedtime

- take over-the-counter (OTC) medicines, such as Alka-Seltzer, Maalox, or Rolaids

How Do Doctors Treat GERD in Children and Teens?

Depending on the severity of the child's symptoms, a doctor may recommend lifestyle changes, medicines, or surgery.

Lifestyle Changes

Helping a child or teen make lifestyle changes can reduce his or her GERD symptoms. A child or teen should:

- lose weight, if needed
- eat smaller meals
- avoid high-fat foods
- wear loose-fitting clothing around the abdomen. Tight clothing can squeeze the stomach area and push the acid up into the esophagus.
- stay upright for three hours after meals and avoid reclining and slouching when sitting
- sleep at a slight angle. Raise the head of the child or teen's bed six to eight inches by safely putting blocks under the bedposts. Just using extra pillows will not help.

If a teen smokes, help them quit smoking and avoid secondhand smoke.

Over-the-Counter (OTC) and Prescription Medicines

If a child or teen has symptoms that won't go away, you should take him or her to see a doctor. The doctor can prescribe medicine to relieve his or her symptoms. Some medicines are available over-the-counter (OTC). All GERD medicines work in different ways. A child or teen may need a combination of GERD medicines to control symptoms.

Antacids

Doctors often first recommend antacids to relieve GER and other mild GERD symptoms. A doctor will tell you which OTC antacids to give a child or teen, such as:

- Alka-Seltzer
- Maalox
- Mylanta
- Riopan
- Rolaids

Antacids can have side effects, including diarrhea and constipation. Don't give your child or teen OTC antacids without first checking with his or her doctor.

H2 Blockers

H2 blockers decrease acid production. They provide short-term or on-demand relief for many people with GERD symptoms. They can also help heal the esophagus, although not as well as other medicines. If a doctor recommends an H2 blocker for the child or teen, you can buy them OTC or a doctor can prescribe one. Types of H2 blockers include:

- Cimetidine (Tagamet HB)

- Famotidine (Pepcid AC)

- Nizatidine (Axid AR)

- Ranitidine (Zantac 75)

If a child or teen develops heartburn after eating, his or her doctor may prescribe an antacid and an H2 blocker. The antacids neutralize stomach acid, and the H2 blockers stop the stomach from creating acid. By the time the antacids wear off, the H2 blockers are controlling the acid in the stomach.

Don't give your child or teen OTC H2 blockers without first checking with his or her doctor.

Proton Pump Inhibitors (PPIs)

PPIs lower the amount of acid the stomach makes. PPIs are better at treating GERD symptoms than H2 blockers. They can heal the esophageal lining in most people with GERD. Doctors often prescribe PPIs for long-term GERD treatment.

However, studies show that people who take PPIs for a long time or in high doses are more likely to have hip, wrist, and spinal fractures. A child or teen should take these medicines on an empty stomach so that his or her stomach acid can make them work correctly.

Several types of PPIs are available by a doctor's prescription, including:

- Esomeprazole (Nexium)

- Lansoprazole (Prevacid)

- Omeprazolc (Prilosec, Zegerid)

- Pantoprazole (Protonix)
- Rabeprazole (AcipHex)

Talk with the child or teen's doctor about taking lower-strength omeprazole or lansoprazole, sold OTC. Don't give a child or teen over-the-counter PPIs without first checking with his or her doctor.

Prokinetics

Prokinetics help the stomach empty faster. Prescription prokinetics include:

- Bethanechol (Urecholine)
- Metoclopramide (Reglan)

Both these medicines have side effects, including:

- Nausea
- Diarrhea
- Fatigue, or feeling tired
- Depression
- Anxiety
- Delayed or abnormal physical movement

Prokinetics can cause problems if a child or teen mixes them with other medicines, so tell the doctor about all the medicines he or she is taking.

Antibiotics

Antibiotics, including erythromycin, can help the stomach empty faster. Erythromycin has fewer side effects than prokinetics; however, it can cause diarrhea.

Surgery

A pediatric gastroenterologist may recommend surgery if a child or teen's GERD symptoms don't improve with lifestyle changes or medicines. A child or teen is more likely to develop complications from surgery than from medicines.

Fundoplication is the most common surgery for GERD. In most cases, it leads to long-term reflux control. A surgeon performs fundoplication using a laparoscope, a thin tube with a tiny video camera.

During the operation, a surgeon sews the top of the stomach around the esophagus to add pressure to the lower end of the esophagus and reduce reflux.

The surgeon performs the operation at a hospital. The child or teen receives general anesthesia and can leave the hospital in one to three days. Most children and teens return to their usual daily activities in two to three weeks.

Endoscopic techniques, such as endoscopic sewing and radiofrequency, help control GERD in a small number of people. Endoscopic sewing uses small stitches to tighten the sphincter muscle. Radiofrequency creates heat lesions, or sores, that help tighten the sphincter muscle. A surgeon performs both operations using an endoscope at a hospital or an outpatient center, and the child or teen receives general anesthesia. The results for endoscopic techniques may not be as good as those for fundoplication. Doctors don't use endoscopic techniques.

How Can Diet Help Prevent or Relieve GER or GERD in Children and Teens?

You can help a child or teen prevent or relieve their symptoms from gastroesophageal reflux (GER) or gastroesophageal reflux disease (GERD) by changing their diet. He or she may need to avoid certain foods and drinks that make his or her symptoms worse. Other dietary changes that can help reduce the child or teen's symptoms include:

- Decreasing fatty foods

- Eating small, frequent meals instead of three large meals

What Should a Child or Teen with GERD Avoid Eating or Drinking?

He or she should avoid eating or drinking the following items that may make GER or GERD worse:

- Chocolate

- Coffee

- Peppermint

- Greasy or spicy foods

- Tomatoes and tomato products

What Can a Child or Teen Eat If They Have GERD?

Eating healthy and balanced amounts of different types of foods is good for your child or teen's overall health. If your child or teen is overweight or obese, talk with a doctor or dietitian about dietary changes that can help with losing weight and decreasing the GERD symptoms.

Section 14.3

Gastroesophageal Reflux (GER) and Gastroesophageal Reflux Disease (GERD) in Adults

This section includes text excerpted from "Acid Reflux (GER and GERD) in Adults," National Institute of Diabetes and Digestive and Kidney Diseases (NIDDK), November 2014. Reviewed September 2018.

What Is Gastroesophageal Reflux (GER)?

Gastroesophageal reflux (GER) happens when your stomach contents come back up into your esophagus. Stomach acid that touches the lining of your esophagus can cause heartburn, also called acid indigestion.

How Common Is GER?

Having GER once in a while is common.

What Is Gastroesophageal Reflux Disease (GERD)?

Gastroesophageal reflux disease (GERD) is a more serious and long-lasting form of GER.

What Is the Difference between GER and GERD?

GER that occurs more than twice a week for a few weeks could be GERD. GERD can lead to more serious health problems over time. If you think you have GERD, you should see your doctor.

How Common Is GERD?

GERD affects about 20 percent of the U.S. population.

Who Is More Likely to Have GERD?

Anyone can develop GERD, some for unknown reasons. You are more likely to have GERD if you are:

- Overweight or obese
- A pregnant woman
- Taking certain medicines
- A smoker or regularly exposed to secondhand smoke

What Are the Complications of GERD?

Without treatment, GERD can sometimes cause serious complications over time, such as:

Esophagitis

Esophagitis is inflammation in the esophagus. Adults who have chronic esophagitis over many years are more likely to develop precancerous changes in the esophagus.

Esophageal Stricture

An esophageal stricture happens when your esophagus becomes too narrow. Esophageal strictures can lead to problems with swallowing.

Respiratory Problems

With GERD you might breathe stomach acid into your lungs. The stomach acid can then irritate your throat and lungs, causing respiratory problems, such as:

- Asthma—a long-lasting disease in your lungs that makes you extra sensitive to things that you're allergic to
- Chest congestion, or extra fluid in your lungs
- A dry, long-lasting cough or a sore throat
- Hoarseness—the partial loss of your voice
- Laryngitis—the swelling of your voice box that can lead to a short-term loss of your voice

- Pneumonia—an infection in one or both of your lungs—that keeps coming back

- Wheezing—a high-pitched whistling sound when you breathe

Barrett Esophagus

GERD can sometimes cause Barrett esophagus. A small number of people with Barrett's esophagus develop a rare yet often deadly type of cancer of the esophagus. If you have GERD, talk with your doctor about how to prevent or treat long-term problems.

What Are the Symptoms of GER and GERD?

If you have gastroesophageal reflux (GER), you may taste food or stomach acid in the back of your mouth. The most common symptom of gastroesophageal reflux disease (GERD) is regular heartburn, a painful, burning feeling in the middle of your chest, behind your breastbone, and in the middle of your abdomen. Not all adults with GERD have heartburn.

Other common GERD symptoms include:

- Bad breath

- Nausea

- Pain in your chest or the upper part of your abdomen

- Problems swallowing or painful swallowing

- Respiratory problems

- Vomiting

- The wearing away of your teeth

Some symptoms of GERD come from its complications, including those that affect your lungs.

What Causes GER and GERD

GER and GERD happen when your lower esophageal sphincter becomes weak or relaxes when it shouldn't, causing stomach contents to rise up into the esophagus. The lower esophageal sphincter becomes weak or relaxes due to certain things, such as:

- Increased pressure on your abdomen from being overweight, obese, or pregnant

- Certain medicines, including:
  - Those that doctors use to treat asthma—a long-lasting disease in your lungs that makes you extra sensitive to things that you're allergic to
  - Calcium channel blockers—medicines that treat high blood pressure
  - Antihistamines—medicines that treat allergy symptoms
  - Painkillers
  - Sedatives—medicines that help put you to sleep
  - Antidepressants—medicines that treat depression
- Smoking or inhaling secondhand smoke

A hiatal hernia can also cause GERD. Hiatal hernia is a condition in which the opening in your diaphragm lets the upper part of the stomach move up into your chest, which lowers the pressure in the esophageal sphincter.

When Should I Seek a Doctor's Help?

You should see a doctor if you have persistent GER symptoms that do not get better with over-the-counter (OTC) medications or change in your diet.

Call a doctor right away if you:

- Vomit large amounts
- Have regular projectile, or forceful, vomiting
- Vomit fluid that is:
  - Green or yellow
  - Looks like coffee grounds
  - Contains blood
- Have problems breathing after vomiting
- Have pain in the mouth or throat when you eat
- Have problems swallowing or painful swallowing

How Do Doctors Diagnose GER?

In most cases, your doctor diagnoses gastroesophageal reflux (GER) by reviewing your symptoms and medical history. If your symptoms don't improve with lifestyle changes and medications, you may need testing.

How Do Doctors Diagnose GERD?

If your GER symptoms don't improve, if they come back frequently, or if you have trouble swallowing, your doctor may recommend testing you for gastroesophageal reflux disease (GERD). Your doctor may refer you to a gastroenterologist to diagnose and treat GERD.

What Tests Do Doctors Use to Diagnose GERD?

Several tests can help a doctor diagnose GERD. Your doctor may order more than one test to make a diagnosis.

Upper Gastrointestinal (GI) Endoscopy and Biopsy

In an upper gastrointestinal (GI) endoscopy, a gastroenterologist, surgeon, or other trained healthcare professional uses an endoscope to see inside your upper GI tract. This procedure takes place at a hospital or an outpatient center.

An intravenous (IV) needle will be placed in your arm to provide a sedative. Sedatives help you stay relaxed and comfortable during the procedure. In some cases, the procedure can be performed without sedation. You will be given a liquid anesthetic to gargle or spray anesthetic on the back of your throat. The doctor carefully feeds the endoscope down your esophagus and into your stomach and duodenum. A small camera mounted on the endoscope sends a video image to a monitor, allowing close examination of the lining of your upper GI tract. The endoscope pumps air into your stomach and duodenum, making them easier to see.

The doctor may perform a biopsy with the endoscope by taking a small piece of tissue from the lining of your esophagus. You won't feel the biopsy. A pathologist examines the tissue in a lab. In most cases, the procedure only diagnoses GERD if you have moderate to severe symptoms.

Upper GI Series

An upper GI series looks at the shape of your upper GI tract. An X-ray technician performs this procedure at a hospital or an outpatient center. A radiologist reads and reports on the X-ray images.

You don't need anesthesia. A healthcare professional will tell you how to prepare for the procedure, including when to stop eating and drinking.

During the procedure, you will stand or sit in front of an X-ray machine and drink barium to coat the inner lining of your upper GI tract. The X-ray technician takes several X-rays as the barium moves through your GI tract. The upper GI series can't show GERD in your esophagus; rather, the barium shows up on the X-ray and can find problems related to GERD, such as:

- Hiatal hernias

- Esophageal strictures

- Ulcers

You may have bloating and nausea for a short time after the procedure. For several days afterward, you may have white or light-colored stools from the barium. A healthcare professional will give you instructions about eating, drinking, and taking your medicines after the procedure.

Esophageal pH and Impedance Monitoring

The most accurate procedure to detect acid reflux is esophageal pH and impedance monitoring. Esophageal pH and impedance monitoring measures the amount of acid in your esophagus while you do normal things, such as eating and sleeping.

A gastroenterologist performs this procedure at a hospital or an outpatient center as a part of an upper GI endoscopy. Most often, you can stay awake during the procedure.

A gastroenterologist will pass a thin tube through your nose or mouth into your stomach. The gastroenterologist will then pull the tube back into your esophagus and tape it to your cheek. The end of the tube in your esophagus measures when and how much acid comes up your esophagus. The other end of the tube attaches to a monitor outside your body that records the measurements.

You will wear a monitor for the next 24 hours. You will return to the hospital or outpatient center to have the tube removed. This procedure is most useful to your doctor if you keep a diary of when, what, and how much food you eat and your GERD symptoms are after you eat. The gastroenterologist can see how your symptoms, certain foods, and certain times of day relate to one another. The procedure can also help show whether acid reflux triggers any respiratory symptoms.

Bravo Wireless Esophageal pH Monitoring

Bravo wireless esophageal pH monitoring also measures and records the pH in your esophagus to determine if you have GERD. A doctor temporarily attaches a small capsule to the wall of your esophagus during an upper endoscopy. The capsule measures pH levels in the esophagus and transmits information to a receiver. The receiver is about the size of a pager, which you wear on your belt or waistband.

You will follow your usual daily routine during monitoring, which usually lasts 48 hours. The receiver has several buttons on it that you will press to record symptoms of GERD such as heartburn. The nurse will tell you what symptoms to record. You will be asked to maintain a diary to record certain events such as when you start and stop eating and drinking, when you lie down, and when you get back up.

To prepare for the test talk to your doctor about medicines you are taking. He or she will tell you whether you can eat or drink before the procedure. After about seven to ten days the capsule will fall off the esophageal lining and pass through your digestive tract.

Esophageal Manometry

Esophageal manometry measures muscle contractions in your esophagus. A gastroenterologist may order this procedure if you're thinking about antireflux surgery.

The gastroenterologist can perform this procedure during an office visit. A healthcare professional will spray a liquid anesthetic on the back of your throat or ask you to gargle a liquid anesthetic.

The gastroenterologist passes a soft, thin tube through your nose and into your stomach. You swallow as the gastroenterologist pulls the tube slowly back into your esophagus. A computer measures and records the pressure of muscle contractions in different parts of your esophagus.

The procedure can show if your symptoms are due to a weak sphincter muscle. A doctor can also use the procedure to diagnose other esophagus problems that might have symptoms similar to heartburn. A healthcare professional will give you instructions about eating, drinking, and taking your medicines after the procedure.

How Do You Control GER and GERD?

You may be able to control gastroesophageal reflux (GER) and gastroesophageal reflux disease (GERD) by:

- not eating or drinking items that may cause GER, such as greasy or spicy foods and alcoholic drinks

- not overeating

- not eating two to three hours before bedtime

- losing weight if you're overweight or obese

- quitting smoking and avoiding secondhand smoke

- taking OTC medicines, such as Maalox, or Rolaids

How Do Doctors Treat GERD?

Depending on the severity of your symptoms, your doctor may recommend lifestyle changes, medicines, surgery, or a combination.

Lifestyle Changes

Making lifestyle changes can reduce your GER and GERD symptoms. You should:

- lose weight, if needed.

- wear loose-fitting clothing around your abdomen. Tight clothing can squeeze your stomach area and push acid up into your esophagus.

- stay upright for three hours after meals. Avoid reclining and slouching when sitting.

- sleep on a slight angle. Raise the head of your bed six to eight inches by safely putting blocks under the bedposts. Just using extra pillows will not help.

- quit smoking and avoid secondhand smoke.

Over-the-Counter (OTC) and Prescription Medicines

You can buy many GERD medicines without a prescription. However, if you have symptoms that will not go away, you should see your doctor. All GERD medicines work in different ways. You may need a combination of GERD medicines to control your symptoms.

Antacids. Doctors often first recommend antacids to relieve heartburn and other mild GER and GERD symptoms. Antacids include OTC medicines such as:

- Maalox

- Mylanta

- Riopan
- Rolaids

Antacids can have side effects, including diarrhea and constipation.

H2 blockers. H2 blockers decrease acid production. They provide short-term or on-demand relief for many people with GER and GERD symptoms. They can also help heal the esophagus, although not as well as other medicines. You can buy H2 blockers OTC or your doctor can prescribe one. Types of H2 blockers include:

- Cimetidine (Tagamet HB)
- Famotidine (Pepcid AC)
- Nizatidine (Axid AR)
- Ranitidine (Zantac 75)

If you get heartburn after eating, your doctor may recommend that you take an antacid and an H2 blocker. The antacid neutralizes stomach acid, and the H2 blocker stops your stomach from creating acid. By the time the antacid stops working, the H2 blocker has stopped the acid.

Proton pump inhibitors (PPIs). PPIs lower the amount of acid your stomach makes. PPIs are better at treating GERD symptoms than H2 blockers. They can heal the esophageal lining in most people with GERD. Doctors often prescribe PPIs for long-term GERD treatment.

However, studies show that people who take PPIs for a long time or in high doses are more likely to have hip, wrist, and spinal fractures. You need to take these medicines on an empty stomach so that your stomach acid can make them work.

Several types of PPIs are available by a doctor's prescription, including:

- Esomeprazole (Nexium)
- Lansoprazole (Prevacid)
- Omeprazole (Prilosec, Zegerid)
- Pantoprazole (Protonix)
- Rabeprazole (AcipHex)

Talk with your doctor about taking lower-strength omeprazole or lansoprazole, sold OTC.

Prokinetics. Prokinetics help your stomach empty faster. Prescription prokinetics include:

- Bethanechol (Urecholine)
- Metoclopramide (Reglan)

Both of these medicines have side effects, including:

- Nausea
- Diarrhea
- Fatigue or feeling tired
- Depression
- Anxiety
- Delayed or abnormal physical movement

Prokinetics can cause problems if you mix them with other medicines, so tell your doctor about all the medicines you're taking.

Antibiotics. Antibiotics, including erythromycin, can help your stomach empty faster. Erythromycin has fewer side effects than prokinetics; however, it can cause diarrhea.

Surgery

Your doctor may recommend surgery if your GERD symptoms don't improve with lifestyle changes or medicines. You're more likely to develop complications from surgery than from medicines.

Fundoplication is the most common surgery for GERD. In most cases, it leads to long-term reflux control.

A surgeon performs fundoplication using a laparoscope, a thin tube with a tiny video camera. During the operation, a surgeon sews the top of your stomach around your esophagus to add pressure to the lower end of your esophagus and reduce reflux. The surgeon performs the operation at a hospital. You receive general anesthesia and can leave the hospital in one to three days. Most people return to their usual daily activities in two to three weeks.

Endoscopic techniques, such as endoscopic sewing and radiofrequency, help control GERD in a small number of people. Endoscopic sewing uses small stitches to tighten your sphincter muscle. Radiofrequency creates heat lesions, or sores, that help tighten your sphincter muscle. A surgeon performs both operations using an endoscope at a hospital or an outpatient center, and you receive general anesthesia. The results for endoscopic techniques may not be as good as those for fundoplication. Doctors don't use endoscopic techniques often.

How Can Your Diet Help Prevent or Relieve GER or GERD?

You can prevent or relieve your symptoms from gastroesophageal reflux (GER) or gastroesophageal reflux disease (GERD) by changing your diet. You may need to avoid certain foods and drinks that make your symptoms worse. Other dietary changes that can help reduce your symptoms include:

- Decreasing fatty foods
- Eating small, frequent meals instead of three large meals

What Should I Avoid Eating If I Have GER or GERD?

Avoid eating or drinking the following items that may make GER or GERD worse:

- Chocolate
- Coffee
- Peppermint
- Greasy or spicy foods
- Tomatoes and tomato products
- Alcoholic drinks

What Can I Eat If I Have GER or GERD?

Eating healthy and balanced amounts of different types of foods is good for your overall health. If you're overweight or obese, talk with your doctor or a dietitian about dietary changes that can help you lose weight and decrease your GERD symptoms.

Chapter 15

Swallowing Disorder: Dysphagia

What Is Dysphagia?

People with dysphagia have difficulty swallowing and may even experience pain while swallowing (odynophagia). Some people may be completely unable to swallow or may have trouble safely swallowing liquids, foods, or saliva. When that happens, eating becomes a challenge. Often, dysphagia makes it difficult to take in enough calories and fluids to nourish the body and can lead to additional serious medical problems.

How Do We Swallow?

Swallowing is a complex process. Some 50 pairs of muscles and many nerves work to receive food into the mouth, prepare it, and move it from the mouth to the stomach. This happens in three stages.

During the first stage, called the oral phase, the tongue collects the food or liquid, making it ready for swallowing. The tongue and jaw move solid food around in the mouth so it can be chewed. Chewing makes solid food the right size and texture to swallow by mixing the food with saliva. Saliva softens and moistens the food to make

---

This chapter includes text excerpted from "Dysphagia," National Institute on Deafness and Other Communication Disorders (NIDCD), March 6, 2017.

swallowing easier. Normally, the only solid we swallow without chewing is in the form of a pill or caplet. Everything else that we swallow is in the form of a liquid, a puree, or a chewed solid.

The second stage begins when the tongue pushes the food or liquid to the back of the mouth. This triggers a swallowing response that passes the food through the pharynx, or throat (see figure 15.1). During this phase, called the pharyngeal phase, the larynx (voice box) closes tightly and breathing stops to prevent food or liquid from entering the airway and lungs.

The third stage begins when food or liquid enters the esophagus, the tube that carries food and liquid to the stomach. The passage through the esophagus, called the esophageal phase, usually occurs in about three seconds, depending on the texture or consistency of the food, but can take slightly longer in some cases, such as when swallowing a pill.

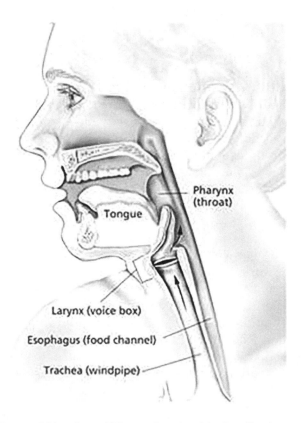

Figure 15.1. *Parts of Mouth and Throat Involved in Swallowing*

How Does Dysphagia Occur?

Dysphagia occurs when there is a problem with the neural control or the structures involved in any part of the swallowing process. Weak tongue or cheek muscles may make it hard to move food around in the mouth for chewing. A stroke or other nervous system disorder may make it difficult to start the swallowing response, a stimulus that allows food and liquids to move safely through the throat. Another difficulty can occur when weak throat muscles, such as after cancer surgery, cannot move all of the food toward the stomach. Dysphagia may also result from disorders of the esophagus.

What Are Some Problems Caused by Dysphagia?

Dysphagia can be serious. Someone who cannot swallow safely may not be able to eat enough of the right foods to stay healthy or maintain an ideal weight.

Food pieces that are too large for swallowing may enter the throat and block the passage of air. In addition, when foods or liquids enter the airway of someone who has dysphagia, coughing or throat clearing sometimes cannot remove it. Food or liquid that stays in the airway may enter the lungs and allow harmful bacteria to grow, resulting in a lung infection called aspiration pneumonia.

Swallowing disorders may also include the development of a pocket outside the esophagus caused by weakness in the esophageal wall. This abnormal pocket traps some food being swallowed. While lying down or sleeping, someone with this problem may draw undigested food into the throat. The esophagus may also be too narrow, causing food to stick. This food may prevent other food or even liquids from entering the stomach.

What Causes Dysphagia

Dysphagia has many possible causes and happens most frequently in older adults. Any condition that weakens or damages the muscles and nerves used for swallowing may cause dysphagia. For example, people with diseases of the nervous system, such as cerebral palsy (CP) or Parkinson disease (PD), often have problems swallowing. Additionally, stroke or head injury may weaken or affect the coordination of the swallowing muscles or limit sensation in the mouth and throat.

People born with abnormalities of the swallowing mechanism may not be able to swallow normally. Infants who are born with an opening in the roof of the mouth (cleft palate) are unable to suck properly, which complicates nursing and drinking from a regular baby bottle.

In addition, cancer of the head, neck, or esophagus may cause swallowing problems. Sometimes the treatment for these types of cancers can cause dysphagia. Injuries of the head, neck, and chest may also create swallowing problems. An infection or irritation can cause narrowing of the esophagus. Finally, for people with dementia, memory loss, and cognitive decline may make it difficult to chew and swallow.

How Is Dysphagia Treated?

There are different treatments for various types of dysphagia. Medical doctors and speech-language pathologists who evaluate and treat swallowing disorders use a variety of tests that allow them to look at the stages of the swallowing process. One test, the Flexible Endoscopic Evaluation of Swallowing with Sensory Testing (FEESST), uses a lighted fiber optic tube, or endoscope, to view the mouth and throat while examining how the swallowing mechanism responds to such stimuli as a puff of air, food, or liquids.

A videofluoroscopic swallow study (VFSS) is a test in which a clinician takes a videotaped X-ray of the entire swallowing process by having you consume several foods or liquids along with the mineral barium to improve visibility of the digestive tract. Such images help identify where in the swallowing process you are experiencing problems. Speech-language pathologists use this method to explore what changes can be made to offer a safe strategy when swallowing. The changes may be in food texture, size, head and neck posture, or behavioral maneuvers, such as "chin tuck," a strategy in which you tuck your chin so that food and other substances do not enter the trachea when swallowing. If you are unable to swallow safely despite rehabilitation strategies, then medical or surgical intervention may be necessary for the short-term as you recover. In progressive conditions such as amyotrophic lateral sclerosis (ALS, or Lou Gehrig disease), a feeding tube in the stomach may be necessary for the long term.

For some people, treatment may involve muscle exercises to strengthen weak facial muscles or to improve coordination. For others, treatment may involve learning to eat. For example, some people may have to eat with their head turned to one side or looking straight ahead. Preparing food in a certain way or avoiding certain foods may help in some situations. For instance, people who cannot swallow thin liquids may need to add special thickeners to their drinks. Other people may have to avoid hot or cold foods or drinks.

For some, however, consuming enough foods and liquids by mouth may no longer be possible. These individuals must use other methods to nourish their bodies. Usually, this involves a feeding system, such as a feeding tube, that bypasses or supplements the part of the swallowing mechanism that is not working normally.

Chapter 16

What You Need to Know about Peptic Ulcers

What Is a Peptic Ulcer?

A peptic ulcer is a sore on the lining of your stomach or duodenum. Rarely, a peptic ulcer may develop just above your stomach in your esophagus. Doctors call this type of peptic ulcer an esophageal ulcer.

Who Is More Likely to Develop Peptic Ulcers Caused By Nonsteroidal Anti-Inflammatory Drugs (NSAIDs)?

People of any age who take NSAIDs every day or multiple times per week are more likely to develop a peptic ulcer than people who do not take them regularly. NSAIDs are a class of painkillers, such as aspirin and ibuprofen. Long-term use of NSAIDs can cause peptic ulcer disease.

Your chance of having a peptic ulcer caused by NSAIDs, also called an NSAID-induced peptic ulcer, is increased if you:

- are age 70 or older

- are female

This chapter includes text excerpted from "Peptic Ulcers (Stomach Ulcers)," National Institute of Diabetes and Digestive and Kidney Diseases (NIDDK), November 2014. Reviewed September 2018.

- are taking more than two types of NSAIDs or have taken NSAIDs regularly for a long time

- have had a peptic ulcer before

- have two or more medical conditions or diseases

- are taking other medicines, such as corticosteroids and medicines to increase your bone mass

- drink alcohol or smoke

Who Is More Likely to Develop Peptic Ulcers Caused by H. pylori?

About 30–40 percent of people in the United States get an *H. pylori* infection. In most cases, the infection remains dormant, or quiet without signs or symptoms, for years. Most people get an *H. pylori* infection as a child.

Adults who have an *H. pylori* infection may get a peptic ulcer, also called an *H. pylori*-induced peptic ulcer. However, most people with an *H. pylori* infection never develop a peptic ulcer. Peptic ulcers caused by *H. pylori* are uncommon in children.

H. pylori are spiral-shaped bacteria that can damage the lining of your stomach and duodenum and cause peptic ulcer disease. Researchers are not certain how *H. pylori* spread. They think the bacteria may spread through:

- Unclean food

- Unclean water

- Unclean eating utensils

- Contact with an infected person's saliva and other bodily fluids, including kissing

Researchers have found *H. pylori* in the saliva of some infected people, which means an *H. pylori* infection could spread through direct contact with saliva or other bodily fluids.

Who Develops Peptic Ulcers Caused by Tumors?

People who have Zollinger-Ellison syndrome (ZES) develop peptic ulcers caused by tumors. Anyone can have ZES, yet it is rare and only occurs in about one in every one million people. However, ZES is more common among men 30–50 years old. A child who has a parent with multiple endocrine neoplasia type 1 is also more likely to have Zollinger-Ellison syndrome.

What Other Problems Can a Peptic Ulcer Cause?

A peptic ulcer can cause other problems, including:

- Bleeding from a broken blood vessel in your stomach or small intestine
- Perforation of your stomach or small intestine
- A blockage that can stop food from moving from your stomach into your duodenum
- Peritonitis

You may need surgery to treat these problems.

What Are the Symptoms of a Peptic Ulcer?

A dull or burning pain in your stomach is the most common symptom of a peptic ulcer. You may feel the pain anywhere between your belly button and breastbone. The pain most often:

- happens when your stomach is empty—such as between meals or during the night
- stops briefly if you eat or if you take antacids
- lasts for minutes to hours
- comes and goes for several days, weeks, or months

Less common symptoms may include:

- Bloating
- Burping
- Feeling sick to your stomach
- Poor appetite
- Vomiting
- Weight loss

Even if your symptoms are mild, you may have a peptic ulcer. You should see your doctor to talk about your symptoms. Without treatment, your peptic ulcer can get worse.

What Causes a Peptic Ulcer

Causes of peptic ulcers include:

- Long-term use of nonsteroidal anti-inflammatory drugs (NSAIDs), such as aspirin and ibuprofen

- An infection with the bacteria *Helicobacter pylori* (*H. pylori*)

- Rare cancerous and noncancerous tumors in the stomach, duodenum, or pancreas—known as Zollinger-Ellison syndrome

Sometimes peptic ulcers are caused by both NSAIDs and *H. pylori*.

How Do NSAIDs Cause a Peptic Ulcer?

To understand how NSAIDs cause peptic ulcer disease, it is important to understand how NSAIDs work. NSAIDs reduce pain, fever, and inflammation, or swelling.

Everyone has two enzymes that produce chemicals in your body's cells that promote pain, inflammation, and fever. NSAIDs work by blocking or reducing the amount of these enzymes that your body makes. However, one of the enzymes also produces another type of chemical that protects the stomach lining from stomach acid and helps control bleeding. When NSAIDs block or reduce the amount of this enzyme in your body, they also increase your chance of developing a peptic ulcer.

How Do H. pylori *Cause a Peptic Ulcer and Peptic Ulcer Disease?*

H. pylori are spiral-shaped bacteria that can cause peptic ulcer disease by damaging the mucous coating that protects the lining of the stomach and duodenum. Once *H. pylori* have damaged the mucous coating, powerful stomach acid can get through to the sensitive lining. Together, the stomach acid and *H. pylori* irritate the lining of the stomach or duodenum and cause a peptic ulcer.

How Do Tumors from Zollinger-Ellison Syndrome (ZES) Cause Peptic Ulcers?

Zollinger-Ellison syndrome (ZES) is a rare disorder that happens when one or more tumors form in your pancreas and duodenum. The tumors release large amounts of gastrin, a hormone that causes your stomach to produce large amounts of acid. The extra acid causes peptic ulcers to form in your duodenum and in the upper intestine.

When Should You Call or See a Doctor?

You should call or see your doctor right away if you:

- feel weak or faint
- have difficulty breathing
- have red blood in your vomit or vomit that looks like coffee grounds
- have red blood in your stool or black stools
- have sudden, sharp stomach pain that doesn't go away

These symptoms could be signs that a peptic ulcer has caused a more serious problem.

How Do Doctors Diagnose a Peptic Ulcer?

Your doctor will use information from your medical history, a physical exam, and tests to diagnose an ulcer and its cause. The presence of an ulcer can only be determined by looking directly at the stomach with endoscopy or an X-ray test.

Medical History

To help diagnose a peptic ulcer, your doctor will ask you questions about your medical history, your symptoms, and the medicines you take.

Be sure to mention medicines that you take without a prescription, especially nonsteroidal anti-inflammatory drugs (NSAIDs), such as:

- Aspirin (Bayer Aspirin)
- Ibuprofen (Motrin, Advil)
- Naproxen (Aleve)

Physical Exam

A physical exam may help a doctor diagnose a peptic ulcer. During a physical exam, a doctor most often:

- checks for bloating in your abdomen

- listens to sounds within your abdomen using a stethoscope
- taps on your abdomen checking for tenderness or pain

Lab Tests

To see if you have a *Helicobacter pylori* (*H. pylori*) infection, your doctor will order these tests:

- Blood test
- Urea breath test
- Stool test

Upper Gastrointestinal (GI) Endoscopy and Biopsy

In an upper GI endoscopy, a gastroenterologist, surgeon, or other trained healthcare professional uses an endoscope to see inside your upper GI tract. This procedure takes place at a hospital or an outpatient center.

An intravenous (IV) needle will be placed in your arm to provide a sedative. Sedatives help you stay relaxed and comfortable during the procedure. In some cases, the procedure can be performed without sedation. You will be given a liquid anesthetic to gargle or spray anesthetic on the back of your throat. The doctor will carefully feed the endoscope down your esophagus and into your stomach and duodenum. A small camera mounted on the endoscope sends a video image to a monitor, allowing close examination of the lining of your upper GI tract. The endoscope pumps air into your stomach and duodenum, making them easier to see.

The doctor may perform a biopsy with the endoscope by taking a small piece of tissue from the lining of your esophagus. You won't feel the biopsy. A pathologist examines the tissue in a lab.

Upper GI Series

An upper GI series looks at the shape of your upper GI tract. An X-ray technician performs this test at a hospital or an outpatient center. A radiologist reads and reports on the X-ray images. You don't need anesthesia. A healthcare professional will tell you how to prepare for the procedure, including when to stop eating and drinking.

During the procedure, you'll stand or sit in front of an X-ray machine and drink barium, a chalky liquid. Barium coats your esophagus, stomach, and small intestine so your doctor can see the shapes of these organs more clearly on X-rays.

You may have bloating and nausea for a short time after the test. For several days afterward, you may have white or light-colored stools from the barium. A healthcare professional will give you instructions about eating and drinking after the test.

Computerized Tomography (CT) Scan

A CT scan uses a combination of X-rays and computer technology to create images. For a CT scan, a healthcare professional may give you a solution to drink and an injection of a special dye, which doctors call contrast medium. You'll lie on a table that slides into a tunnel-shaped device that takes the X-rays. An X-ray technician performs the procedure in an outpatient center or a hospital, and a radiologist interprets the images. You don't need anesthesia.

CT scans can help diagnose a peptic ulcer that has created a hole in the wall of your stomach or small intestine.

How Do Doctors Treat Peptic Ulcer Disease?

There are several types of medicines used to treat a peptic ulcer. Your doctor will decide the best treatment based on the cause of your peptic ulcer.

How Do Doctors Treat an NSAID-Induced Peptic Ulcer?

If NSAIDs are causing your peptic ulcer and you don't have an *H. pylori* infection, your doctor may tell you to:

- stop taking the NSAID

- reduce how much of the NSAID you take

- switch to another medicine that won't cause a peptic ulcer

Your doctor may also prescribe medicines to reduce stomach acid and coat and protect your peptic ulcer. Proton pump inhibitors (PPIs), histamine receptor blockers, and protectants can help relieve pain and help your ulcer heal.

Proton Pump Inhibitors (PPIs)

PPIs reduce stomach acid and protect the lining of your stomach and duodenum. While PPIs can't kill *H. pylori*, they do help fight the *H. pylori* infection.

PPIs include:

- Esomeprazole (Nexium)

- Dexlansoprazole (Dexilant)

- Lansoprazole (Prevacid)

- Omeprazole (Prilosec, Zegerid)

- Pantoprazole (Protonix)

- Rabeprazole (AcipHex)

Histamine Receptor Blockers

Histamine receptor blockers work by blocking histamine, a chemical in your body that signals your stomach to produce acid. Histamine receptor blockers include:

- Cimetidine (Tagamet)

- Famotidine (Pepcid)

- Ranitidine (Zantac)

- Nizatidine (Axid) Protectants

Protectants

Protectants coat ulcers and protect them against acid and enzymes so that healing can occur. Doctors only prescribe one protectant—sucralfate (Carafate)—for peptic ulcer disease. Tell your doctor if the medicines make you feel sick or dizzy or cause diarrhea or headaches. Your doctor can change your medicines. If you smoke, quit. You also should avoid alcohol. Drinking alcohol and smoking slows the healing of a peptic ulcer and can make it worse.

What If I Still Need to Take NSAIDs?

If you take NSAIDs for other conditions, such as arthritis, you should talk with your doctor about the benefits and risks of using NSAIDs. Your doctor can help you determine how to continue using an NSAID safely after your peptic ulcer symptoms go away. Your doctor may prescribe a medicine used to prevent NSAID-induced ulcers called Misoprostol.

Tell your doctor about all the prescription and over-the-counter (OTC) medicines you take. Your doctor can then decide if you may safely take NSAIDs or if you should switch to a different medicine. In either case, your doctor may prescribe a PPI or histamine receptor blocker to protect the lining of your stomach and duodenum.

If you need NSAIDs, you can reduce the chance of a peptic ulcer returning by:

- taking the NSAID with a meal
- using the lowest effective dose possible
- quitting smoking
- avoiding alcohol

How Do Doctors Treat an NSAID-Induced Peptic Ulcer When You Have an H. pylori Infection?

If you have an *H. pylori* infection, a doctor will treat your NSAID-induced peptic ulcer with PPIs or histamine receptor blockers and other medicines, such as antibiotics, bismuth subsalicylate, or antacids.

PPIs reduce stomach acid and protect the lining of your stomach and duodenum. While PPIs can't kill *H. pylori*, they do help fight the *H. pylori* infection.

PPIs include:

- Esomeprazole (Nexium)
- Dexlansoprazole (Dexilant)
- Lansoprazole (Prevacid)
- Omeprazole (Prilosec, Zegerid)
- Pantoprazole (Protonix)
- Rabeprazole (AcipHex)

Histamine Receptor Blockers

Histamine receptor blockers work by blocking histamine, a chemical in your body that signals your stomach to produce acid. Histamine receptor blockers include:

- Cimetidine (Tagamet)
- Famotidine (Pepcid)
- Ranitidine (Zantac)
- Nizatidine (Axid)

Antibiotics

A doctor will prescribe antibiotics to kill *H. pylori*. How doctors prescribe antibiotics may differ throughout the world. Over time, some types of antibiotics can no longer destroy certain types of *H. pylori*. Antibiotics can cure most peptic ulcers caused by *H. pylori* or *H. pylori*-induced peptic ulcers. However, getting rid of the bacteria can be difficult. Take all doses of your antibiotics exactly as your doctor prescribes, even if the pain from a peptic ulcer is gone.

Bismuth Subsalicylate

Medicines containing bismuth subsalicylate, such as Pepto-Bismol, coat a peptic ulcer and protect it from stomach acid. Although bismuth subsalicylate can kill *H. pylori*, doctors sometimes prescribe it with antibiotics, not in place of antibiotics.

Antacids

An antacid may make the pain from a peptic ulcer go away temporarily, yet it will not kill *H. pylori*. If you receive treatment for an *H. pylori*-induced peptic ulcer, check with your doctor before taking antacids. Some of the antibiotics may not work as well if you take them with an antacid.

How Do Doctors Treat an H. pylori-*Induced Peptic Ulcer?*

Doctors may prescribe triple therapy, quadruple therapy, or sequential therapy to treat an *H. pylori*-induced peptic ulcer.

Triple Therapy

For triple therapy, your doctor will prescribe that you take the following for 7–14 days:

- The antibiotic clarithromycin
- The antibiotic metronidazole or the antibiotic amoxicillin
- A PPI

Quadruple Therapy

For quadruple therapy, your doctor will prescribe that you take the following for 14 days:

- A PPI

- Bismuth subsalicylate

- The antibiotics tetracycline and metronidazole

Doctors prescribe quadruple therapy to treat patients who:

- can't take amoxicillin because of an allergy to penicillin. Penicillin and amoxicillin are similar

- have previously received a macrolide antibiotic, such as clarithromycin

- are still infected with *H. pylori* after triple therapy treatment

Doctors prescribe quadruple therapy after the first treatment has failed. In the second round of treatment, the doctor may prescribe different antibiotics than those that he or she prescribed the first time.

Sequential Therapy

For sequential therapy, your doctor will prescribe that you take the following for five days:

- A PPI

- Amoxicillin

Then the doctor will prescribe you the following for another five days:

- A PPI

- Clarithromycin

- The antibiotic tinidazole

Triple therapy, quadruple therapy, and sequential therapy may cause nausea and other side effects, including:

- An altered sense of taste

- Darkened stools

- A darkened tongue

- Diarrhea

- Headaches

- Temporary reddening of the skin when drinking alcohol

- Vaginal yeast infections

Talk with your doctor about any side effects that bother you. He or she may prescribe you other medicines.

How Do Doctors Treat Peptic Ulcers Caused by ZES?

Doctors use medicines, surgery, and chemotherapy to treat Zollinger-Ellison syndrome (ZES).

What If a Peptic Ulcer Doesn't Heal?

Most often, medicines heal a peptic ulcer. If an *H. pylori* infection caused your peptic ulcer, you should finish all of your antibiotics and take any other medicines your doctor prescribes. The infection and peptic ulcer will heal only if you take all medicines as your doctor prescribes. When you have finished your medicines, your doctor may do another breath or stool test in four weeks or more to be sure the *H. pylori* infection is gone. Sometimes, *H. pylori* bacteria are still present, even after you have taken all the medicines correctly. If the infection is still present, your peptic ulcer could return or, rarely, stomach cancer could develop. Your doctor will prescribe different antibiotics to get rid of the infection and cure your peptic ulcer.

Can a Peptic Ulcer Come Back?

Yes, a peptic ulcer can come back. If you smoke or take NSAIDs, peptic ulcers are more likely to come back. If you need to take an NSAID, your doctor may switch you to a different medicine or add medicines to help prevent a peptic ulcer. Peptic ulcer disease can return, even if you have been careful to reduce your risk.

How Can I Prevent a Peptic Ulcer?

To help prevent a peptic ulcer caused by NSAIDs, ask your doctor if you should:

- stop using NSAIDs
- take NSAIDs with a meal if you still need NSAIDs
- take a lower dose of NSAIDs
- take medicines to protect your stomach and duodenum while taking NSAIDs

- switch to a medicine that won't cause ulcers

To help prevent a peptic ulcer caused by *H. pylori*, your doctor may recommend that you avoid drinking alcohol.

How Can Your Diet Help Prevent or Relieve a Peptic Ulcer?

Researchers have not found that diet and nutrition play an important role in causing or preventing peptic ulcers. Before acid-blocking drugs became available, milk was used to treat ulcers. However, milk is not an effective way to prevent or relieve a peptic ulcer. Alcohol and smoking contribute to ulcers and should be avoided.

Chapter 17

Gastroparesis

What Is Gastroparesis?

Gastroparesis, also called delayed gastric emptying, is a disorder that slows or stops the movement of food from your stomach to your small intestine. Normally, after you swallow food, the muscles in the wall of your stomach grind the food into smaller pieces and push them into your small intestine to continue digestion. When you have gastroparesis, your stomach muscles work poorly or not at all, and your stomach takes too long to empty its contents. Gastroparesis can delay digestion, which can lead to various symptoms and complications.

How Common Is Gastroparesis?

Gastroparesis is not common. Out of 100,000 people, about 10 men and about 40 women have gastroparesis. However, symptoms that are similar to those of gastroparesis occur in about one out of four adults in the United States.

Who Is More Likely to Get Gastroparesis?

You are more likely to get gastroparesis if you:

- have diabetes

This chapter includes text excerpted from "Gastroparesis," National Institute of Diabetes and Digestive and Kidney Diseases (NIDDK), January 2018

- had surgery on your esophagus, stomach, or small intestine, which may injure the vagus nerve. The vagus nerve controls the muscles of the stomach and small intestine.

- had certain cancer treatments, such as radiation therapy on your chest or stomach area

What Other Health Problems Do People with Gastroparesis Have?

People with gastroparesis may have other health problems, such as:

- Diabetes

- Scleroderma

- Hypothyroidism

- Nervous system disorders, such as migraine, Parkinson disease (PD), and multiple sclerosis (MS)

- Gastroesophageal reflux disease (GERD)

- Eating disorders

- Amyloidosis

What Are the Complications of Gastroparesis?

Complications of gastroparesis may include:

- Dehydration due to repeated vomiting

- Malnutrition due to poor absorption of nutrients

- Blood glucose, also called blood sugar, levels that are harder to control, which can worsen diabetes

- Low-calorie intake

- Bezoars

- Losing weight without trying

- Lower quality of life

What Are the Symptoms of Gastroparesis?

The symptoms of gastroparesis may include:

- Feeling full soon after starting a meal

- Feeling full long after eating a meal
- Nausea
- Vomiting
- Too much bloating
- Too much belching
- Pain in your upper abdomen
- Heartburn
- Poor appetite

Certain medicines may delay gastric emptying or affect motility, resulting in symptoms that are similar to those of gastroparesis. If you have been diagnosed with gastroparesis, these medicines may make your symptoms worse. Medicines that may delay gastric emptying or make symptoms worse include the following:

- Narcotic pain medicines, such as codeine, hydrocodone, morphine, oxycodone, and tapentadol
- Some antidepressants, such as amitriptyline, nortriptyline, and venlafaxine
- Some anticholinergics—medicines that block certain nerve signals
- Some medicines used to treat overactive bladder
- Pramlintide

These medicines do not cause gastroparesis.

When Should I Seek a Doctor's Help?

You should seek a doctor's help right away if you have any of the following signs or symptoms:

- Severe pain or cramping in your abdomen
- Blood glucose levels that are too high or too low
- Red blood in your vomit, or vomit that looks like coffee grounds
- Sudden, sharp stomach pain that doesn't go away
- Vomiting for more than an hour
- Feeling extremely weak or fainting

- Difficulty breathing

- Fever

You should seek a doctor's help if you have any signs or symptoms of dehydration, which may include:

- Extreme thirst and dry mouth

- Urinating less than usual

- Feeling tired

- Dark-colored urine

- Decreased skin turgor, meaning that when your skin is pinched and released, the skin does not flatten back to normal right away

- Sunken eyes or cheeks

- Lightheadedness or fainting

You should seek a doctor's help if you have any signs or symptoms of malnutrition, which may include:

- Feeling tired or weak all the time

- Losing weight without trying

- Feeling dizzy

- Loss of appetite

- Abnormal paleness of the skin

What Causes Gastroparesis

In most cases, doctors aren't able to find the underlying cause of gastroparesis, even with medical tests. Gastroparesis without a known cause is called idiopathic gastroparesis. Diabetes is the most common known underlying cause of gastroparesis. Diabetes can damage nerves, such as the vagus nerve and nerves and special cells, called pacemaker cells, in the wall of the stomach. The vagus nerve controls the muscles of the stomach and small intestine. If the vagus nerve is damaged or stops working, the muscles of the stomach and small intestine do not work normally. The movement of food through the digestive tract is then slowed or stopped. Similarly, if nerves or pacemaker cells in the wall of the stomach are damaged or do not work normally, the stomach does not empty.

In addition to diabetes, other known causes of gastroparesis include:

- Injury to the vagus nerve due to surgery on your esophagus, stomach, or small intestine

- Hypothyroidism

- Certain autoimmune diseases, such as scleroderma

- Certain nervous system disorders, such as Parkinson disease (PD) and multiple sclerosis (MS)

- Viral infections of your stomach

How Do Doctors Diagnose Gastroparesis?

Doctors diagnose gastroparesis based on your medical history, a physical exam, your symptoms, and medical tests. Your doctor may also perform medical tests to look for signs of gastroparesis complications and to rule out other health problems that may be causing your symptoms.

Medical History

Your doctor will ask about your medical history. He or she will ask for details about your current symptoms and medicines, and current and past health problems such as diabetes, scleroderma, nervous system disorders, and hypothyroidism.

Your doctor may also ask about:

- the types of medicines you are taking. Be sure to tell your doctor about all prescription medicines, over-the-counter (OTC) medicines, and dietary supplements you are taking.

- whether you've had surgery on your esophagus, stomach, or small intestine

- whether you've had radiation therapy on your chest or stomach area

Physical Exam

During a physical exam, your doctor will:

- check your blood pressure, temperature, and heart rate

- check for signs of dehydration and malnutrition

- check your abdomen for unusual sounds, tenderness, or pain

What Medical Tests Do Doctors Use to Diagnose Gastroparesis?

Doctors use lab tests, upper gastrointestinal (GI) endoscopy, imaging tests, and tests to measure how fast your stomach is emptying its contents to diagnose gastroparesis.

Lab Tests

Your doctor may use the following lab tests:

- Blood tests can show signs of dehydration, malnutrition, inflammation, and infection. Blood tests can also show whether your blood glucose levels are too high or too low.

- Urine tests can show signs of diabetes, dehydration, infection, and kidney problems.

Upper Gastrointestinal (GI) Endoscopy

Your doctor may perform an upper GI endoscopy to look for problems in your upper digestive tract that may be causing your symptoms.

Imaging Tests

Imaging tests can show problems, such as stomach blockage or intestinal obstruction, that may be causing your symptoms. Your doctor may perform the following imaging tests:

- Upper GI Series

- Ultrasound of your abdomen

Tests to Measure Stomach Emptying

Your doctor may perform one or more of the following tests to see how fast your stomach is emptying its contents.

- **Gastric emptying scan, also called gastric emptying scintigraphy.** For this test, you eat a bland meal—such as eggs or an egg substitute—that contains a small amount of radioactive material. A camera outside your body scans your abdomen to show where the radioactive material is located. By tracking the radioactive material, a healthcare professional can measure how fast your stomach empties after the meal. The scan usually takes about four hours.

- **Gastric emptying breath test.** For this test, you eat a meal that contains a substance that is absorbed in your intestines and eventually passed into your breath. After you eat the meal, a healthcare professional collects samples of your breath over a period of a few hours—usually about four hours. The test can show how fast your stomach empties after the meal by measuring the amount of the substance in your breath.

- **Wireless motility capsule, also called a SmartPill.** The SmartPill is a small electronic device that you swallow. The capsule moves through your entire digestive tract and sends information to a recorder hung around your neck or clipped to your belt. A healthcare professional uses the information to find out how fast or slow your stomach empties, and how fast liquid and food move through your small intestine and large intestine. The capsule will pass naturally out of your body with a bowel movement.

How Do Doctors Treat Gastroparesis?

How doctors treat gastroparesis depends on the cause, how severe your symptoms and complications are, and how well you respond to different treatments. Sometimes, treating the cause may stop gastroparesis. If diabetes is causing your gastroparesis, your healthcare professional will work with you to help control your blood glucose levels. When the cause of your gastroparesis is not known, your doctor will provide treatments to help relieve your symptoms and treat complications.

Changing Eating Habits

Changing your eating habits can help control gastroparesis and make sure you get the right amount of nutrients, calories, and liquids. Getting the right amount of nutrients, calories, and liquids can also treat the disorder's two main complications: malnutrition and dehydration.

Your doctor may recommend that you:

- eat foods low in fat and fiber

- eat five or six small, nutritious meals a day instead of two or three large meals

- chew your food thoroughly

- eat soft, well-cooked foods

- avoid carbonated, or fizzy, beverages

- avoid alcohol

- drink plenty of water or liquids that contain glucose and electrolytes, such as:

  - low-fat broths or clear soups

  - naturally sweetened, low-fiber fruit and vegetable juices

  - sports drinks

  - oral rehydration solutions

- do some gentle physical activity after a meal, such as taking a walk

- avoid lying down for two hours after a meal

- take a multivitamin each day

If your symptoms are moderate to severe, your doctor may recommend drinking only liquids or eating well-cooked solid foods that have been processed into very small pieces or paste in a blender.

Controlling Blood Glucose Levels

If you have gastroparesis and diabetes, you will need to control your blood glucose levels, especially hyperglycemia. Hyperglycemia may further delay the emptying of food from your stomach. Your doctor will work with you to make sure your blood glucose levels are not too high or too low and don't keep going up or down. Your doctor may recommend:

- Taking insulin more often, or changing the type of insulin you take

- Taking insulin after, instead of before, meals

- Checking your blood glucose levels often after you eat, and taking insulin when you need it

Your doctor will give you specific instructions for taking insulin based on your needs and the severity of your gastroparesis.

Medicines

Your doctor may prescribe medicines that help the muscles in the wall of your stomach work better. He or she may also prescribe medicines to control nausea and vomiting and reduce pain.

Your doctor may prescribe one or more of the following medicines:

- **Metoclopramide.** This medicine increases the tightening, or contraction, of the muscles in the wall of your stomach and may improve gastric emptying. Metoclopramide may also help relieve nausea and vomiting.

- **Domperidone.** This medicine also increases the contraction of the muscles in the wall of your stomach and may improve gastric emptying. However, this medicine is available for use only under a special program administered by the U.S. Food and Drug Administration (FDA).

- **Erythromycin.** This medicine also increases stomach muscle contraction and may improve gastric emptying.

- **Antiemetics.** Antiemetics are medicines that help relieve nausea and vomiting. Prescription antiemetics include ondansetron, prochlorperazine, and promethazine. Over-the-counter (OTC) antiemetics include bismuth subsalicylate and diphenhydramine. Antiemetics do not improve gastric emptying.

- **Antidepressants.** Certain antidepressants, such as mirtazapine, may help relieve nausea and vomiting. These medicines may not improve gastric emptying.

- **Pain medicines.** Pain medicines that are not narcotic pain medicines may reduce pain in your abdomen due to gastroparesis.

Oral or Nasal Tube Feeding

In some cases, your doctor may recommend oral or nasal tube feeding to make sure you're getting the right amount of nutrients and calories. A healthcare professional will put a tube either into your mouth or nose, through your esophagus and stomach, to your small intestine. Oral and nasal tube feeding bypass your stomach and deliver a special liquid food directly into your small intestine.

Jejunostomy Tube Feeding

If you aren't getting enough nutrients and calories from other treatments, your doctor may recommend jejunostomy tube feeding. Jejunostomy feedings are a longer-term method of feeding, compared to oral or nasal tube feeding.

Jejunostomy tube feeding is a way to feed you through a tube placed into part of your small intestine called the jejunum. To place the tube into the jejunum, a doctor creates an opening, called a jejunostomy, in your abdominal wall that goes into your jejunum. The feeding tube bypasses your stomach and delivers a liquid food directly into your jejunum.

Parenteral Nutrition

Your doctor may recommend parenteral, or intravenous (IV), nutrition if your gastroparesis is so severe that other treatments are not helping. Parenteral nutrition delivers liquid nutrients directly into your bloodstream. Parenteral nutrition may be short term, until you can eat again. Parenteral nutrition may also be used until a tube can be placed for oral, nasal, or jejunostomy tube feeding. In some cases, parental nutrition may be long term.

Venting Gastrostomy

Your doctor may recommend a venting gastrostomy to relieve pressure inside your stomach. A doctor creates an opening, called a gastrostomy, in your abdominal wall and into your stomach. The doctor then places a tube through the gastrostomy into your stomach. Stomach contents can then flow out of the tube and relieve pressure inside your stomach.

Gastric Electrical Stimulation (GES)

Gastric electrical stimulation (GES) uses a small, battery-powered device to send mild electrical pulses to the nerves and muscles in the lower stomach. A surgeon puts the device under the skin in your lower abdomen and attaches wires from the device to the muscles in the wall of your stomach. GES can help decrease long-term nausea and vomiting. GES is used to treat people with gastroparesis due to diabetes or unknown causes only, and only in people whose symptoms can't be controlled with medicines.

How Can I Prevent Gastroparesis?

Gastroparesis without a known cause, called idiopathic gastroparesis, cannot be prevented. If you have diabetes, you can prevent or delay nerve damage that can cause gastroparesis by keeping your blood glucose levels within the target range that your doctor thinks is best for you. Meal planning, physical activity, and medicines, if needed, can help you keep your blood glucose levels within your target range. What you eat can help prevent or relieve your gastroparesis symptoms. If you have diabetes, following a healthy meal plan can help you manage your blood glucose levels. What you eat can also help make sure you get the right amount of nutrients, calories, and liquids if you are malnourished or dehydrated from gastroparesis.

How Can My Diet Help Prevent or Relieve Gastroparesis?

What you eat can help prevent or relieve your gastroparesis symptoms. If you have diabetes, following a healthy meal plan can help you manage your blood glucose levels. What you eat can also help make sure you get the right amount of nutrients, calories, and liquids if you are malnourished or dehydrated from gastroparesis.

What Should I Eat and Drink If I Have Gastroparesis?

If you have gastroparesis, your doctor may recommend that you eat or drink:

- Foods and beverages that are low in fat
- Foods and beverages that are low in fiber
- Five or six small, nutritious meals a day instead of two or three large meals
- Soft, well-cooked foods

If you are unable to eat solid foods, your doctor may recommend that you drink:

- Liquid nutrition meals
- Solid foods puréed in a blender

Your doctor may also recommend that you drink plenty of water or liquids that contain glucose and electrolytes, such as:

- Low-fat broths and clear soups
- Low-fiber fruit and vegetable juices
- Sports drinks
- Oral rehydration solutions

If your symptoms are moderate to severe, your doctor may recommend drinking only liquids or eating well-cooked solid foods that have been processed into very small pieces or paste in a blender.

What Should I Avoid Eating and Drinking If I Have Gastroparesis?

If you have gastroparesis, you should avoid:

- Foods and beverages that are high in fat
- Foods and beverages that are high in fiber
- Foods that can't be chewed easily
- Carbonated, or fizzy, beverages
- Alcohol

Your doctor may refer you to a dietitian to help you plan healthy meals that are easy for you to digest and give you the right amount of nutrients, calories, and liquids.

Chapter 18

Whipple Disease

What Is Whipple Disease?

Whipple disease is a rare bacterial infection that primarily affects the small intestine. The infection may spread to any organ in the body.

Left untreated, Whipple disease gets worse and is usually life-threatening.

The small intestine is part of the upper gastrointestinal (GI) tract and is a tube-shaped organ between the stomach and large intestine. The upper GI tract also includes the mouth, esophagus, stomach, and duodenum, or the first part of the small intestine. Most food digestion and nutrient absorption take place in the small intestine. The small intestine measures about 20 feet long and includes the duodenum, jejunum, and ileum. Villi—tiny, finger-like protrusions—line the inside of the small intestine. Villi normally let nutrients from food be absorbed through the walls of the small intestine into the bloodstream.

What Causes Whipple Disease

Bacteria called *Tropheryma whipplei* (*T. whipplei*) cause Whipple disease. *T. whipplei* infection can cause internal sores, also called lesions, and thickening of tissues in the small intestine. The villi take on an abnormal, clublike appearance and the damaged intestinal lining

This chapter includes text excerpted from "Whipple Disease," National Institute of Diabetes and Digestive and Kidney Diseases (NIDDK), August 2014. Reviewed September 2018.

does not properly absorb nutrients, causing diarrhea and malnutrition. Diarrhea is frequent, loose, and watery bowel movements. Malnutrition is a condition that develops when the body does not get the right amount of vitamins, minerals, and other nutrients it needs to maintain healthy tissues and organ function. Over time, the infection spreads to other parts of the person's body and will damage other organs.

Who Is More Likely to Develop Whipple Disease?

Anyone can get Whipple disease. However, it is more common in Caucasian men between 40 and 60 years old. Whipple disease is rare, and fewer than one in one million people get this disease each year. The condition appears to be more common in farmers and other people who work outdoors and have frequent contact with soil and sewage wastewater.

Experts are not sure how *T. whipplei* infects people; however, scientists have noted:

- the bacteria are found in soil and sewage wastewater

- the bacteria are also found in people who are carriers of the disease—healthy individuals who have the bacteria, yet do not get sick

- Whipple disease is not transmitted from person to person

Some people may be more likely to develop Whipple disease because of genetic factors—related to genes, or traits passed from parent to child—that influence the body's immune system. The immune system normally protects people from infection by identifying and destroying bacteria, viruses, and other potentially harmful foreign substances.

What Are the Signs and Symptoms of Whipple Disease?

Signs and symptoms of Whipple disease can vary widely from person to person. The most common symptoms of Whipple disease are:

- Diarrhea

- Weight-loss caused by malabsorption

A person may not have diarrhea. Instead, other signs and symptoms of Whipple disease may appear, such as:

- Abnormal yellow and white patches on the lining of the small intestine

- Joint pain, with or without inflammation, that may appear off and on for years before other symptoms
- Fatty or bloody stools
- Abdominal cramps or bloating felt between the chest and groin
- Enlarged lymph nodes—the small glands that make infection-fighting white blood cells (WBCs)
- Loss of appetite
- Fever
- Fatigue, or feeling tired
- Weakness
- Darkening of the skin

People with a more advanced stage of Whipple disease may have neurologic symptoms—those related to the central nervous system—such as:

- Vision problems
- Memory problems or personality changes
- Facial numbness
- Headaches
- Muscle weakness or twitching
- Difficulty walking
- Hearing loss or ringing in the ears
- Dementia—the name for a group of symptoms caused by disorders that affect the brain. People with dementia may not be able to think well enough to do normal activities such as getting dressed or eating.

Less common symptoms of Whipple disease may include:

- Chronic cough
- Chest pain
- Pericarditis—inflammation of the membrane surrounding the heart.
- Heart failure—a long-lasting condition in which the heart cannot pump enough blood to meet the body's needs. Heart failure does not mean the heart suddenly stops working.

What Are the Complications of Whipple Disease?

People with Whipple disease may have complications caused by malnutrition, which is due to damaged villi in the small intestine. As a result of delayed diagnosis or treatment, people may experience the following complications in other areas of the body:

- Long-lasting nutritional deficiencies

- Heart and heart valve damage

- Brain damage

A person with Whipple disease may experience a relapse—a return of symptoms. Relapse can happen years after treatment and requires repeat treatments.

How Is Whipple Disease Diagnosed?

A healthcare provider may use several tests and exams to diagnose Whipple disease, including the following:

- Medical and family history

- Physical exam

- Blood tests

- Upper GI endoscopy and enteroscopy

A patient may be referred to a gastroenterologist—a doctor who specializes in digestive diseases. A healthcare provider may first try to rule out more common conditions with similar symptoms, including:

- Inflammatory rheumatic disease—characterized by inflammation and loss of function in one or more connecting or supporting structures of the body

- Celiac disease—a digestive disease that damages the small intestine and interferes with the absorption of nutrients from food. People who have celiac disease cannot tolerate gluten, a protein in wheat, rye, and barley.

- Neurologic diseases—disorders of the central nervous system

- Intra-abdominal lymphoma—abdominal cancer in part of the immune system called the lymphatic system

- *Mycobacterium avium* complex (MAC)—an infection that affects people with acquired immunodeficiency syndrome (AIDS)

Medical and Family History

Taking a family and medical history can help a healthcare provider diagnose Whipple disease.

Physical Exam

A physical exam may help diagnose Whipple disease. During a physical exam, a healthcare provider usually:

- Examines a patient's body

- Uses a stethoscope to listen to sounds related to the abdomen

- Taps on specific areas of the patient's body checking for pain or tenderness

Blood Tests

A technician or nurse draws a blood sample during an office visit or at a commercial facility and sends the sample to a lab for analysis. The healthcare provider may use blood tests to check for:

- **Malabsorption.** When the damaged villi do not absorb certain nutrients from food, the body has a shortage of protein, calories, and vitamins. Blood tests can show shortages of protein, calories, and vitamins in the body.

- **Abnormal levels of electrolytes.** Electrolytes—chemicals in body fluids, including sodium, potassium, magnesium, and chloride—regulate a person's nerve and muscle function. A patient who has malabsorption or a lot of diarrhea may lose fluids and electrolytes, causing an imbalance in the body.

- **Anemia.** Anemia is a condition in which the body has fewer red blood cells (RBCs) than normal. A patient with Whipple disease does not absorb the proper nutrients to make enough red blood cells in the body, leading to anemia.

- *T. whipplei* **deoxyribonucleic acid (DNA).** Although not yet approved, rapid polymerase chain reaction diagnostic tests have been developed to detect *T. whipplei* DNA and may be useful in diagnosis.

Upper Gastrointestinal Endoscopy and Enteroscopy

An upper GI endoscopy and enteroscopy are procedures that use an endoscope—a small, flexible tube with a light—to see the upper

GI tract. A healthcare provider performs these tests at a hospital or an outpatient center. The healthcare provider carefully feeds the endoscope down the esophagus and into the stomach and duodenum.

Once the endoscope is in the duodenum, the healthcare provider will use smaller tools and a smaller scope to see more of the small intestine. These additional procedures may include:

- Push enteroscopy, which uses a long endoscope to examine the upper portion of the small intestine.

- Double-balloon enteroscopy, which uses balloons to help move the endoscope through the entire small intestine.

- Capsule enteroscopy, during which the patient swallows a capsule containing a tiny camera. As the capsule passes through the GI tract, the camera will transmit images to a video monitor. Using this procedure, the healthcare provider can examine the entire digestive tract.

A small camera mounted on the endoscope transmits a video image to a monitor, allowing close examination of the intestinal lining. A healthcare provider may give a patient a liquid anesthetic to gargle or may spray anesthetic on the back of the patient's throat. A healthcare provider will place an intravenous (IV) needle in a vein in the arm or hand to administer sedation. Sedatives help patients stay relaxed and comfortable. The test can show changes in the lining of the small intestine that can occur with Whipple disease.

The healthcare provider can use tiny tools passed through the endoscope to perform biopsies. A biopsy is a procedure that involves taking a piece of tissue for examination with a microscope. A pathologist—a doctor who specializes in examining tissues to diagnose diseases—examines the tissue from the stomach lining in a lab. The pathologist applies a special stain to the tissue and examines it for *T. whipplei*-infected cells with a microscope. Once the pathologist completes the examination of the tissue, he or she sends a report to the gastroenterologist for review.

How Is Whipple Disease Treated?

The healthcare provider prescribes antibiotics to destroy the *T. whipplei* bacteria and treat Whipple disease. Healthcare providers choose antibiotics that treat the infection in the small intestine and cross the blood–brain barrier (BBB)—a layer of tissue around the brain. Using antibiotics that cross the blood-brain barrier ensures destruction of any bacteria that may have entered the patient's brain and central nervous system.

The healthcare provider usually prescribes IV antibiotics for the first two weeks of treatment. Most patients feel relief from symptoms within the first week or two. A nurse or technician places an IV in the patient's arm to give the antibiotics. IV antibiotics used to treat Whipple disease may include:

- Ceftriaxone (Rocephin)

- Meropenem (Merrem I.V.)

- Penicillin G (Pfizerpen)

- Streptomycin (Streptomycin)

After a patient completes the IV antibiotics, the healthcare provider will prescribe long-term oral antibiotics. Patients receive long-term treatment—at least one to two years—to cure the infection anywhere in the body. Oral antibiotics may include:

- Trimethoprim with sulfamethoxazole (Septra, Bactrim)—a combination antibiotic

- Doxycycline (Vibramycin)

Patients should finish the prescribed course of antibiotics to ensure the medication destroyed all *T. whipplei* bacteria in the body. Patients who feel better may still have the bacteria in the small intestine or other areas of the body for one to two years. A healthcare provider will monitor the patient closely, repeat the blood tests, and repeat the upper GI endoscopy with biopsy during and after treatment to determine whether *T. whipplei* is still present.

People may relapse during or after treatment. A healthcare provider will prescribe additional or new antibiotics if a relapse occurs. Some people will relapse years after treatment, so it is important for patients to schedule routine follow-ups with the healthcare provider. Most patients have good outcomes with an early diagnosis and complete treatment.

Healthcare providers treat patients with neurologic symptoms at diagnosis or during relapse more aggressively. Treatment may include:

- A combination of antibiotics

- Hydroxychloroquine (Plaquenil)—an antimalarial medication

- Weekly injections of interferon gamma—a substance made by the body that activates the immune system

253

- Corticosteroids—medications that decrease inflammation

How Can Whipple Disease Be Prevented?

Experts have not yet found a way to prevent Whipple disease.

Eating, Diet, and Nutrition

A person with Whipple disease and malabsorption may need:

- A diet high in calories and protein
- Vitamins
- Nutritional supplements

People with Whipple disease should discuss their nutritional needs with a dietitian or other healthcare professional and meet regularly with him or her to monitor changing nutritional needs.

Chapter 19

Other Diseases of the Upper Gastrointestinal Tract

Chapter Contents

Section 19.1

Gastritis

This section includes text excerpted from "Gastritis,"
National Institute of Diabetes and Digestive and
Kidney Diseases (NIDDK), July 2015.

What Is Gastritis?

Gastritis is a condition in which the stomach lining—known as the mucosa—is inflamed, or swollen. The stomach lining contains glands that produce stomach acid and an enzyme called pepsin. The stomach acid breaks down food and pepsin digests protein. A thick layer of mucus coats the stomach lining and helps prevent the acidic digestive juice from dissolving the stomach tissue. When the stomach lining is inflamed, it produces less acid and fewer enzymes. However, the stomach lining also produces less mucus and other substances that normally protect the stomach lining from acidic digestive juice.

Gastritis may be acute or chronic:

- Acute gastritis starts suddenly and lasts for a short time.

- Chronic gastritis is long lasting. If chronic gastritis is not treated, it may last for years or even a lifetime.

Gastritis can be erosive or nonerosive:

- Erosive gastritis can cause the stomach lining to wear away, causing erosions—shallow breaks in the stomach lining—or ulcers—deep sores in the stomach lining.

- Nonerosive gastritis causes inflammation in the stomach lining; however, erosions or ulcers do not accompany nonerosive gastritis.

What Causes Gastritis

Common causes of gastritis include:

- *Helicobacter pylori* (*H. pylori*) infection

- Damage to the stomach lining, which leads to reactive gastritis

- An autoimmune response

H. pylori infection. *H. pylori* is a type of bacteria—organisms that may cause an infection. *H. pylori* infection:

- causes most cases of gastritis

- typically causes nonerosive gastritis

- may cause acute or chronic gastritis

H. pylori infection is common, particularly in developing countries, and the infection often begins in childhood. Many people who are infected with *H. pylori* never have any symptoms. Adults are more likely to show symptoms when symptoms do occur. Researchers are not sure how the *H. pylori* infection spreads, although they think contaminated food, water, or eating utensils may transmit the bacteria. Some infected people have *H. pylori* in their saliva, which suggests that infection can spread through direct contact with saliva or other body fluids.

Damage to the stomach lining, which leads to reactive gastritis. Some people who have damage to the stomach lining can develop reactive gastritis.

Reactive gastritis:

- may be acute or chronic

- may cause erosions

- may cause little or no inflammation

Reactive gastritis may also be called reactive gastropathy when it causes little or no inflammation.

The causes of reactive gastritis may include:

- Nonsteroidal anti-inflammatory drugs (NSAIDs), a type of over-the-counter (OTC) medication. Aspirin and ibuprofen are common types of NSAIDs.

- Drinking alcohol

- Using cocaine

- Exposure to radiation or having radiation treatments

- Reflux of bile from the small intestine into the stomach. Bile reflux may occur in people who have had part of their stomach removed.

- A reaction to stress caused by traumatic injuries, critical illness, severe burns, and major surgery. This type of reactive gastritis is called stress gastritis.

An autoimmune response. In autoimmune gastritis, the immune system attacks healthy cells in the stomach lining. The immune system normally protects people from infection by identifying and destroying bacteria, viruses, and other potentially harmful foreign substances. Autoimmune gastritis is chronic and typically nonerosive.

Less common causes of gastritis may include:

- Crohn disease, which causes inflammation and irritation of any part of the gastrointestinal (GI) tract

- Sarcoidosis, a disease that causes inflammation that will not go away. The chronic inflammation causes tiny clumps of abnormal tissue to form in various organs in the body. The disease typically starts in the lungs, skin, and lymph nodes.

- Allergies to food, such as cow's milk and soy, especially in children

- Infections with viruses, parasites, fungi, and bacteria other than *H. pylori*, typically in people with weakened immune systems

What Are the Signs and Symptoms of Gastritis?

Some people who have gastritis have pain or discomfort in the upper part of the abdomen—the area between the chest and hips. However, many people with gastritis do not have any signs and symptoms. The relationship between gastritis and a person's symptoms is not clear. The term "gastritis" is sometimes mistakenly used to describe any symptoms of pain or discomfort in the upper abdomen.

When symptoms are present, they may include:

- Upper abdominal discomfort or pain

- Nausea

- Vomiting

What Are the Complications of Chronic and Acute Gastritis?

The complications of chronic gastritis may include:

- **Peptic ulcers.** Peptic ulcers are sores involving the lining of the stomach or duodenum, the first part of the small intestine. NSAID use and *H. pylori* gastritis increase the chance of developing peptic ulcers.

- **Atrophic gastritis.** Atrophic gastritis happens when chronic inflammation of the stomach lining causes the loss of the stomach lining and glands. Chronic gastritis can progress to atrophic gastritis.

- **Anemia.** Erosive gastritis can cause chronic bleeding in the stomach, and the blood loss can lead to anemia. Anemia is a condition in which red blood cells (RBCs) are fewer or smaller than normal, which prevents the body's cells from getting enough oxygen. Red blood cells contain hemoglobin, an iron-rich protein that gives blood its red color and enables the red blood cells to transport oxygen from the lungs to the tissues of the body. Research suggests that *H. pylori* gastritis and autoimmune atrophic gastritis can interfere with the body's ability to absorb iron from food, which may also cause anemia.

- **Vitamin B$_{12}$ deficiency and pernicious anemia.** People with autoimmune atrophic gastritis do not produce enough intrinsic factor. Intrinsic factor is a protein made in the stomach and helps the intestines absorb vitamin B$_{12}$. The body needs vitamin B$_{12}$ to make red blood cells and nerve cells. Poor absorption of vitamin B$_{12}$ may lead to a type of anemia called pernicious anemia.

- **Growths in the stomach lining.** Chronic gastritis increases the chance of developing benign, or noncancerous, and malignant, or cancerous, growths in the stomach lining. Chronic *H. pylori* gastritis increases the chance of developing a type of cancer called gastric mucosa-associated lymphoid tissue (MALT) lymphoma.

In most cases, acute gastritis does not lead to complications. In rare cases, acute stress gastritis can cause severe bleeding that can be life-threatening.

How Is Gastritis Diagnosed?

A healthcare provider diagnoses gastritis based on the following:

- Medical history
- Physical exam
- Upper GI endoscopy
- Other tests

Medical History

Taking a medical history may help the healthcare provider diagnose gastritis. He or she will ask the patient to provide a medical history. The history may include questions about chronic symptoms and travel to developing countries.

Physical Exam

A physical exam may help diagnose gastritis. During a physical exam, a healthcare provider usually:

- examines a patient's body

- uses a stethoscope to listen to sounds in the abdomen

- taps on the abdomen checking for tenderness or pain

Upper Gastrointestinal (GI) Endoscopy

Upper GI endoscopy is a procedure that uses an endoscope—a small, flexible camera with a light—to see the upper GI tract. A healthcare provider performs the test at a hospital or an outpatient center. The healthcare provider carefully feeds the endoscope down the esophagus and into the stomach and duodenum. The small camera built into the endoscope transmits a video image to a monitor, allowing close examination of the GI lining. A healthcare provider may give a patient a liquid anesthetic to gargle or may spray anesthetic on the back of the patient's throat before inserting the endoscope. A healthcare provider will place an intravenous (IV) needle in a vein in the arm to administer sedation. Sedatives help patients stay relaxed and comfortable. The test may show signs of inflammation or erosions in the stomach lining.

The healthcare provider can use tiny tools passed through the endoscope to perform biopsies. A biopsy is a procedure that involves taking a piece of tissue for examination with a microscope by a pathologist—a doctor who specializes in examining tissues to diagnose diseases. A healthcare provider may use the biopsy to diagnose gastritis, find the cause of gastritis, and find out if chronic gastritis has progressed to atrophic gastritis.

Other Tests

A healthcare provider may have a patient complete other tests to identify the cause of gastritis or any complications. These tests may include the following:

- **Upper GI series.** Upper GI series is an X-ray exam that provides a look at the shape of the upper GI tract. An X-ray technician performs this test at a hospital or an outpatient center, and a radiologist—a doctor who specializes in medical imaging—interprets the images. This test does not require anesthesia. A patient should not eat or drink before the procedure, as directed by the healthcare provider. Patients should check with their healthcare provider about what to do to prepare for an upper GI series. During the procedure, the patient will stand or sit in front of an X-ray machine and drink barium, a chalky liquid. Barium coats the esophagus, stomach, and small intestine so the radiologist and healthcare provider can see these organs' shapes more clearly on X-rays. A patient may experience bloating and nausea for a short time after the test. For several days afterward, barium liquid in the GI tract may cause white or light-colored stools. A healthcare provider will give the patient specific instructions about eating and drinking after the test.

- **Blood tests.** A healthcare provider may use blood tests to check for anemia or *H. pylori*. A healthcare provider draws a blood sample during an office visit or at a commercial facility and sends the sample to a lab for analysis.

- **Stool test.** A healthcare provider may use a stool test to check for blood in the stool, another sign of bleeding in the stomach, and for *H. pylori* infection. A stool test is an analysis of a sample of stool. The healthcare provider will give the patient a container for catching and storing the stool. The patient returns the sample to the healthcare provider or a commercial facility that will send the sample to a lab for analysis.

- **Urea breath test.** A healthcare provider may use a urea breath test to check for *H. pylori* infection. The patient swallows a capsule, liquid, or pudding that contains urea—a waste product the body produces as it breaks down protein. The urea is "labeled" with a special carbon atom. If *H. pylori* are present, the bacteria will convert the urea into carbon dioxide. After a few minutes, the patient breathes into a container, exhaling carbon dioxide. A nurse or technician will perform this test at a healthcare provider's office or a commercial facility and send the samples to a lab. If the test detects the labeled carbon atoms in the exhaled breath, the healthcare provider will confirm an *H. pylori* infection in the GI tract.

How Is Gastritis Treated?

Healthcare providers treat gastritis with medications to:

- reduce the amount of acid in the stomach
- treat the underlying cause

Reduce the Amount of Acid in the Stomach

The stomach lining of a person with gastritis may have less protection from acidic digestive juice. Reducing acid can promote healing of the stomach lining. Medications that reduce acid include:

- **Antacids,** such as Alka-Seltzer, Maalox, Mylanta, Rolaids, and Riopan. Many brands use different combinations of three basic salts—magnesium, aluminum, and calcium—along with hydroxide or bicarbonate ions to neutralize stomach acid. Antacids, however, can have side effects. Magnesium salt can lead to diarrhea, and aluminum salt can cause constipation. Magnesium and aluminum salts are often combined in a single product to balance these effects. Calcium carbonate antacids, such as Tums, Titralac, and Alka-2, can cause constipation.

- **H2 blockers,** such as cimetidine (Tagamet HB), famotidine (Pepcid AC), nizatidine (Axid AR), and ranitidine (Zantac 75). H2 blockers decrease acid production. They are available in both over-the-counter (OTC) and prescription strengths.

- **Proton pump inhibitors (PPIs)** include omeprazole (Prilosec, Zegerid), lansoprazole (Prevacid), dexlansoprazole (Dexilant), pantoprazole (Protonix), rabeprazole (AcipHex), and esomeprazole (Nexium). PPIs decrease acid production more effectively than H2 blockers. All of these medications are available by prescription. Omeprazole and lansoprazole are also available in OTC strength.

Treat the Underlying Cause

Depending on the cause of gastritis, a healthcare provider may recommend additional treatments.

- Treating *H. pylori* infection with antibiotics is important, even if a person does not have symptoms from the infection. Curing the infection often cures the gastritis and decreases the chance of developing complications, such as peptic ulcer disease, MALT lymphoma, and gastric cancer.

- Avoiding the cause of reactive gastritis can provide some people with a cure. For example, if prolonged NSAID use is the cause of the gastritis, a healthcare provider may advise the patient to stop taking the NSAIDs, reduce the dose, or change pain medications.

- Healthcare providers may prescribe medications to prevent or treat stress gastritis in a patient who is critically ill or injured. Medications to protect the stomach lining include sucralfate (Carafate), H2 blockers, and PPIs. Treating the underlying illness or injury most often cures stress gastritis.

- Healthcare providers may treat people with pernicious anemia due to autoimmune atrophic gastritis with vitamin B_{12} injections.

How Can Gastritis Be Prevented?

People may be able to reduce their chances of getting gastritis by preventing *H. pylori* infection. No one knows for sure how *H. pylori* infection spreads, so prevention is difficult. To help prevent infection, healthcare providers advise people to:

- wash their hands with soap and water after using the bathroom and before eating

- eat food that has been washed well and cooked properly

- drink water from a clean, safe source

Eating, Diet, and Nutrition

Researchers have not found that eating, diet, and nutrition play a major role in causing or preventing gastritis.

Section 19.2

Ménétrier Disease

This section includes text excerpted from "Ménétrier's Disease," National Institute of Diabetes and Digestive and Kidney Diseases (NIDDK), March 2014. Reviewed September 2018.

What Is Ménétrier Disease?

Ménétrier disease causes the ridges along the inside of the stomach wall—called rugae—to enlarge, forming giant folds in the stomach lining. The rugae enlarge because of an overgrowth of mucous cells in the stomach wall. In a normal stomach, mucous cells in the rugae release protein-containing mucus. The mucous cells in enlarged rugae release too much mucus, causing proteins to leak from the blood into the stomach. This shortage of protein in the blood is known as hypoproteinemia. Ménétrier disease also reduces the number of acid-producing cells in the stomach, which decreases stomach acid. Ménétrier disease is also called hypoproteinemic hypertrophic gastropathy.

What Causes Ménétrier Disease

Scientists are unsure about what causes Ménétrier disease; however, researchers think that most people acquire, rather than inherit, the disease. In extremely rare cases, siblings have developed Ménétrier disease as children, suggesting a genetic link.

Studies suggest that people with Ménétrier disease have stomachs that make abnormally high amounts of a protein called transforming growth factor-alpha (TGF-α).

TGF-α binds to and activates a receptor called epidermal growth factor receptor. Growth factors are proteins in the body that tell cells what to do, such as grow larger, change shape, or divide to make more cells. Researchers have not yet found a cause for the overproduction of TGF-α.

Some studies have found cases of people with Ménétrier disease who also had *Helicobacter pylori* (*H. pylori*) infection. *H. pylori* is a bacterium that is a cause of peptic ulcers, or sores on the lining of the stomach or the duodenum, the first part of the small intestine. In these cases, treatment for *H. pylori* reversed and improved the symptoms of Ménétrier disease.

Researchers have linked some cases of Ménétrier disease in children to infection with cytomegalovirus (CMV). CMV is one of the herpes viruses. This group of viruses includes the herpes simplex viruses, which cause chickenpox, shingles, and infectious mononucleosis, also known as mono. Most healthy children and adults infected with CMV have no symptoms and may not even know they have an infection. However, in people with a weakened immune system, CMV can cause serious disease, such as retinitis, which can lead to blindness. Researchers are not sure how *H. pylori* and CMV infections contribute to the development of Ménétrier disease.

Who Gets Ménétrier Disease?

Ménétrier disease is rare. The disease is more common in men than in women. The average age at diagnosis is 55.

What Are the Signs and Symptoms of Ménétrier Disease?

The most common symptom of Ménétrier disease is pain in the upper middle part of the abdomen. The abdomen is the area between the chest and hips.

Other signs and symptoms of Ménétrier disease may include:

- Nausea and frequent vomiting

- Diarrhea

- Loss of appetite

- Extreme weight loss

- Malnutrition

- Low levels of protein in the blood

- Swelling of the face, abdomen, limbs, and feet due to low levels of protein in the blood

- Anemia—too few red blood cells in the body, which prevents the body from getting enough oxygen—due to bleeding in the stomach

People with Ménétrier disease have a higher chance of developing stomach cancer, also called gastric cancer.

How Is Ménétrier Disease Diagnosed?

Healthcare providers base the diagnosis of Ménétrier disease on a combination of symptoms, lab findings, findings on upper gastrointestinal (GI) endoscopy, and stomach biopsy results. A healthcare provider will begin the diagnosis of Ménétrier disease by taking a patient's medical and family history and performing a physical exam. However, a healthcare provider will confirm the diagnosis of Ménétrier disease through a computerized tomography (CT) scan, an upper GI endoscopy, and a biopsy of stomach tissue. A healthcare provider also may order blood tests to check for infection with *H. pylori* or CMV.

Medical and family history. Taking a medical and family history is one of the first things a healthcare provider may do to help diagnose Ménétrier disease. He or she will ask the patient to provide a medical and family history.

Physical exam. A physical exam may help diagnose Ménétrier disease. During a physical exam, a healthcare provider usually:

- examines a patient's body

- uses a stethoscope to listen to bodily sounds

- taps on specific areas of the patient's body

Computed tomography (CT) scan. CT scans use a combination of X-rays and computer technology to create images. For a CT scan, a healthcare provider may give the patient a solution to drink and an injection of a special dye, called contrast medium. CT scans require the patient to lie on a table that slides into a tunnel-shaped device where an X-ray technician takes X-rays. An X-ray technician performs the procedure in an outpatient center or a hospital, and a radiologist—a doctor who specializes in medical imaging—interprets them. The patient does not need anesthesia. CT scans can show enlarged folds in the stomach wall.

Upper gastrointestinal (GI) endoscopy. This procedure involves using an endoscope—a small, flexible tube with a light—to see the upper GI tract, which includes the esophagus, stomach, and duodenum. A gastroenterologist—a doctor who specializes in digestive diseases—performs the test at a hospital or an outpatient center. The gastroenterologist carefully feeds the endoscope down the esophagus and into the stomach. A small camera mounted on the endoscope transmits a video image to a monitor, allowing close examination of the stomach lining. The gastroenterologist also can take a biopsy of the stomach tissue during the endoscopy. A healthcare provider may give a patient a liquid anesthetic to gargle or may spray anesthetic on the back of the patient's throat. A healthcare provider will place an intravenous (IV) needle in a vein in the arm to administer sedation. Sedatives help patients stay relaxed and comfortable. The test can show enlarged folds in the stomach wall.

Biopsy. Biopsy is a procedure that involves taking a piece of stomach tissue for examination with a microscope. A gastroenterologist performs the biopsy at the time of upper GI endoscopy. A pathologist—a doctor who specializes in diagnosing diseases—examines the stomach tissue in a lab. The test can diagnose Ménétrier disease by showing changes in the stomach's mucous cells and acid-producing cells.

Blood test. A healthcare provider will take a blood sample that can show the presence of infection with *H. pylori* or CMV. A blood test involves drawing blood at a healthcare provider's office or a commercial facility and sending the sample to a lab for analysis.

How Is Ménétrier Disease Treated?

Treatment may include medications, IV protein, blood transfusions, and surgery.

Medications

Healthcare providers may prescribe the anticancer medication cetuximab (Erbitux) to treat Ménétrier disease. Studies have shown that cetuximab blocks the activity of epidermal growth factor receptor and can significantly improve a person's symptoms, as well as decrease the thickness of the stomach wall from the overgrowth of mucous cells. A person receives cetuximab by IV in a healthcare provider's office or an outpatient center. Studies to assess the effectiveness of cetuximab to treat Ménétrier disease are ongoing. A healthcare provider also may prescribe medications to relieve nausea and abdominal pain.

In people with Ménétrier disease who also have *H. pylori* or CMV infection, treatment of the infection may improve symptoms. Healthcare providers prescribe antibiotics to kill *H. pylori*. Antibiotic regimens may differ throughout the world because some strains of *H. pylori* have become resistant to certain antibiotics—meaning that an antibiotic that once destroyed the bacterium is no longer effective. Healthcare providers use antiviral medications to treat CMV infection in a person with a weakened immune system in order to prevent a serious disease from developing as a result of CMV. Antiviral medications cannot kill CMV; however, they can slow down the virus reproduction.

Intravenous Protein and Blood Transfusions

A healthcare provider may recommend an IV treatment of protein and a blood transfusion to a person who is malnourished or anemic because of Ménétrier disease. In most cases of children with Ménétrier disease who also have had CMV infection, treatment with protein and a blood transfusion led to a full recovery.

Surgery

If a person has severe Ménétrier disease with significant protein loss, a surgeon may need to remove part or all of the stomach in a surgery called gastrectomy.

Surgeons perform gastrectomy in a hospital. The patient will require general anesthesia. Some surgeons perform a gastrectomy through laparoscopic surgery rather than through a wide incision in the abdomen. In laparoscopic surgery, the surgeon uses several smaller incisions and feeds special surgical tools through the incisions to remove the diseased part of the stomach. After gastrectomy, the surgeon may reconstruct the changed portions of the GI tract so that it may continue to function. Usually, the surgeon attaches the small intestine to any remaining portion of the stomach or to the esophagus if he or she removed the entire stomach.

Eating, Diet, and Nutrition

Researchers have not found that eating, diet, and nutrition play a role in causing or preventing Ménétrier disease. In some cases, a healthcare provider may prescribe a high-protein diet to offset the loss of protein due to Ménétrier disease. Some people with severe malnutrition may require IV nutrition, which is called total parenteral nutrition (TPN). TPN is a method of providing an IV liquid food mixture through a special tube in the chest.

Section 19.3

Dumping Syndrome (Rapid Gastric Emptying)

This section includes text excerpted from "Dumping Syndrome," National Institute of Diabetes and Digestive and Kidney Diseases (NIDDK), September 2013. Reviewed September 2018.

What Is Dumping Syndrome?

Dumping syndrome occurs when food, especially sugar, moves too fast from the stomach to the duodenum—the first part of the small intestine—in the upper gastrointestinal (GI) tract. This condition is also called rapid gastric emptying. Dumping syndrome has two forms, based on when symptoms occur:

* Early dumping syndrome—occurs 10–30 minutes after a meal

* Late dumping syndrome—occurs two to three hours after a meal

What Is the Gastrointestinal Tract (GI) Tract?

The GI tract is a series of hollow organs joined in a long, twisting tube from the mouth to the anus—the opening where stool leaves the body. The body digests food using the movement of muscles in the GI tract, along with the release of hormones and enzymes. The upper GI tract includes the mouth, esophagus, stomach, duodenum, and small intestine. The esophagus carries food and liquids from the mouth to the stomach. The stomach slowly pumps the food and liquids into the intestine, which then absorbs needed nutrients. Two digestive organs, the liver and the pancreas, produce digestive juices that reach the small intestine through small tubes called ducts.

The last part of the GI tract—called the lower GI tract—consists of the large intestine and anus. The large intestine is about five feet long in adults and absorbs water and any remaining nutrients from partially digested food passed from the small intestine. The large intestine then changes waste from liquid to a solid matter called stool. Stool passes from the colon to the rectum. The rectum is located between the last part of the colon—called the sigmoid colon—and the anus. The rectum stores stool prior to a bowel movement. During a bowel movement, stool moves from the rectum to the anus.

What Causes Dumping Syndrome

Dumping syndrome is caused by problems with the storage of food particles in the stomach and emptying of particles into the duodenum. Early dumping syndrome results from rapid movement of fluid into the intestine following a sudden addition of a large amount of food from the stomach. Late dumping syndrome results from rapid movement of sugar into the intestine, which raises the body's blood glucose level and causes the pancreas to increase its release of the hormone insulin. The increased release of insulin causes a rapid drop in blood glucose levels, a condition known as hypoglycemia, or low blood sugar.

Who Is More Likely to Develop Dumping Syndrome?

People who have had surgery to remove or bypass a significant part of the stomach are more likely to develop dumping syndrome. Some types of gastric surgery, such as bariatric surgery, reduce the size of the stomach. As a result, dietary nutrients pass quickly into the small intestine. Other conditions that impair how the stomach stores and empties itself of food, such as nerve damage caused by esophageal surgery, can also cause dumping syndrome.

What Are the Symptoms of Dumping Syndrome?

The symptoms of early and late dumping syndrome are different and vary from person to person. Early dumping syndrome symptoms may include:

- Nausea
- Vomiting
- Abdominal pain and cramping
- Diarrhea
- Feeling uncomfortably full or bloated after a meal
- Sweating
- Weakness
- Dizziness
- Flushing, or blushing of the face or skin
- Rapid or irregular heartbeat

The symptoms of late dumping syndrome may include:

- Hypoglycemia
- Sweating
- Weakness
- Rapid or irregular heartbeat
- Flushing
- Dizziness

About 75 percent of people with dumping syndrome report symptoms of early dumping syndrome and about 25 percent report symptoms of late dumping syndrome. Some people have symptoms of both types of dumping syndrome.

How Is Dumping Syndrome Diagnosed?

A healthcare provider will diagnose dumping syndrome primarily on the basis of symptoms. A scoring system helps differentiate dumping syndrome from other GI problems. The scoring system assigns points to each symptom and the total points result in a score. A person with a score above seven likely has dumping syndrome.

The following tests may confirm dumping syndrome and exclude other conditions with similar symptoms:

- A modified oral glucose tolerance test checks how well insulin works with tissues to absorb glucose. A healthcare provider performs the test during an office visit or in a commercial facility and sends the blood samples to a lab for analysis. The person should fast—eat or drink nothing except water—for at least eight hours before the test. The healthcare provider will measure blood glucose concentration, hematocrit—the amount of red blood cells in the blood—pulse rate, and blood pressure before the test begins. After the initial measurements, the person drinks a glucose solution. The healthcare provider repeats the initial measurements immediately and at 30-minute intervals for up to 180 minutes. A healthcare provider often confirms dumping syndrome in people with:

  - low blood sugar between 120 and 180 minutes after drinking the solution

  - an increase in hematocrit of more than three percent at 30 minutes

- a rise in pulse rate of more than 10 beats per minute after 30 minutes

- A gastric emptying scintigraphy test involves eating a bland meal—such as eggs or an egg substitute—that contains a small amount of radioactive material. A specially trained technician performs this test in a radiology center or hospital, and a radiologist—a doctor who specializes in medical imaging— interprets the results. Anesthesia is not needed. An external camera scans the abdomen to locate the radioactive material. The radiologist measures the rate of gastric emptying at one, two, three, and four hours after the meal. The test can help confirm a diagnosis of dumping syndrome.

The healthcare provider may also examine the structure of the esophagus, stomach, and upper small intestine with the following tests:

- An upper GI endoscopy involves using an endoscope—a small, flexible tube with a light—to see the upper GI tract. A gastroenterologist—a doctor who specializes in digestive diseases—performs the test at a hospital or an outpatient center. The gastroenterologist carefully feeds the endoscope down the esophagus and into the stomach and duodenum. A small camera mounted on the endoscope transmits a video image to a monitor, allowing close examination of the intestinal lining. A person may receive general anesthesia or a liquid anesthetic that is gargled or sprayed on the back of the throat. If the person receives general anesthesia, a healthcare provider will place an intravenous (IV) needle in a vein in the arm. The test may show ulcers, swelling of the stomach lining, or cancer.

- An upper GI series examines the small intestine. An X-ray technician performs the test at a hospital or an outpatient center and a radiologist interprets the images. Anesthesia is not needed. No eating or drinking is allowed before the procedure, as directed by the healthcare staff. During the procedure, the person will stand or sit in front of an X-ray machine and drink barium, a chalky liquid. Barium coats the small intestine, making signs of a blockage or other complications of gastric surgery show up more clearly on X-rays.

A person may experience bloating and nausea for a short time after the test. For several days afterward, barium liquid in the GI tract causes white or light-colored stools. A healthcare provider will give the person specific instructions about eating and drinking after the test.

How Is Dumping Syndrome Treated?

Treatment for dumping syndrome includes changes in eating, diet, and nutrition; medication; and, in some cases, surgery. Many people with dumping syndrome have mild symptoms that improve over time with simple dietary changes.

Eating, Diet, and Nutrition

The first step to minimizing symptoms of dumping syndrome involves changes in eating, diet, and nutrition, and may include:

- Eating five or six small meals a day instead of three larger meals

- Delaying liquid intake until at least 30 minutes after a meal

- Increasing intake of protein, fiber, and complex carbohydrates— found in starchy foods such as oatmeal and rice

- Avoiding simple sugars such as table sugar, which can be found in candy, syrup, sodas, and juice beverages

- Increasing the thickness of food by adding pectin or guar gum— plant extracts used as thickening agents

Some people find that lying down for 30 minutes after meals also helps reduce symptoms.

Medication

A healthcare provider may prescribe octreotide acetate (Sandostatin) to treat dumping syndrome symptoms. The medication works by slowing gastric emptying and inhibiting the release of insulin and other GI hormones. Octreotide comes in short- and long-acting formulas. The short-acting formula is injected subcutaneously—under the skin—or intravenously—into a vein—two to four times a day. A healthcare provider may perform the injections or may train the patient or patient's friend or relative to perform the injections. A healthcare provider injects the long-acting formula into the buttocks muscles once every four weeks. Complications of octreotide treatment include increased or decreased blood glucose levels, pain at the injection site, gallstones, and fatty, foul-smelling stools.

Surgery

A person may need surgery if dumping syndrome is caused by previous gastric surgery or if the condition is not responsive to other treatments. For most people, the type of surgery depends on the type of gastric surgery performed previously. However, surgery to correct dumping syndrome often has unsuccessful results.

Section 19.4

Zollinger-Ellison Syndrome

This section includes text excerpted from "Zollinger-Ellison Syndrome," National Institute of Diabetes and Digestive and Kidney Diseases (NIDDK), December 2013. Reviewed September 2018.

What Is Zollinger-Ellison Syndrome?

Zollinger-Ellison syndrome (ZES) is a rare disorder that occurs when one or more tumors form in the pancreas and duodenum. The tumors, called gastrinomas, release large amounts of gastrin that cause the stomach to produce large amounts of acid. Normally, the body releases small amounts of gastrin after eating, which triggers the stomach to make gastric acid that helps break down food and liquid in the stomach. The extra acid causes peptic ulcers to form in the duodenum and elsewhere in the upper intestine. The tumors seen with Zollinger-Ellison syndrome are sometimes cancerous and may spread to other areas of the body.

What Are the Stomach, Duodenum, and Pancreas?

The stomach, duodenum, and pancreas are digestive organs that break down food and liquid.

- The stomach stores swallowed food and liquid. The muscle action of the lower part of the stomach mixes the food and liquid with digestive juice. Partially digested food and liquid slowly move into the duodenum and are further broken down.

- The duodenum is the first part of the small intestine—the tube-shaped organ between the stomach and the large intestine—where digestion of the food and liquid continues.

- The pancreas is an organ that makes the hormone insulin and enzymes for digestion. A hormone is a natural chemical produced in one part of the body and released into the blood to trigger or regulate particular functions of the body. Insulin helps cells throughout the body remove glucose, also called sugar, from blood and use it for energy. The pancreas is located behind the stomach and close to the duodenum.

What Causes Zollinger-Ellison Syndrome

Experts do not know the exact cause of Zollinger-Ellison syndrome. About 25–30 percent of gastrinomas are caused by an inherited genetic disorder called multiple endocrine neoplasia type 1 (MEN1). MEN1 causes hormone-releasing tumors in the endocrine glands and the duodenum. Symptoms of MEN1 include increased hormone levels in the blood, kidney stones, diabetes, muscle weakness, weakened bones, and fractures.

How Common Is Zollinger-Ellison Syndrome?

Zollinger-Ellison syndrome is rare and only occurs in about one in every one million people. Although anyone can get Zollinger-Ellison syndrome, the disease is more common among men 30–50 years old. A child who has a parent with MEN1 is also at increased risk for Zollinger-Ellison syndrome.

What Are the Signs and Symptoms of Zollinger-Ellison Syndrome?

Zollinger-Ellison syndrome signs and symptoms are similar to those of peptic ulcers. A dull or burning pain felt anywhere between the navel and midchest is the most common symptom of a peptic ulcer. This discomfort usually:

- occurs when the stomach is empty—between meals or during the night—and may be briefly relieved by eating food

- lasts for minutes to hours

- comes and goes for several days, weeks, or months

Other symptoms include:

- Diarrhea
- Bloating
- Burping
- Nausea
- Vomiting
- Weight loss
- Poor appetite

Some people with Zollinger-Ellison syndrome have only diarrhea, with no other symptoms. Others develop gastroesophageal reflux (GER), which occurs when stomach contents flow back up into the esophagus—a muscular tube that carries food and liquids to the stomach. In addition to nausea and vomiting, reflux symptoms include a painful, burning feeling in the midchest.

Seek Help for Emergency Symptoms

A person who has any of the following emergency symptoms should call or see a healthcare provider right away:

- Chest pain
- Sharp, sudden, persistent, and severe stomach pain
- Red blood in stool or black stools
- Red blood in vomit or vomit that looks like coffee grounds

These symptoms could be signs of a serious problem, such as:

- Internal bleeding—when gastric acid or a peptic ulcer breaks a blood vessel
- Perforation—when a peptic ulcer forms a hole in the duodenal wall
- Obstruction—when a peptic ulcer blocks the path of food trying to leave the stomach

How Is Zollinger-Ellison Syndrome Diagnosed?

A healthcare provider diagnoses Zollinger-Ellison syndrome based on the following:

- Medical history
- Physical exam
- Signs and symptoms
- Blood tests
- Upper gastrointestinal (GI) endoscopy
- Imaging tests to look for gastrinomas
- Measurement of stomach acid

Medical History

Taking a medical and family history is one of the first things a healthcare provider may do to help diagnose Zollinger-Ellison syndrome. The healthcare provider may ask about family cases of MEN1 in particular.

Physical Exam

A physical exam may help diagnose Zollinger-Ellison syndrome. During a physical exam, a healthcare provider usually:

- examines a person's body
- uses a stethoscope to listen to bodily sounds
- taps on specific areas of the person's body

Signs and Symptoms

A healthcare provider may suspect Zollinger-Ellison syndrome if:

- diarrhea accompanies peptic ulcer symptoms or if peptic ulcer treatment fails
- a person has peptic ulcers without the use of nonsteroidal anti-inflammatory drugs (NSAIDs) such as aspirin and ibuprofen or a bacterial *Helicobacter pylori* (*H. pylori*) infection. NSAID use and *H. pylori* infection may cause peptic ulcers.
- a person has severe ulcers that bleed or cause holes in the duodenum or stomach
- a healthcare provider diagnoses a person or the person's family member with MEN1 or a person has symptoms of MEN1

Blood Tests

The healthcare provider may use blood tests to check for an elevated gastrin level. A technician or nurse draws a blood sample during an office visit or at a commercial facility and sends the sample to a lab for analysis. A healthcare provider will ask the person to fast for several hours prior to the test and may ask the person to stop acid-reducing medications for a period of time before the test. A gastrin level that is 10 times higher than normal suggests Zollinger-Ellison syndrome.

A healthcare provider may also check for an elevated gastrin level after an infusion of secretin. Secretin is a hormone that causes gastrinomas to release more gastrin. A technician or nurse places an intravenous (IV) needle in a vein in the arm to give an infusion of secretin. A healthcare provider may suspect Zollinger-Ellison syndrome if blood drawn after the infusion shows an elevated gastrin level.

Upper Gastrointestinal (GI) Endoscopy

The healthcare provider uses an upper GI endoscopy to check the esophagus, stomach, and duodenum for ulcers and esophagitis—a general term used to describe irritation and swelling of the esophagus. This procedure involves using an endoscope—a small, flexible tube with a light—to see the upper GI tract, which includes the esophagus, stomach, and duodenum. A gastroenterologist—a doctor who specializes in digestive diseases—performs the test at a hospital or an outpatient center. The gastroenterologist carefully feeds the endoscope down the esophagus and into the stomach and duodenum. A small camera mounted on the endoscope transmits a video image to a monitor, allowing close examination of the intestinal lining. A person may receive a liquid anesthetic that is gargled or sprayed on the back of the throat. A technician or nurse inserts an IV needle in a vein in the arm if anesthesia is given.

Imaging Tests

To help find gastrinomas, a healthcare provider may order one or more of the following imaging tests:

- **Computerized tomography (CT) scan.** CT scans require the person to lie on a table that slides into a tunnel-shaped device where an X-ray technician takes X-rays. A computer puts the different views together to create a model of the pancreas, stomach, and duodenum. The X-ray technician performs the procedure in an outpatient center or a hospital, and a radiologist—a doctor who specializes in medical imaging— interprets the images. The person does not need anesthesia. CT scans can show tumors and ulcers.

- **Magnetic resonance imaging (MRI).** During an MRI, the person, although usually awake, remains perfectly still while the technician takes the images, which usually takes only a few minutes. The technician will take a sequence of images from different angles to create a detailed picture of the upper GI tract. During sequencing, the person will hear loud mechanical knocking and humming noises.

- **Endoscopic ultrasound.** The gastroenterologist carefully feeds the endo-echoscope down the esophagus, through the stomach and duodenum, until it is near the pancreas. A person may receive a liquid anesthetic that is gargled or sprayed on the back of the throat. A sedative helps the person stay relaxed and comfortable. The images can show gastrinomas in the pancreas.

- **Angiogram.** An angiogram is a special kind of X-ray in which an interventional radiologist—a specially trained radiologist— threads a thin, flexible tube called a catheter through the large arteries, often from the groin, to the artery of interest. The radiologist injects contrast medium through the catheter so the images show up more clearly on the X-ray. The interventional radiologist performs the procedure and interprets the images in a hospital or an outpatient center. A person does not need anesthesia, though a light sedative may help reduce a person's anxiety during the procedure. This test can show gastrinomas in the pancreas.

- **Somatostatin receptor scintigraphy.** An X-ray technician performs this test, also called OctreoScan, at a hospital or an outpatient center, and a radiologist interprets the images. A person does not need anesthesia. A radioactive compound called a radiotracer, when injected into the bloodstream, selectively labels tumor cells. The labeled cells light up when scanned with a device called a gamma camera. The test can show gastrinomas in the duodenum, pancreas, and other parts of the body.

Small gastrinomas may be hard to see; therefore, healthcare providers may order several types of imaging tests to find gastrinomas.

279

Stomach-Acid Measurement

Using a sample of stomach juices for analysis, a healthcare provider may measure the amount of stomach acid a person produces. During the exam, a healthcare provider puts in a nasogastric tube—a tiny tube inserted through the nose and throat that reaches into the stomach. A person may receive a liquid anesthetic that is gargled or sprayed on the back of the throat. Once the tube is placed, a healthcare provider takes samples of the stomach acid. High acid levels in the stomach indicate Zollinger-Ellison syndrome.

How Is Zollinger-Ellison Syndrome Treated?

A healthcare provider treats Zollinger-Ellison syndrome with medications to reduce gastric acid secretion and with surgery to remove gastrinomas. A healthcare provider sometimes uses chemotherapy—medications to shrink tumors—when tumors are too widespread to remove with surgery.

Medications

A class of medications called proton pump inhibitors (PPIs) includes:

- Esomeprazole (Nexium)
- Lansoprazole (Prevacid)
- Pantoprazole (Protonix)
- Omeprazole (Prilosec or Zegerid)
- Dexlansoprazole (Dexilant)

PPIs stop the mechanism that pumps acid into the stomach, helping to relieve peptic ulcer pain and promote healing. A healthcare provider may prescribe people who have Zollinger-Ellison syndrome higher-than-normal doses of PPIs to control the acid production. Studies show that PPIs may increase the risk of hip, wrist, and spine fractures when a person takes them long term or in high doses, so it's important for people to discuss risks versus benefits with their healthcare provider.

Surgery

Surgical removal of gastrinomas is the only cure for Zollinger-Ellison syndrome. Some gastrinomas spread to other parts of the body, especially the liver and bones. Finding and removing all gastrinomas before they spread is often challenging because many of the tumors are small.

Chemotherapy

Healthcare providers sometimes use chemotherapy drugs to treat gastrinomas that cannot be surgically removed, including:

- Streptozotocin (Zanosar)
- 5-fluorouracil (Adrucil)
- Doxorubicin (Doxil)

Eating, Diet, and Nutrition

Researchers have not found that eating, diet, and nutrition play a role in causing or preventing Zollinger-Ellison syndrome.

Part Four

Disorders of the Lower Gastrointestinal Tract

Chapter 20

Irritable Bowel Syndrome (IBS)

What Is Irritable Bowel Syndrome (IBS)?

Irritable bowel syndrome (IBS) is a group of symptoms that occur together, including repeated pain in your abdomen and changes in your bowel movements, which may be diarrhea, constipation, or both. With IBS, you have these symptoms without any visible signs of damage or disease in your digestive tract. IBS is a functional gastrointestinal (GI) disorder. Functional GI disorders, which doctors now call disorders of gut–brain interactions, are related to problems with how your brain and your gut work together. These problems can cause your gut to be more sensitive and change how the muscles in your bowel contract. If your gut is more sensitive, you may feel more abdominal pain and bloating. Changes in how the muscles in your bowel contract lead to diarrhea, constipation, or both. In the past, doctors called IBS colitis, mucous colitis, spastic colon, nervous colon, and spastic bowel.

Are There Different Types of IBS?

Three types of IBS are based on different patterns of changes in your bowel movements or abnormal bowel movements. Sometimes, it

---

This chapter includes text excerpted from "Irritable Bowel Syndrome (IBS)," National Institute of Diabetes and Digestive and Kidney Diseases (NIDDK), November 2017.

is important for your doctor to know which type of IBS you have. Some medicines work only for some types of IBS or make other types worse. Your doctor might diagnose IBS even if your bowel movement pattern does not fit one particular type. Many people with IBS have normal bowel movements on some days and abnormal bowel movements on other days.

IBS with Constipation (IBS-C)

With IBS-C, on days when you have at least one abnormal bowel movement

- more than a quarter of your stools are hard or lumpy and
- less than a quarter of your stools are loose or watery

IBS with Diarrhea (IBS-D)

In IBS-D, on days when you have at least one abnormal bowel movement

- more than a quarter of your stools are loose or watery and
- less than a quarter of your stools are hard or lumpy

IBS with Mixed Bowel Habits (IBS-M)

In IBS-M, on days when you have at least one abnormal bowel movement

- more than a quarter of your stools are hard or lumpy and
- more than a quarter of your stools are loose or watery

How Common Is IBS?

Studies suggest that about 12 percent of people in the United States have IBS.

Who Is More Likely to Develop IBS?

Women are up to two times more likely than men to develop IBS. People younger than age 50 are more likely to develop IBS than people older than age 50.

Factors that can increase your chance of having IBS include:

- Having a family member with IBS

- A history of stressful or difficult life events, such as abuse in childhood

- Having a severe infection in your digestive tract

What Other Health Problems Do People with IBS Have?

People with IBS often have other health problems, including:

- Certain conditions that involve chronic pain, such as fibromyalgia, chronic fatigue syndrome, and chronic pelvic pain

- Certain digestive diseases, such as dyspepsia and gastroesophageal reflux disease (GERD)

- Certain mental disorders, such as anxiety, depression, and somatic symptom disorder

What Are the Symptoms of IBS?

The most common symptoms of irritable bowel syndrome (IBS) are pain in your abdomen, often related to your bowel movements, and changes in your bowel movements. These changes may be diarrhea, constipation, or both, depending on what type of IBS you have.

Other symptoms of IBS may include:

- Bloating

- The feeling that you haven't finished a bowel movement

- Whitish mucus in your stool

Women with IBS often have more symptoms during their periods. IBS can be painful but doesn't lead to other health problems or damage your digestive tract.

To diagnose IBS, your doctor will look for a certain pattern in your symptoms over time. IBS is a chronic disorder, meaning it lasts a long time, often years. However, the symptoms may come and go.

What Causes IBS

Doctors aren't sure what causes IBS. Experts think that a combination of problems may lead to IBS. Different factors may cause IBS in different people. Functional gastrointestinal (GI) disorders such as IBS are problems with brain–gut interaction—how your brain and gut work together. Experts think that problems with brain–gut interaction may affect how your body works and cause IBS symptoms. For example, in some people with IBS, food may move too slowly or too quickly through the digestive tract, causing changes in bowel movements. Some people with IBS may feel pain when a normal amount of gas or stool is in the gut.

Certain problems are more common in people with IBS. Experts think these problems may play a role in causing IBS. These problems include:

- Stressful or difficult early life events, such as physical or sexual abuse

- Certain mental disorders, such as depression, anxiety, and somatic symptom disorder

- Bacterial infections in your digestive tract

- Small intestinal bacterial overgrowth, an increase in the number or a change in the type of bacteria in your small intestine

- Food intolerances or sensitivities, in which certain foods cause digestive symptoms

Research suggests that genes may make some people more likely to develop IBS.

How Do Doctors Diagnose IBS?

To diagnose IBS, doctors review your symptoms and medical and family history and perform a physical exam. In some cases, doctors may order tests to rule out other health problems.

Review of Your Symptoms

Your doctor will ask about your symptoms and look for a certain pattern in your symptoms to diagnose IBS. Your doctor may diagnose IBS if you have pain in your abdomen along with two or more of the following symptoms:

- Your pain is related to your bowel movements. For example, your pain may improve or get worse after bowel movements.

- You notice a change in how often you have a bowel movement.

- You notice a change in the way your stools look.

Your doctor will ask how long you've had symptoms. Your doctor may diagnose IBS if:

- You've had symptoms at least once a week in the last three months and

- Your symptoms first started at least six months ago

Your doctor may diagnose IBS even if you've had symptoms for a shorter length of time. You should talk to your doctor if your symptoms are like the symptoms of IBS.

Your doctor will also ask about other symptoms. Certain symptoms may suggest that you have another health problem instead of IBS. These symptoms include:

- Anemia

- Bleeding from your rectum

- Bloody stools or stools that are black and tarry

- Weight loss

Medical and Family History

Your doctor will ask about:

- A family history of digestive diseases, such as celiac disease, colon cancer, or inflammatory bowel disease (IBD)

- Medicines you take

- Recent infections

- Stressful events related to the start of your symptoms

- What you eat

- Your history of other health problems that are more common in people who have IBS

Physical Exam

During a physical exam, your doctor usually:

- Checks for abdominal bloating

- Listens to sounds within your abdomen using a stethoscope

- Taps on your abdomen checking for tenderness or pain

What Tests Do Doctors Use to Diagnose IBS?

In most cases, doctors don't use tests to diagnose IBS. Your doctor may order blood tests, stool tests, and other tests to check for other health problems.

Blood Test

A healthcare professional will take a blood sample from you and send the sample to a lab. Doctors use blood tests to check for conditions other than IBS, including anemia, infection, and digestive diseases.

Stool Test

Your doctor will give you a container for catching and holding a stool sample. You will receive instructions on where to send or take the kit for testing. Doctors use stool tests to check for blood in your stool or other signs of infections or diseases. Your doctor may also check for blood in your stool by examining your rectum during your physical exam.

Other Tests

Doctors may perform other tests to rule out health problems that cause symptoms similar to IBS symptoms. Your doctor will decide whether you need other tests based on:

- Blood or stool test results
- Whether you have a family history of digestive diseases, such as celiac disease, colon cancer, or IBD
- Whether you have symptoms that could be signs of another condition or disease

Other tests may include:

- Hydrogen breath test to check for small intestinal bacterial overgrowth or problems digesting certain carbohydrates, such as lactose intolerance
- Upper GI endoscopy with a biopsy to check for celiac disease
- Colonoscopy to check for conditions such as colon cancer or IBD

How Do Doctors Treat IBS?

Doctors may treat IBS by recommending changes in what you eat and other lifestyle changes, medicines, probiotics, and mental health therapies. You may have to try a few treatments to see what works best for you. Your doctor can help you find the right treatment plan.

Changes to What You Eat and Other Lifestyle Changes

Changes in what you eat may help treat your symptoms. Your doctor may recommend trying one of the following changes:

- Eat more fiber

- Avoid gluten

- Follow a special eating plan called the low FODMAP diet

Research suggests that other lifestyle changes may help IBS symptoms, including:

- Increasing your physical activity

- Reducing stressful life situations as much as possible

- Getting enough sleep

Medicines

Your doctor may recommend medicine to relieve your IBS symptoms. To treat IBS with diarrhea, your doctor may recommend:

- Loperamide

- Rifaximin (Xifaxan), an antibiotic

- Eluxadoline (Viberzi)

- Alosetron (Lotronex), which is prescribed only to women and is prescribed with special warnings and precautions

To treat IBS with constipation, your doctor may recommend:

- Fiber supplements, when increasing fiber in your diet doesn't help

- Laxatives

- Lubiprostone (Amitiza)

- Linaclotide (Linzess)

- Plecanatide (Trulance)

Other medicines may help treat pain in your abdomen, including:

- Antispasmodics

- Antidepressants, such as low doses of tricyclic antidepressants and selective serotonin reuptake inhibitors

- Coated peppermint oil capsules

Follow your doctor's instructions when you use medicine to treat IBS. Talk with your doctor about possible side effects and what to do if you have them.

Probiotics

Your doctor may also recommend probiotics. Probiotics are live microorganisms, most often bacteria, that are similar to microorganisms you normally have in your digestive tract. Researchers are still studying the use of probiotics to treat IBS.

To be safe, talk with your doctor before using probiotics or any other complementary or alternative medicines or practices. If your doctor recommends probiotics, talk with him or her about how much probiotics you should take and for how long.

Mental Health Therapies

Your doctor may recommend mental health therapies to help improve your IBS symptoms. Therapies used to treat IBS include:

- **Cognitive behavioral therapy (CBT)**, which focuses on helping you change thought and behavior patterns to improve IBS symptoms

- **Gut-directed hypnotherapy**, in which a therapist uses hypnosis—a trance-like state in which you are relaxed or focused—to help improve your IBS symptoms

- **Relaxation training**, which can help you relax your muscles or reduce stress

How Can My Diet Help Treat the Symptoms of IBS?

Your doctor may recommend changes in your diet to help treat symptoms of irritable bowel syndrome (IBS). Your doctor may suggest that you:

- Eat more fiber

- Avoid gluten

- Follow a special diet called the low FODMAP diet

Different changes may help different people with IBS. You may need to change what you eat for several weeks to see if your symptoms improve. Your doctor may also recommend talking with a dietitian.

Eat More Fiber

Fiber may improve constipation in IBS because it makes stool soft and easier to pass. The *2015–2020 Dietary Guidelines for Americans* recommends that adults should get 22–34 grams of fiber a day.

Two types of fiber are:

- Soluble fiber, which is found in beans, fruit, and oat products

- Insoluble fiber, which is found in whole-grain products and vegetables

Research suggests that soluble fiber is more helpful in relieving IBS symptoms.

To help your body get used to more fiber, add foods with fiber to your diet a little at a time. Too much fiber at once can cause gas, which can trigger IBS symptoms. Adding fiber to your diet slowly, by two to three grams a day, may help prevent gas and bloating.

Avoid Gluten

Your doctor may recommend avoiding foods that contain gluten—a protein found in wheat, barley, and rye—to see if your IBS symptoms improve. Foods that contain gluten include most cereal, grains, and pasta, and many processed foods. Some people with IBS have more symptoms after eating gluten, even though they do not have celiac disease.

Low FODMAP Diet

Your doctor may recommend that you try a special diet—called the low FODMAP diet—to reduce or avoid certain foods that contain carbohydrates that are hard to digest. These carbohydrates are called FODMAPs.

Examples of foods that contain FODMAPs include:

- Fruits such as apples, apricots, blackberries, cherries, mango, nectarines, pears, plums, and watermelon, or juice containing any of these fruits

- Canned fruit in natural fruit juice, or large amounts of fruit juice or dried fruit

- Vegetables such as artichokes, asparagus, beans, cabbage, cauliflower, garlic and garlic salts, lentils, mushrooms, onions, and sugar snap or snow peas

- Dairy products such as milk, milk products, soft cheeses, yogurt, custard, and ice cream

- Wheat and rye products

- Honey and foods with high-fructose corn syrup

- Products, including candy and gum, with sweeteners ending in "–ol," such as sorbitol, mannitol, xylitol, and maltitol

Your doctor may suggest that you try the low FODMAP diet for a few weeks to see if it helps with your symptoms. If your symptoms improve, your doctor may recommend slowly adding foods that contain FODMAPs back into your diet. You may be able to eat some foods with FODMAPs without having IBS symptoms.

Chapter 21

Inflammatory Bowel Disease

Chapter Contents

Section 21.1

Inflammatory Bowel Disease (IBD): An Overview

This section includes text excerpted from "Inflammatory Bowel Disease (IBD): What Is It?" Centers for Disease Control and Prevention (CDC), May 18, 2018.

The number of U.S. adults who have been diagnosed with inflammatory bowel disease (IBD) has increased greatly since 1999—from two to three million. However, these estimates do not include people younger than 18 who may also have the disease.

What Is Inflammatory Bowel Disease (IBD)?

IBD which is characterized by chronic inflammation of the gastrointestinal (GI) tract includes Crohn disease and ulcerative colitis (UC). The GI tract extends from the mouth to the anus and includes the organs that digest food, absorb nutrients, and process wastes. Long-term inflammation results in damage to the GI tract.

What Are the Symptoms of IBD?

Some common symptoms are:

- Persistent diarrhea
- Abdominal pain
- Rectal bleeding or bloody stools
- Weight loss
- Fatigue

Some of the differences between Crohn disease and ulcerative colitis:

Crohn Disease

Can affect any part of the GI tract (from the mouth to the anus). Most often it affects the portion of the small intestine before the large intestine/colon.

Damaged areas appear in patches that are next to areas of healthy tissue.

Inflammation may reach through the multiple layers of the walls of the GI tract.

Ulcerative Colitis (UC)

- Occurs in the large intestine (colon) and the rectum.

- Damaged areas are continuous (not patchy)—usually starting at the rectum and spreading further into the colon.

- Inflammation is present only in the innermost layer of the lining of the colon.

IBD Is Not Irritable Bowel Syndrome (IBS)

IBD should not be confused with irritable bowel syndrome or IBS. Although people with IBS may have symptoms similar to IBD, IBD and IBS are very different. IBS is not caused by inflammation and does not damage the bowel. Treatment is also different.

IBD Is Not Celiac Disease

Celiac disease is another condition with similar symptoms to IBD. However, the cause of celiac disease is known and is very specific. It is an inflammatory response to gluten, a group of proteins found in wheat and similar grains. The symptoms of celiac disease will go away after starting a gluten-free diet, usually after a few months.

How Common Is IBD in the United States?

In 2015 and 2016, about three million U.S. adults (1.3%) reported being diagnosed with IBD (either Crohn disease or ulcerative colitis). This was a large increase from 1999 (two million, or 0.9% adults reported IBD).

Some groups were more likely to report IBD, including those:

- Aged 45 or older

- Women

- Non-Hispanic white

- With less than a high school level of education

- Divorced, separated, or widowed

- Not currently employed

- Born in the United States

- Living in poverty

- Living in suburban areas

This estimate does not include children younger than 18 years, who may also have IBD. Most people with IBD are diagnosed in their 20s and 30s.

What Causes IBD

We do not yet know the exact cause of IBD, but it is the result of an improper immune response. A normal immune system attacks foreign organisms, such as viruses and bacteria, to protect the body. In IBD, the immune system responds incorrectly to environmental triggers such as smoking, viruses, or bacteria, which may cause inflammation of the GI tract. There also seems to be a genetic component—someone with a family history of IBD is more likely to develop this inappropriate immune response.

How Is IBD Diagnosed?

IBD is diagnosed using a combination of endoscopy and colonoscopy (both of which let your doctor see inside your body by inserting an instrument with a very small camera), radiologic imaging (such as X-rays, computed tomography (CT) scans, or magnetic resonance imaging (MRIs), and blood or stool tests.

How Is IBD Treated?

Several types of medicines may be used to treat IBD. Some vaccinations are also recommended for patients with IBD to prevent infections. For some patients, surgery may be required to remove damaged portions of the GI tract, but advances in treatment with medicines mean that surgery is less common than it was a few decades ago. Since Crohn disease and ulcerative colitis affect different parts of the GI tract, the surgical procedures are different for the two conditions.

Section 21.2

Understanding Crohn Disease

This section includes text excerpted from "Crohn's Disease," National Institute of Diabetes and Digestive and Kidney Diseases (NIDDK), September 2017.

What Is Crohn Disease?

Crohn disease is a chronic disease that causes inflammation and irritation in your digestive tract. Most commonly, Crohn affects your small intestine and the beginning of your large intestine. However, the disease can affect any part of your digestive tract, from your mouth to your anus. Crohn disease is an inflammatory bowel disease (IBD). Ulcerative colitis (UC) and microscopic colitis are other common types of IBD. Crohn disease most often begins gradually and can become worse over time. You may have periods of remission that can last for weeks or years.

How Common Is Crohn Disease?

Researchers estimate that more than half a million people in the United States have Crohn disease. Studies show that, over time, Crohn disease has become more common in the United States and other parts of the world. Experts do not know the reason for this increase.

Who Is More Likely to Develop Crohn Disease?

Crohn disease can develop in people of any age and is more likely to develop in people:

- Between the ages of 20 and 29
- Who has a family member, most often a sibling or parent, with IBD
- Who smoke cigarettes

What Are the Complications of Crohn Disease?

Complications of Crohn disease can include the following:

- Intestinal obstruction
- Fistulas

- Abscesses
- Anal fissures
- Ulcers
- Malnutrition
- Inflammation in other areas of your body

What Other Health Problems Do People with Crohn Disease Have?

If you have Crohn disease in your large intestine, you may be more likely to develop colon cancer. If you receive ongoing treatment for Crohn disease and stay in remission, you may reduce your chances of developing colon cancer. Talk with your doctor about how often you should get screened for colon cancer. Screening is testing for diseases when you have no symptoms. Screening for colon cancer can include colonoscopy with biopsies. Although screening does not reduce your chances of developing colon cancer, it may help to find cancer at an early stage and improve the chance of curing the cancer.

What Are the Symptoms of Crohn Disease?

The most common symptoms of Crohn disease are:

- Diarrhea
- Cramping and pain in your abdomen
- Weight loss

Other symptoms include:

- Anemia
- Eye redness or pain
- Feeling tired
- Fever
- Joint pain or soreness
- Nausea or loss of appetite
- Skin changes that involve red, tender bumps under the skin

Your symptoms may vary depending on the location and severity of your inflammation. Some research suggests that stress, including the stress of living with Crohn disease, can make symptoms worse. Also, some people may find that certain foods can trigger or worsen their symptoms.

What Causes Crohn Disease

Doctors aren't sure what causes Crohn disease. Experts think the following factors may play a role in causing Crohn disease.

Autoimmune Reaction

One cause of Crohn disease may be an autoimmune reaction—when your immune system attacks healthy cells in your body. Experts think bacteria in your digestive tract can mistakenly trigger your immune system. This immune system response causes inflammation, leading to symptoms of Crohn disease.

Genes

Crohn disease sometimes runs in families. Research has shown that if you have a parent or sibling with Crohn disease, you may be more likely to develop the disease. Experts continue to study the link between genes and Crohn disease.

Other Factors

Some studies suggest that other factors may increase your chance of developing Crohn disease:

- Smoking may double your chance of developing Crohn disease.
- Nonsteroidal anti-inflammatory drugs (NSAIDs) such as aspirin or ibuprofen, antibiotics, and birth-control pills may slightly increase the chance of developing Crohn disease.
- A high-fat diet may also slightly increase your chance of getting Crohn disease.

Stress and eating certain foods do not cause Crohn disease.

How Do Doctors Diagnose Crohn Disease?

Doctors typically use a combination of tests to diagnose Crohn disease. Your doctor will also ask you about your medical history—including medicines you are taking—and your family history and will perform a physical exam.

Physical Exam

During a physical exam, a doctor most often:

- Checks for bloating in your abdomen
- Listens to sounds within your abdomen using a stethoscope
- Taps on your abdomen to check for tenderness and pain and to see if your liver or spleen is abnormal or enlarged

Diagnostic Tests

Your doctor may use the following tests to help diagnose Crohn disease:

- Lab tests
- Intestinal endoscopy
- Upper gastrointestinal (GI) series
- Computed tomography (CT) scan

Your doctor may also perform tests to rule out other diseases, such as ulcerative colitis, diverticular disease, or cancer, that cause symptoms similar to those of Crohn disease.

What Tests Do Doctors Use to Diagnose Crohn Disease?

Your doctor may perform the following tests to help diagnose Crohn disease.

Lab Tests

Lab tests to help diagnose Crohn disease include:

- Blood tests
- Stool tests

Intestinal Endoscopy

Intestinal endoscopies are the most accurate methods for diagnosing Crohn disease and ruling out other possible conditions, such as ulcerative colitis, diverticular disease, or cancer. Intestinal endoscopies include the following:

- Colonoscopy

- Upper GI endoscopy and enteroscopy

- Capsule endoscopy

Upper GI Series

An upper GI series is a procedure in which a doctor uses X-rays, fluoroscopy, and a chalky liquid called barium to view your upper GI tract.

CT Scan

A CT scan uses a combination of X-rays and computer technology to create images of your digestive tract. For a CT scan, a healthcare professional may give you a solution to drink and an injection of a special dye, called contrast medium. Contrast medium makes the structures inside your body easier to see during the procedure. You'll lie on a table that slides into a tunnel-shaped device that takes the X-rays. CT scans can diagnose both Crohn disease and the complications of the disease.

How Do Doctors Treat Crohn Disease?

Doctors treat Crohn disease with medicines, bowel rest, and surgery. No single treatment works for everyone with Crohn disease. The goals of treatment are to decrease the inflammation in your intestines, to prevent flare-ups of your symptoms, and to keep you in remission.

Medicines

Many people with Crohn disease need medicines. Which medicines your doctor prescribes will depend on your symptoms. Although no medicine cures Crohn disease, many can reduce symptoms.

- Aminosalicylates

- Corticosteroids

- Immunomodulators

- Biologic therapies

Other medicines doctors prescribe for symptoms or complications may include:

- Acetaminophen for mild pain. You should avoid using ibuprofen, naproxen, and aspirin because these medicines can make your symptoms worse.

- Antibiotics to prevent or treat complications that involve infection, such as abscesses and fistulas.

- Loperamide to help slow or stop severe diarrhea. In most cases, people only take this medicine for short periods of time because it can increase the chance of developing megacolon.

Bowel Rest

If your Crohn disease symptoms are severe, you may need to rest your bowel for a few days to several weeks. Bowel rest involves drinking only certain liquids or not eating or drinking anything. During bowel rest, your doctor may:

- Ask you to drink a liquid that contains nutrients

- Give you a liquid that contains nutrients through a feeding tube inserted into your stomach or small intestine

- Give you intravenous (IV) nutrition through a special tube inserted into a vein in your arm

You may stay in the hospital, or you may be able to receive the treatment at home. In most cases, your intestines will heal during bowel rest.

Surgery

Even with medicines, many people will need surgery to treat their Crohn disease. One study found that nearly 60 percent of people had surgery within 20 years of having Crohn disease. Although surgery will not cure Crohn disease, it can treat complications and improve symptoms. Doctors most often recommend surgery to treat:

- Fistulas

- Bleeding that is life threatening

- Intestinal obstructions

- Side effects from medicines when they threaten your health

- Symptoms when medicines do not improve your condition

A surgeon can perform different types of operations to treat Crohn disease.

For any surgery, you will receive general anesthesia. You will most likely stay in the hospital for three to seven days following the surgery. Full recovery may take four to six weeks.

Small bowel resection. Small bowel resection is surgery to remove part of your small intestine. When you have an intestinal obstruction or severe Crohn disease in your small intestine, a surgeon may need to remove that section of your intestine. The two types of small bowel resection are:

- **Laparoscopic**—when a surgeon makes several small, half-inch incisions in your abdomen. The surgeon inserts a laparoscope—a thin tube with a tiny light and video camera on the end— through the small incisions. The camera sends a magnified image from inside your body to a video monitor, giving the surgeon a close-up view of your small intestine. While watching the monitor, the surgeon inserts tools through the small incisions and removes the diseased or blocked section of small intestine. The surgeon will reconnect the ends of your intestine.

- **Open surgery**—when a surgeon makes one incision about six inches long in your abdomen. The surgeon will locate the diseased or blocked section of small intestine and remove or repair that section. The surgeon will reconnect the ends of your intestine.

Subtotal colectomy. A subtotal colectomy, also called a large bowel resection, is surgery to remove part of your large intestine. When you have an intestinal obstruction, a fistula, or severe Crohn disease in your large intestine, a surgeon may need to remove that section of intestine. A surgeon can perform a subtotal colectomy by:

- **Laparoscopic colectomy**—when a surgeon makes several small, half-inch incisions in your abdomen. While watching the monitor, the surgeon removes the diseased or blocked section of your large intestine. The surgeon will reconnect the ends of your intestine.

- **Open surgery**—when a surgeon makes one incision about six to eight inches long in your abdomen. The surgeon will locate the diseased or blocked section of large intestine and remove that section. The surgeon will reconnect the ends of your intestine.

Proctocolectomy and ileostomy. A proctocolectomy is a surgery to remove your entire colon and rectum. An ileostomy is a stoma, or opening in your abdomen, that a surgeon creates from a part of your ileum. The surgeon brings the end of your ileum through an opening in your abdomen and attaches it to your skin, creating an opening outside your body. The stoma is about three-quarters of an inch to a little less than two inches wide and is most often located in the lower part of your abdomen, just below the beltline.

A removable external collection pouch, called an ostomy pouch or ostomy appliance, connects to the stoma and collects stool outside your body. Stool passes through the stoma instead of passing through your anus. The stoma has no muscle, so it cannot control the flow of stool, and the flow occurs whenever occurs.

If you have this type of surgery, you will have the ileostomy for the rest of your life.

How Do Doctors Treat the Complications of Crohn Disease?

Your doctor may recommend treatments for the following complications of Crohn disease:

- Intestinal obstruction

- Fistulas

- Abscesses

- Anal fissures

- Ulcers

- Malnutrition

- Inflammation in other areas of your body

How Can My Diet Help the Symptoms of Crohn Disease?

Changing your diet can help reduce symptoms. Your doctor may recommend that you make changes to your diet such as:

- Avoiding carbonated, or "fizzy," drinks

- Avoiding popcorn, vegetable skins, nuts, and other high-fiber foods

- Drinking more liquids

- Eating smaller meals more often

- Keeping a food diary to help identify foods that cause problems

Depending on your symptoms or medicines, your doctor may recommend a specific diet, such as a diet that is:

- High calorie

- Lactose free

- Low fat

- Low fiber

- Low salt

Talk with your doctor about specific dietary recommendations and changes. Your doctor may recommend nutritional supplements and vitamins if you do not absorb enough nutrients. For safety reasons, talk with your doctor before using dietary supplements, such as vitamins, or any complementary or alternative medicines or medical practices.

Section 21.3

Understanding Ulcerative Colitis

This section includes text excerpted from "Ulcerative Colitis,"
National Institute of Diabetes and Digestive and Kidney Diseases
(NIDDK), September 2014. Reviewed September 2018.

What Is Ulcerative Colitis?

Ulcerative colitis (UC) is a chronic, or long lasting, disease that causes inflammation—irritation or swelling—and sores called ulcers on the inner lining of the large intestine.

Ulcerative colitis is a chronic inflammatory disease of the gastrointestinal (GI) tract, called inflammatory bowel disease (IBD). Crohn disease and microscopic colitis are the other common IBDs.

Ulcerative colitis most often begins gradually and can become worse over time. Symptoms can be mild to severe. Most people have periods of remission—times when symptoms disappear—that can last for weeks or years. The goal of care is to keep people in remission long term. Most people with ulcerative colitis receive care from a gastroenterologist, a doctor who specializes in digestive diseases.

What Is the Large Intestine?

The large intestine is part of the GI tract, a series of hollow organs joined in a long, twisting tube from the mouth to the anus—an opening through which stool leaves the body. The last part of the GI tract, called the lower GI tract, consists of the large intestine—which includes the appendix, cecum, colon, and rectum—and anus. The intestines are sometimes called the bowel.

The large intestine is about five feet long in adults and absorbs water and any remaining nutrients from partially digested food passed from the small intestine. The large intestine changes waste from liquid to a solid matter called stool. Stool passes from the colon to the rectum. The rectum is located between the lower, or sigmoid, colon, and the anus. The rectum stores stool prior to a bowel movement, when stool moves from the rectum to the anus and out of a person's body.

What Causes Ulcerative Colitis

The exact cause of ulcerative colitis is unknown. Researchers believe the following factors may play a role in causing ulcerative colitis:

- Overactive intestinal immune system

- Genes

- Environment

Overactive intestinal immune system. Scientists believe one cause of ulcerative colitis may be an abnormal immune reaction in the intestine. Normally, the immune system protects the body from infection by identifying and destroying bacteria, viruses, and other potentially harmful foreign substances. Researchers believe bacteria or viruses can mistakenly trigger the immune system to attack the inner lining of the large intestine. This immune system response causes the inflammation, leading to symptoms.

Genes. Ulcerative colitis sometimes runs in families. Research studies have shown that certain abnormal genes may appear in people with ulcerative colitis. However, researchers have not been able to show a clear link between the abnormal genes and ulcerative colitis.

Environment. Some studies suggest that certain things in the environment may increase the chance of a person getting ulcerative colitis, although the overall chance is low. Nonsteroidal anti-inflammatory drugs, antibiotics, and oral contraceptives may slightly increase the chance of developing ulcerative colitis. A high-fat diet may also slightly increase the chance of getting ulcerative colitis.

Some people believe eating certain foods, stress, or emotional distress can cause ulcerative colitis. Emotional distress does not seem to cause ulcerative colitis. A few studies suggest that stress may increase a person's chance of having a flare-up of ulcerative colitis. Also, some people may find that certain foods can trigger or worsen symptoms.

Who Is More Likely to Develop Ulcerative Colitis?

Ulcerative colitis can occur in people of any age. However, it is more likely to develop in people:

- Between the ages of 15 and 30

- Older than 60

- Who has a family member with IBD

- Of Jewish descent

What Are the Signs and Symptoms of Ulcerative Colitis?

The most common signs and symptoms of ulcerative colitis are diarrhea with blood or pus and abdominal discomfort. Other signs and symptoms include:

- An urgent need to have a bowel movement

- Feeling tired

- Nausea or loss of appetite

- Weight loss

- Fever

- Anemia—a condition in which the body has fewer red blood cells than normal

Less common symptoms include:

- Joint pain or soreness

- Rye irritation
- Certain rashes

The symptoms a person experiences can vary depending on the severity of the inflammation and where it occurs in the intestine. When symptoms first appear,

- Most people with ulcerative colitis have mild to moderate symptoms
- About 10 percent of people can have severe symptoms, such as frequent, bloody bowel movements; fevers; and severe abdominal cramping

How Is Ulcerative Colitis Diagnosed?

A healthcare provider diagnoses ulcerative colitis with the following:

- Medical and family history
- Physical exam
- Lab tests
- Endoscopies of the large intestine

The healthcare provider may perform a series of medical tests to rule out other bowel disorders, such as irritable bowel syndrome (IBS), Crohn disease, or celiac disease, that may cause symptoms similar to those of ulcerative colitis.

Medical and Family History

Taking a medical and family history can help the healthcare provider diagnose ulcerative colitis and understand a patient's symptoms. The healthcare provider will also ask the patient about current and past medical conditions and medications.

Physical Exam

A physical exam may help diagnose ulcerative colitis. During a physical exam, the healthcare provider most often:

- Checks for abdominal distension, or swelling
- Listens to sounds within the abdomen using a stethoscope
- Taps on the abdomen to check for tenderness and pain

Lab Tests

A healthcare provider may order lab tests to help diagnose ulcerative colitis, including blood and stool tests.

Blood tests. A blood test involves drawing blood at a healthcare provider's office or a lab. A lab technologist will analyze the blood sample. A healthcare provider may use blood tests to look for:

- Anemia

- Inflammation or infection somewhere in the body

- Markers that show ongoing inflammation

- Low albumin, or protein—common in patients with severe ulcerative colitis

Stool tests. A stool test is the analysis of a sample of stool. A healthcare provider will give the patient a container for catching and storing the stool at home. The patient returns the sample to the healthcare provider or to a lab. A lab technologist will analyze the stool sample. healthcare providers commonly order stool tests to rule out other causes of GI diseases, such as infection.

Endoscopies of the Large Intestine

Endoscopies of the large intestine are the most accurate methods for diagnosing ulcerative colitis and ruling out other possible conditions, such as Crohn disease, diverticular disease, or cancer. Endoscopies of the large intestine include:

- Colonoscopy

- Flexible sigmoidoscopy

How Is Ulcerative Colitis Treated?

A healthcare provider treats ulcerative colitis with:

- Medications

- Surgery

Which treatment a person needs depends on the severity of the disease and the symptoms. Each person experiences ulcerative colitis differently, so healthcare providers adjust treatments to improve the person's symptoms and induce, or bring about, remission.

Medications

While no medication cures ulcerative colitis, many can reduce symptoms. The goals of medication therapy are:

- Inducing and maintaining remission

- Improving the person's quality of life (QOL)

Many people with ulcerative colitis require medication therapy indefinitely, unless they have their colon and rectum surgically removed.

Healthcare providers will prescribe the medications that best treat a person's symptoms:

- Aminosalicylates

- Corticosteroids

- Immunomodulators

- Biologics, also called anti-tumor necrosis factor (anti-TNF) therapies

- Other medications

Depending on the location of the symptoms in the colon, healthcare providers may recommend a person take medications by:

- Enema, which involves flushing liquid medication into the rectum using a special wash bottle. The medication directly treats inflammation of the large intestine.

- Rectal foam—a foamy substance the person puts into the rectum like an enema. The medication directly treats inflammation of the large intestine.

- Suppository—a solid medication the person inserts into the rectum to dissolve. The intestinal lining absorbs the medication.

- Mouth

- Intravenous (IV)

Surgery

Some people will need surgery to treat their ulcerative colitis when they have:

- Colon cancer

- Dysplasia, or precancerous cells in the colon

- Complications that are life threatening, such as megacolon or bleeding

- No improvement in symptoms or condition despite treatment

- Continued dependency on steroids

- Side effects from medications that threaten their health

Removal of the entire colon, including the rectum, "cures" ulcerative colitis. A surgeon performs the procedure at a hospital. A surgeon can perform two different types of surgery to remove a patient's colon and treat ulcerative colitis:

- Proctocolectomy and ileostomy

- Proctocolectomy and ileoanal reservoir

- Full recovery from both operations may take four to six weeks.

- **Proctocolectomy and ileostomy.** A proctocolectomy is a surgery to remove a patient's entire colon and rectum. An ileostomy is a stoma, or opening in the abdomen, that a surgeon creates from a part of the ileum—the last section of the small intestine. The surgeon brings the end of the ileum through an opening in the patient's abdomen and attaches it to the skin, creating an opening outside of the patient's body. The stoma most often is located in the lower part of the patient's abdomen, just below the beltline.

- A removable external collection pouch, called an ostomy pouch or ostomy appliance, connects to the stoma and collects intestinal contents outside the patient's body. Intestinal contents pass through the stoma instead of passing through the anus. The stoma has no muscle, so it cannot control the flow of intestinal contents, and the flow occurs whenever peristalsis occurs. Peristalsis is the movement of the organ walls that propels food and liquid through the GI tract.

- People who have this type of surgery will have the ileostomy for the rest of their lives.

- **Proctocolectomy and ileoanal reservoir.** An ileoanal reservoir is an internal pouch made from the patient's ileum. This surgery is a common alternative to an ileostomy and does

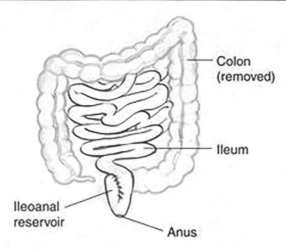

Figure 21.1. *Ileostomy*

not have a permanent stoma. Ileoanal reservoir is also known as a J-pouch, a pelvic pouch, or an ileoanal pouch anastamosis. The ileoanal reservoir connects the ileum to the anus. The surgeon preserves the outer muscles of the patient's rectum during the proctocolectomy. Next, the surgeon creates the ileal pouch and attaches it to the end of the rectum. Waste is stored in the pouch and passes through the anus.

- After surgery, bowel movements may be more frequent and watery than before the procedure. People may have fecal incontinence—the accidental passing of solid or liquid stool or mucus from the rectum. Medications can be used to control pouch function. Women may be infertile following the surgery.

- Many people develop pouchitis in the ileoanal reservoir. Pouchitis is an irritation or inflammation of the lining of the ileoanal reservoir. A healthcare provider treats pouchitis with antibiotics. Rarely, pouchitis can become chronic and require long-term antibiotics or other medications.

- The surgeon will recommend one of the operations based on a person's symptoms, severity of disease, expectations, age, and lifestyle. Before making a decision, the person should get as much information as possible by talking with:

- Healthcare providers

- Enterostomal therapists, nurses who work with colon-surgery patients

- People who have had one of the surgeries

Patient-advocacy organizations can provide information about support groups and other resources.

Eating, Diet, and Nutrition

Researchers have not found that eating, diet, and nutrition play a role in causing ulcerative colitis symptoms. Good nutrition is important in the management of ulcerative colitis, however. Dietary changes can help reduce symptoms. A healthcare provider may recommend dietary changes such as:

- Avoiding carbonated drinks

- Avoiding popcorn, vegetable skins, nuts, and other high-fiber foods while a person has symptoms

- Drinking more liquids

- Eating smaller meals more often

- Keeping a food diary to help identify troublesome foods

Healthcare providers may recommend nutritional supplements and vitamins for people who do not absorb enough nutrients.

To help ensure coordinated and safe care, people should discuss their use of complementary and alternative medical practices, including their use of dietary supplements and probiotics, with their healthcare provider.

Depending on a person's symptoms or medications, a healthcare provider may recommend a specific diet, such as:

- High-calorie diet

- Lactose-free diet

- Low-fat diet

- Low-fiber diet

- Low-salt diet

People should speak with a healthcare provider about specific dietary recommendations and changes.

What Are the Complications of Ulcerative Colitis?

Complications of ulcerative colitis can include:

- Rectal bleeding

- Dehydration and malabsorption

- Changes in bones

Healthcare providers will monitor people for bone loss and can recommend calcium and vitamin D supplements and medications to help prevent or slow bone loss.

- **Inflammation in other areas of the body.** The immune system can trigger inflammation in the:

  - Joints

  - Eyes

  - Skin

  - Liver

  Healthcare providers can treat inflammation by adjusting medications or prescribing new medications.

- **Megacolon**—a serious complication that occurs when inflammation spreads to the deep tissue layers of the large intestine. The large intestine swells and stops working. Megacolon can be a life-threatening complication and most often requires surgery. Megacolon is a rare complication of ulcerative colitis.

Section 21.4

Microscopic Colitis

This section includes text excerpted from "Microscopic Colitis," National Institute of Diabetes and Digestive and Kidney Diseases (NIDDK), June 2014. Reviewed September 2018.

What Is Microscopic Colitis?

Microscopic colitis is an inflammation of the colon that a healthcare provider can see only with a microscope. Inflammation is the body's normal response to injury, irritation, or infection of tissues. Microscopic colitis is a type of inflammatory bowel disease—the general name for diseases that cause irritation and inflammation in the intestines.

The two types of microscopic colitis are collagenous colitis and lymphocytic colitis. Healthcare providers often use the term microscopic colitis to describe both types because their symptoms and treatments are the same. Some scientists believe that collagenous colitis and lymphocytic colitis may be different phases of the same condition rather than separate conditions.

In both types of microscopic colitis, an increase in the number of lymphocytes, a type of white blood cell (WBC), can be seen in the epithelium—the layer of cells that lines the colon. An increase in the number of white blood cells is a sign of inflammation. The two types of colitis affect the colon tissue in slightly different ways:

- **Lymphocytic colitis.** The number of lymphocytes is higher, and the tissues and lining of the colon are of normal thickness.

- **Collagenous colitis.** The layer of collagen, a threadlike protein, underneath the epithelium builds up and becomes thicker than normal.

When looking through a microscope, the healthcare provider may find variations in lymphocyte numbers and collagen thickness in different parts of the colon. These variations may indicate an overlap of the two types of microscopic colitis.

What Is the Colon?

The colon is part of the gastrointestinal (GI) tract, a series of hollow organs joined in a long, twisting tube from the mouth to the anus—a one-inch-long opening through which stool leaves the body. Organs that make up the GI tract are the:

- Mouth
- Esophagus
- Stomach
- Small intestine
- Large intestine
- Anus

The first part of the GI tract, called the upper GI tract, includes the mouth, esophagus, stomach, and small intestine. The last part of the GI tract, called the lower GI tract, consists of the large intestine and anus. The intestines are sometimes called the bowel.

The large intestine is about five feet long in adults and includes the colon and rectum. The large intestine changes waste from liquid to a solid matter called stool. Stool passes from the colon to the rectum. The rectum is six to eight inches long in adults and is between the last part of the colon—called the sigmoid colon—and the anus. During a bowel movement, stool moves from the rectum to the anus and out of the body.

What Causes Microscopic Colitis

The exact cause of microscopic colitis is unknown. Several factors may play a role in causing microscopic colitis. However, most scientists believe that microscopic colitis results from an abnormal immune-system response to bacteria that normally live in the colon. Scientists have proposed other causes, including:

- Autoimmune diseases
- Medications
- Infections
- Genetic factors
- Bile acid malabsorption

Who Is More Likely to Get Microscopic Colitis?

People are more likely to get microscopic colitis if they:

- Are 50 years of age or older

- Are female
- Have an autoimmune disease
- Smoke cigarettes, especially people ages 16–44
- Use medications that have been linked to the disease

What Are the Signs and Symptoms of Microscopic Colitis?

The most common symptom of microscopic colitis is chronic, watery, nonbloody diarrhea. Episodes of diarrhea can last for weeks, months, or even years. However, many people with microscopic colitis may have long periods without diarrhea. Other signs and symptoms of microscopic colitis can include:

- A strong urge to have a bowel movement or a need to go to the bathroom quickly
- Pain, cramping, or bloating in the abdomen—the area between the chest and the hips—that is usually mild
- Weight loss
- Fecal incontinence—accidental passing of stool or fluid from the rectum—especially at night
- Nausea
- Dehydration—a condition that results from not taking in enough liquids to replace fluids lost through diarrhea

The symptoms of microscopic colitis can come and go frequently. Sometimes, the symptoms go away without treatment.

How Is Microscopic Colitis Diagnosed?

A pathologist—a doctor who specializes in examining tissues to diagnose diseases—diagnoses microscopic colitis based on the findings of multiple biopsies taken throughout the colon. Biopsy is a procedure that involves taking small pieces of tissue for examination with a microscope. The pathologist examines the colon tissue samples in a lab. Many patients can have both lymphocytic colitis and collagenous colitis in different parts of their colon. To help diagnose microscopic colitis, a gastroenterologist—a doctor who specializes in digestive diseases—begins with:

- A medical and family history
- A physical exam

The gastroenterologist may perform a series of medical tests to rule out other bowel diseases—such as irritable bowel syndrome, celiac disease, Crohn disease, ulcerative colitis, and infectious colitis—that cause symptoms similar to those of microscopic colitis. These medical tests include:

- Lab tests

- Imaging tests of the intestines

- Endoscopy of the intestines

Medical and Family History

The gastroenterologist will ask the patient to provide a medical and family history, a review of the symptoms, a description of eating habits, and a list of prescription and over-the-counter (OTC) medications in order to help diagnose microscopic colitis. The gastroenterologist will also ask the patient about current and past medical conditions.

Physical Exam

A physical exam may help diagnose microscopic colitis and rule out other diseases. During a physical exam, the gastroenterologist usually:

- Examines the patient's body

- Taps on specific areas of the patient's abdomen

Lab Tests

Lab tests may include:

- Blood tests

- Stool tests

Imaging Tests of the Intestines

Imaging tests of the intestines may include the following:

- Computerized tomography (CT) scan

- Magnetic resonance imaging (MRI)

- Upper GI series

Specially trained technicians perform these tests at an outpatient center or a hospital, and a radiologist—a doctor who specializes in medical imaging—interprets the images. A patient does not need anesthesia. Healthcare providers use imaging tests to show physical abnormalities and to diagnose certain bowel diseases, in some cases.

Endoscopy of the Intestines

Endoscopy of the intestines may include:

- Colonoscopy with biopsy
- Flexible sigmoidoscopy with biopsy
- Upper GI endoscopy with biopsy

A gastroenterologist performs these tests at a hospital or an outpatient center.

Chapter 22

Appendicitis

What Is Appendicitis?

Appendicitis is inflammation of your appendix.

How Common Is Appendicitis?

In the United States, appendicitis is the most common cause of acute abdominal pain requiring surgery. Over five percent of the population develops appendicitis at some point.

Who Is More Likely to Develop Appendicitis?

Appendicitis most commonly occurs in the teens and twenties but may occur at any age.

What Are the Complications of Appendicitis?

If appendicitis is not treated, it may lead to complications. The complications of a ruptured appendix are:

- Peritonitis, which can be a dangerous condition. Peritonitis happens if your appendix bursts and infection spreads in your

This chapter includes text excerpted from "Appendicitis," National Institute of Diabetes and Digestive and Kidney Diseases (NIDDK), November 2014. Reviewed September 2018.

abdomen. If you have peritonitis, you may be very ill and have:

- Fever
- Nausea
- Severe tenderness in your abdomen
- Vomiting
- An abscess of the appendix called an appendiceal abscess

What Are the Symptoms of Appendicitis?

The most common symptom of appendicitis is pain in your abdomen. If you have appendicitis, you'll most often have pain in your abdomen that:

- Begins near your belly button and then moves lower and to your right
- Gets worse in a matter of hours
- Gets worse when you move around, take deep breaths, cough, or sneeze
- Is severe and often described as different from any pain you've felt before
- Occurs suddenly and may even wake you up if you're sleeping
- Occurs before other symptoms

Other symptoms of appendicitis may include:

- Loss of appetite
- Nausea
- Vomiting
- Constipation or diarrhea
- An inability to pass gas
- A low-grade fever
- Swelling in your abdomen
- The feeling that having a bowel movement will relieve discomfort

Symptoms can be different for each person and can seem like the following conditions that also cause pain in the abdomen:

- Abdominal adhesions

- Constipation

- Inflammatory bowel disease, which includes Crohn disease and ulcerative colitis, long-lasting disorders that cause irritation and ulcers in the gastrointestinal (GI) tract

- Intestinal obstruction

- Pelvic inflammatory disease (PID)

What Causes Appendicitis

Appendicitis can have more than one cause, and in many cases, the cause is not clear. Possible causes include:

- Blockage of the opening inside the appendix

- Enlarged tissue in the wall of your appendix, caused by an infection in the gastrointestinal (GI) tract or elsewhere in your body

- Inflammatory bowel disease (IBD)

- Stool, parasites, or growths that can clog your appendiceal lumen

- Trauma to your abdomen

When Should I Seek a Doctor's Help?

Appendicitis is a medical emergency that requires immediate care. See a healthcare professional or go to the emergency room right away if you think you or a child has appendicitis. A doctor can help treat appendicitis and reduce symptoms and the chance of complications.

How Do Doctors Diagnose Appendicitis?

Most often, healthcare professionals suspect the diagnosis of appendicitis based on your symptoms, your medical history, and a physical exam. A doctor can confirm the diagnosis with an ultrasound, X-ray, or magnetic resonance imaging (MRI) exam.

Medical History

A healthcare professional will ask specific questions about your symptoms and health history to help rule out other health problems. The healthcare professional will want to know:

- When your abdominal pain began

- The exact location and severity of your pain

- When your other symptoms appeared

- Your other medical conditions, previous illnesses, and surgical procedures

- Whether you use medicines, alcohol, or illegal drugs

Physical Exam

Healthcare professionals need specific details about the pain in your abdomen to diagnose appendicitis correctly. A healthcare professional will assess your pain by touching or applying pressure to specific areas of your abdomen. The following responses to touch or pressure may indicate that you have appendicitis:

- Rovsing sign (If palpation of the left lower quadrant of a person's abdomen increases the pain felt in the right lower quadrant, the patient is said to have a positive Rovsing sign.)

- Psoas sign (A medical sign that indicates irritation to the iliopsoas group of hip flexors in the abdomen, and consequently indicates that the inflamed appendix is retrocaecal in orientation)

- Obturator sign (An indicator of irritation to the obturator internus muscle)

- Guarding

- Rebound tenderness

- Digital rectal exam

- Pelvic exam

- Lab tests

Doctors use lab tests to help confirm the diagnosis of appendicitis or find other causes of abdominal pain.

Blood tests. A healthcare professional draws your blood for a blood test at a doctor's office or a commercial facility. The healthcare professional sends the blood sample to a lab for testing. Blood tests can show a high white blood cell (WBC) count, a sign of infection. Blood tests also may show dehydration or fluid and electrolyte imbalances.

Urinalysis. Urinalysis is testing of a urine sample. You will provide a urine sample in a special container in a doctor's office, a commercial facility, or a hospital. Healthcare professionals can test the urine in the same location or send it to a lab for testing. Doctors use urinalysis to rule out a urinary tract infection or a kidney stone.

Pregnancy test. For women, healthcare professionals also may order blood or urine samples to check for pregnancy.

Imaging Tests

Doctors use imaging tests to confirm the diagnosis of appendicitis or find other causes of pain in the abdomen. The following imaging tests are done:

- Abdominal ultrasound

- Magnetic resonance imaging (MRI)

- Computerized tomography (CT) scan

How Do Doctors Treat Appendicitis?

Doctors typically treat appendicitis with surgery to remove the appendix. Surgeons perform the surgery in a hospital with general anesthesia. Your doctor will recommend surgery if you have continuous abdominal pain and fever, or signs of a burst appendix and infection. Prompt surgery decreases the chance that your appendix will burst. Healthcare professionals call the surgery to remove the appendix an appendectomy. A surgeon performs the surgery using one of the following methods:

Laparoscopic surgery. During laparoscopic surgery, surgeons use several smaller incisions and special surgical tools that they feed through the incisions to remove your appendix. Laparoscopic surgery leads to fewer complications, such as hospital-related infections, and has a shorter recovery time.

Laparotomy. Surgeons use laparotomy to remove the appendix through a single incision in the lower right area of your abdomen.

After surgery, most patients completely recover from appendicitis and don't need to make changes to their diet, exercise, or lifestyle. Surgeons recommend that you limit physical activity for the first 10–14 days after a laparotomy and for the first three to five days after laparoscopic surgery.

What If the Surgeon Finds a Normal Appendix?

In some cases, a surgeon finds a normal appendix during surgery. In this case, many surgeons will remove it to eliminate the future possibility of appendicitis. Sometimes surgeons find a different problem, which they may correct during surgery.

Can Doctors Treat Appendicitis without Surgery?

Some cases of mild appendicitis may be cured with antibiotics alone. All patients suspected of having appendicitis are treated with antibiotics before surgery, and some patients may improve completely before surgery is performed.

How Do Doctors Treat Complications of a Burst Appendix?

Treating the complications of a burst appendix will depend on the type of complication. In most cases of peritonitis, a surgeon will remove your appendix immediately with surgery. The surgeon will use laparotomy to clean the inside of your abdomen to prevent infection and then remove your appendix. Without prompt treatment, peritonitis can cause death.

A surgeon may drain the pus from an appendiceal abscess during surgery or, more commonly, before surgery. To drain an abscess, the surgeon places a tube in the abscess through the abdominal wall. You leave the drainage tube in place for about two weeks while you take antibiotics to treat the infection. When the infection and inflammation are under control, about six to eight weeks later, surgeons operate to remove what remains of the burst appendix.

How Can Your Diet Help Prevent or Relieve Appendicitis?

Researchers have not found that eating, diet, and nutrition cause or prevent appendicitis.

Chapter 23

Gallstones

What Are Gallstones?

Gallstones are hard, pebble-like pieces of material, usually made of cholesterol or bilirubin, that form in your gallbladder. Gallstones can range in size from a grain of sand to a golf ball. The gallbladder can make one large gallstone, hundreds of tiny stones, or both small and large stones. When gallstones block the bile ducts of your biliary tract, the gallstones can cause sudden pain in your upper right abdomen. This pain is called a gallbladder attack, or biliary colic. If your symptoms continue and they're left untreated, gallstones can cause serious complications. However, most gallstones don't cause blockages and are painless, also called "silent" gallstones. Silent gallstones usually don't need medical treatment.

What Are the Types of Gallstones?

The two main types of gallstones are:

- Cholesterol stones
- Pigment stones

Cholesterol stones are usually yellow-green in color and are made of mostly hardened cholesterol. In some countries, cholesterol stones

---

This chapter includes text excerpted from "Gallstones," National Institute of Diabetes and Digestive and Kidney Diseases (NIDDK), November 2017.

make up about 75 percent of gallstones. Pigment stones are dark in color and are made of bilirubin. Some people have a mix of both kinds of stones. Cholelithiasis is the name doctors sometimes call gallstones.

What Is the Biliary Tract?

Your biliary tract, which is made up of your gallbladder and bile ducts, helps with digestion by releasing bile. The gallbladder is a small, pear-shaped organ that stores bile and is located in your upper right abdomen, below your liver. The bile ducts of your biliary tract include the hepatic ducts, common bile duct, and cystic duct. Bile ducts also carry waste and digestive juices from the liver and pancreas to the duodenum. Your liver produces bile, which is mostly made of cholesterol, bile salts, and bilirubin. Your gallbladder stores the bile until it's needed. When you eat, your body signals your gallbladder to empty bile into your duodenum to mix with food. The bile ducts carry the bile from your gallbladder to the duodenum.

How Common Are Gallstones?

Gallstones are very common, affecting 10–15 percent of the U.S. population, which is almost 25 million people. About a quarter of the nearly one million people diagnosed with gallstones each year will need to be treated, usually with surgery.

Who Is More Likely to Develop Gallstones?

Certain groups of people have a higher risk of developing gallstones than others:

- Women are more likely to develop gallstones than men. Women who have extra estrogen in their body due to pregnancy, hormone replacement therapy, or birth control pills may be more likely to produce gallstones.
- Older people are more likely to develop gallstones. As you age, the chance that you'll develop gallstones becomes higher.
- People with a family history of gallstones have a higher risk.
- American Indians have genes that raise the amount of cholesterol in their bile, and have the highest rate of gallstones in the United States.
- Mexican Americans are also at higher risk of developing gallstones.

People with Certain Health Conditions

You are more likely to develop gallstones if you have one of the following health conditions:

- Cirrhosis, a condition in which your liver slowly breaks down and stops working due to chronic, or long-lasting, injury
- Infections in the bile ducts, which can also be a complication of gallstones
- Hemolytic anemias, conditions in which red blood cells are continuously broken down, such as sickle cell anemia
- Some intestinal diseases that affect normal absorption of nutrients, such as Crohn disease
- High triglyceride levels
- Low high-density lipoprotein (HDL) cholesterol
- Metabolic syndrome, which can also raise the risk of gallstone complications
- Diabetes and insulin resistance

People with Diet- and Weight-Related Health Concerns

You are more likely to develop gallstones if you:

- Have obesity, especially if you are a woman
- Have had fast weight loss, like from weight-loss surgery
- Have been on a diet high in calories and refined carbohydrates and low in fiber

What Are the Complications of Gallstones?

Complications of gallstones can include:

- Inflammation of the gallbladder
- Severe damage to or infection of the gallbladder, bile ducts, or liver
- Gallstone pancreatitis, which is inflammation of the pancreas due to a gallstone blockage

Many people do not have symptoms of gallstones until they have complications. If left untreated, gallstones can be deadly. Treatment for gallstones usually involves gallstone surgery.

What Are the Symptoms of Gallstones?

If gallstones block your bile ducts, bile could build up in your gallbladder, causing a gallbladder attack, sometimes called biliary colic. Gallbladder attacks usually cause pain in your upper right abdomen, sometimes lasting several hours. Gallbladder attacks often follow heavy meals and usually occur in the evening or during the night. If you've had one gallbladder attack, more attacks will likely follow.

Gallbladder attacks usually stop when gallstones move and no longer block the bile ducts. However, if any of your bile ducts stay blocked for more than a few hours, you may develop gallstone complications. Gallstones that do not block your bile ducts do not cause symptoms.

Silent Gallstones

Most people with gallstones do not have symptoms. Gallstones that do not cause symptoms are called silent gallstones. Silent gallstones don't stop your gallbladder, liver, or pancreas from working, so they do not need treatment.

Seek Care Right Away for a Gallbladder Attack

See a doctor right away if you are having these symptoms during or after a gallbladder attack:

- Pain in your abdomen lasting several hours

- Nausea and vomiting

- Fever—even a low-grade fever—or chills

- Yellowish color of your skin or whites of your eyes, called jaundice

- Tea-colored urine and light-colored stools

These symptoms may be signs of a serious infection or inflammation of the gallbladder, liver, or pancreas. Gallstone symptoms may be similar to symptoms of other conditions, such as appendicitis, ulcers, pancreatitis, and gastroesophageal reflux disease (GERD), all of which should be treated by a doctor as soon as possible.

Gallstone complications can occur if your bile ducts stay blocked. Left untreated, blockages of the bile ducts or pancreatic duct can be fatal.

What Causes Gallstones

Gallstones may form if bile contains too much cholesterol, too much bilirubin, or not enough bile salts. Researchers do not fully understand why these changes in bile occur. Gallstones also may form if the gallbladder does not empty completely or often enough. Certain people are more likely to have gallstones than others because of their risk factors for gallstones, including obesity and certain kinds of dieting.

How Does Weight Affect Gallstones?

Being overweight or having obesity may make you more likely to develop gallstones, especially if you are a woman. Researchers have found that people who have obesity may have higher levels of cholesterol in their bile, which can cause gallstones. People who have obesity may also have large gallbladders that do not work well. Some studies have shown that people who carry large amounts of fat around their waist may be more likely to develop gallstones than those who carry fat around their hips and thighs. Losing weight very quickly may raise your chances of forming gallstones, however. Talk with your healthcare professional about how to lose weight safely.

Is Weight Cycling a Problem?

Weight cycling, or losing and regaining weight repeatedly, may also lead to gallstones. The more weight you lose and regain during a cycle, the greater your chances of developing gallstones. Stay away from "crash diets" that promise to help you drop the pounds quickly. Aim for losing weight at a slower pace and keeping it off over time.

How Can I Safely Lose Weight to Lower My Chances of Getting Gallstones?

Losing weight at a slow pace may make it less likely that you will develop gallstones. For people who are overweight or have obesity, experts recommend beginning with a weight loss of 5–10 percent of your starting weight over a period of 6 months. In addition, weight loss may bring you other benefits such as better mood, more energy, and positive self-image.

When making healthy food choices to help you lose weight, you can choose food that may also lower your chances of developing gallstones. Regular physical activity, which will improve your overall health, may also lower your chances of developing gallstones. To improve health or prevent weight gain, aim for two hours and 30 minutes of physical activity each week. Talk with your doctor before you start an eating and physical activity plan to improve your health or maintain your weight loss.

How Do Doctors Diagnose Gallstones?

Doctors use your medical history, a physical exam, and lab and imaging tests to diagnose gallstones. A healthcare professional will ask you about your symptoms. He or she will ask if you have a history of health conditions or health concerns that make you more likely to get gallstones. The healthcare professional also may ask if you have a family history of gallstones and what you typically eat. During a physical exam, the healthcare professional examines your body and checks for pain in your abdomen.

What Tests Do Healthcare Professionals Use to Diagnose Gallstones?

Healthcare professionals may use lab or imaging tests to diagnose gallstones.

Lab Tests

A healthcare professional may take a blood sample from you and send the sample to a lab to test. The blood test can show signs of infection or inflammation of the bile ducts, gallbladder, pancreas, or liver.

Imaging Tests

Healthcare professionals use imaging tests to find gallstones. A technician performs these tests in your doctor's office, an outpatient center, or a hospital. A radiologist reads and reports on the images. You usually don't need anesthesia or a medicine to keep you calm for most of these tests. However, a doctor may give you anesthesia or a medicine to keep you calm for endoscopic retrograde cholangiopancreatography (ERCP). The following imaging tests are done:

- Ultrasound
- Computed tomography (CT) scan
- Magnetic resonance imaging (MRI)

- Cholescintigraphy
- Endoscopic retrograde cholangiopancreatography (ERCP)

How Do Healthcare Professionals Treat Gallstones?

If your gallstones are not causing symptoms, you probably don't need treatment. However, if you are having a gallbladder attack or other symptoms, contact your doctor. Although your symptoms may go away, they may appear again and you may need treatment. Your doctor may refer to you a gastroenterologist or surgeon for treatment. The usual treatment for gallstones is surgery to remove the gallbladder. Doctors sometimes can use nonsurgical treatments to treat cholesterol stones, but pigment stones usually require surgery.

Surgery

Surgery to remove the gallbladder, called cholecystectomy, is one of the most common operations performed on adults in the United States. The gallbladder is not an essential organ, which means you can live normally without a gallbladder. A healthcare professional will usually give you general anesthesia for surgery. Once the surgeon removes your gallbladder, bile flows out of your liver through the hepatic duct and the common bile duct and directly into the duodenum, instead of being stored in the gallbladder.

Surgeons perform two types of cholecystectomy:

- Laparoscopic cholecystectomy
- Open cholecystectomy

What Happens after Gallbladder Removal?

A small number of people have softer and more frequent stools after gallbladder removal, because bile now flows into your duodenum more often. Changes in bowel habits are usually temporary; however, discuss them with your doctor. All surgeries come with a possible risk of complications; however, gallbladder surgery complications are very rare. The most common complication is injury to the bile ducts, which can cause infection. You may need one or more additional operations to repair the bile ducts.

Nonsurgical Treatments

Doctors use nonsurgical treatments for gallstones only in special situations, like if you have cholesterol stones and you have a serious medical condition that prevents surgery. Even with treatment, gallstones can return. Therefore, you may have to be regularly treated for gallstones for a very long time, or even for the rest of your life.

A doctor may use the following types of nonsurgical treatments to remove or break up cholesterol gallstones:

- Endoscopic retrograde cholangiopancreatography (ERCP)
- Oral dissolution therapy
- Shockwave lithotripsy

How Can I Help Prevent Gallstones?

You can help prevent gallstones by:

- Adjusting your eating plan to include more foods high in fiber and healthy fats, fewer refined carbohydrates, and less sugar
- Losing weight safely if you are overweight or have obesity
- Maintaining a healthy weight through healthy eating and regular physical activity

Can What I Eat Help Prevent Gallstones?

You can lower your risk of gallstones by following a healthy eating plan and getting regular physical activity to help you reach and maintain a healthy weight.

Experts recommend the following to help prevent gallstones:

- Eat more foods that are high in fiber, such as:
  - Fruits, vegetables, beans, and peas
  - Whole grains, including brown rice, oats, and whole wheat bread
- Eat fewer refined carbohydrates and less sugar.
- Eat healthy fats, like fish oil and olive oil, to help your gallbladder contract and empty on a regular basis.
- Avoid unhealthy fats, like those often found in desserts and fried foods.

Talk with your healthcare professional before you make any changes to your eating plan. Losing weight too quickly may cause health problems. Very low-calorie diets and weight-loss surgery can lead to rapid weight loss and raise your risk of gallstones.

Chapter 24

Diverticulosis and Diverticulitis

What Is Diverticulosis?

Diverticulosis is a condition that occurs when small pouches, or sacs, form and push outward through weak spots in the wall of your colon. These pouches are most common in the lower part of your colon, called the sigmoid colon. One pouch is called a diverticulum. Multiple pouches are called diverticula. Most people with diverticulosis do not have symptoms or problems. When diverticulosis does cause symptoms or problems, doctors call this diverticular disease. For some people, diverticulosis causes symptoms such as changes in bowel movement patterns or pain in the abdomen. Diverticulosis may also cause problems such as diverticular bleeding and diverticulitis.

Diverticular Bleeding

Diverticular bleeding occurs when a small blood vessel within the wall of a pouch, or diverticulum, bursts.

This chapter includes text excerpted from "Diverticular Disease," National Institute of Diabetes and Digestive and Kidney Diseases (NIDDK), May 2016.

Diverticulitis

- Diverticulitis occurs when you have diverticulosis and one or a few of the pouches in the wall of your colon become inflamed. Diverticulitis can lead to serious complications.

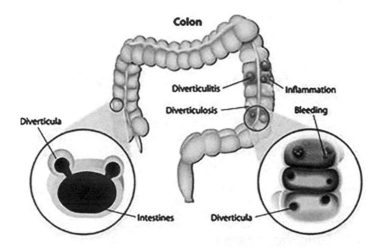

Figure 24.1. *Diverticulosis and Diverticulitis*

What Are the Complications of Diverticulitis?

Diverticulitis can come on suddenly and cause other problems, such as the following:

Abscess

An abscess is a painful, swollen, infected, and pus-filled area just outside your colon wall that may make you ill with nausea, vomiting, fever, and severe tenderness in your abdomen.

Perforation

A perforation is a small tear or hole in a pouch in your colon.

Peritonitis

Peritonitis is inflammation or infection of the lining of your abdomen. Pus and stool that leak through a perforation can cause peritonitis.

Fistula

A fistula is an abnormal passage, or tunnel, between two organs or between an organ and the outside of your body. The most common types of fistula with diverticulitis occur between the colon and the bladder or between the colon and the vagina in women.

Intestinal Obstruction

An intestinal obstruction is a partial or total blockage of the movement of food or stool through your intestines.

How Common Are Diverticulosis and Diverticulitis?

Diverticulosis is quite common, especially as people age. Research suggests that about 35 percent of U.S. adults age 50 years or younger have diverticulosis, while about 58 percent of those older than age 60 have diverticulosis. Most people with diverticulosis will never develop symptoms or problems. Experts used to think that 10–25 percent of people with diverticulosis would develop diverticulitis. However, newer research suggests that the percentage who develop diverticulitis may be much lower—less than five percent. In the United States, about 200,000 people are hospitalized for diverticulitis each year. About 70,000 people are hospitalized for diverticular bleeding each year.

Who Is More Likely to Have Diverticulosis and Diverticulitis?

People are more likely to develop diverticulosis and diverticulitis as they age. Among people ages 50 and older, women are more likely than men to develop diverticulitis. However, among people younger than age 50, men are more likely to develop diverticulitis.

What Are the Symptoms of Diverticulosis?

Most people with diverticulosis do not have symptoms. If your diverticulosis causes symptoms, they may include:

- Bloating
- Constipation or diarrhea
- Cramping or pain in your lower abdomen

Other conditions, such as irritable bowel syndrome (IBS) and peptic ulcers, cause similar symptoms, so these symptoms may not mean you have diverticulosis. If you have these symptoms, see your doctor. If you have diverticulosis and develop diverticular bleeding or diverticulitis, these conditions also cause symptoms.

What Are the Symptoms of Diverticular Bleeding?

In most cases, when you have diverticular bleeding, you will suddenly have a large amount of red or maroon-colored blood in your stool. Diverticular bleeding may also cause dizziness or lightheadedness, or weakness. See your doctor right away if you have any of these symptoms.

What Are the Symptoms of Diverticulitis?

When you have diverticulitis, the inflamed pouches most often cause pain in the lower left side of your abdomen. The pain is usually severe and comes on suddenly, though it can also be mild and get worse over several days. The intensity of the pain can change over time.

Diverticulitis may also cause:

- Constipation or diarrhea
- Fevers and chills
- Nausea or vomiting

What Causes Diverticulosis and Diverticulitis

Experts are not sure what causes diverticulosis and diverticulitis. Researchers are studying several factors that may play a role in causing these conditions.

Fiber

For more than 50 years, experts thought that following a low-fiber diet led to diverticulosis. However, recent research has found that a low-fiber diet may not play a role. This study also found that a high-fiber diet with more frequent bowel movements may be linked with a greater chance of having diverticulosis. Talk with your doctor about how much fiber you should include in your diet.

Genes

Some studies suggest that genes may make some people more likely to develop diverticulosis and diverticulitis. Experts are still studying the role genes play in causing these conditions.

Other Factors

Studies have found links between diverticular disease—diverticulosis that causes symptoms or problems such as diverticular bleeding or diverticulitis—and the following factors:

- Certain medicines—including nonsteroidal anti-inflammatory drugs (NSAIDs), such as aspirin, and steroids

- Lack of exercise

- Obesity

- Smoking

Diverticulitis may begin when bacteria or stool get caught in a pouch in your colon. A decrease in healthy bacteria and an increase in disease-causing bacteria in your colon may also lead to diverticulitis.

How Do Doctors Diagnose Diverticulosis and Diverticulitis?

If your doctor suspects you may have diverticulosis or diverticulitis, your doctor may use your medical history, a physical exam, and tests to diagnose these conditions.

Doctors may also diagnose diverticulosis if they notice pouches in the colon wall while performing tests, such as routine X-rays or colonoscopy, for other reasons.

Medical History

Your doctor will ask about your medical history, including your:

- Bowel movement patterns
- Diet
- Health
- Medicines
- Symptoms

Physical Exam

Your doctor will perform a physical exam, which may include a digital rectal exam. During a digital rectal exam, your doctor will have you bend over a table or lie on your side while holding your knees close to your chest. After putting on a glove, the doctor will slide a lubricated finger into your anus to check for pain, bleeding, hemorrhoids, or other problems.

What Tests Do Doctors Use to Diagnose Diverticulosis and Diverticulitis?

Your doctor may use the following tests to help diagnose diverticulosis and diverticulitis:

Blood Test

A healthcare professional may take a blood sample from you and send the sample to a lab to test for inflammation or anemia.

Computerized Tomography (CT) Scan

A computerized tomography (CT) scan uses a combination of X-rays and computer technology to create images of your gastrointestinal (GI) tract. A CT scan of your colon is the most common test doctors use to diagnose diverticulosis and diverticulitis.

Lower GI Series

A lower GI series, also called a barium enema, is a procedure in which a doctor uses X-rays and a chalky liquid called barium to view your large intestine. The barium will make your large intestine more visible on an X-ray. If pouches are present in your colon, they will appear on the X-ray.

Colonoscopy

Colonoscopy is a procedure in which a doctor uses a long, flexible, narrow tube with a light and tiny camera on one end, called a colonoscope or endoscope, to look inside your rectum and colon. Doctors may use colonoscopy to confirm a diagnosis of diverticulosis or diverticulitis and rule out other conditions, such as cancer.

How Do Doctors Treat Diverticulosis?

The goal of treating diverticulosis is to prevent the pouches from causing symptoms or problems. Your doctor may recommend the following treatments.

High-Fiber Diet

Although a high-fiber diet may not prevent diverticulosis, it may help prevent symptoms or problems in people who already have diverticulosis. A doctor may suggest that you increase fiber in your diet slowly to reduce your chances of having gas and pain in your abdomen.

Fiber Supplements

Your doctor may suggest you take a fiber product such as methylcellulose (Citrucel) or psyllium (Metamucil) one to three times a day. These products are available as powders, pills, or wafers and provide 0.5–3.5 grams of fiber per dose. You should take fiber products with at least eight ounces of water.

Medicines

Some studies suggest that mesalazine (Asacol) taken every day or in cycles may help reduce symptoms that may occur with diverticulosis, such as pain in your abdomen or bloating. Studies suggest that the antibiotic rifaximin (Xifaxan) may also help with diverticulosis symptoms.

Probiotics

Some studies show that probiotics may help with diverticulosis symptoms and may help prevent diverticulitis. However, researchers are still studying this subject. Probiotics are live bacteria like those that occur normally in your stomach and intestines. You can find probiotics in dietary supplements—in capsule, tablet, and powder form—and in some foods, such as yogurt. For safety reasons, talk with your doctor before using probiotics or any complementary or alternative medicines or medical practices.

How Do Doctors Treat Diverticular Bleeding?

Diverticular bleeding is rare. If you have bleeding, it can be severe. In some people, the bleeding may stop by itself and may not require treatment. However, if you have bleeding from your rectum—even a small amount—you should see a doctor right away.

To find the site of the bleeding and stop it, a doctor may perform a colonoscopy. Your doctor may also use a computerized tomography

(CT) scan or an angiogram to find the bleeding site. An angiogram is a special kind of X-ray in which your doctor threads a thin, flexible tube through a large artery, often from your groin, to the bleeding area.

Colon Resection

If your bleeding does not stop, a surgeon may perform abdominal surgery with a colon resection. In a colon resection, the surgeon removes the affected part of your colon and joins the remaining ends of your colon together. You will receive general anesthesia for this procedure. In some cases, during a colon resection, it may not be safe for the surgeon to rejoin the ends of your colon right away. In this case, the surgeon performs a temporary colostomy. Several months later, in a second surgery, the surgeon rejoins the ends of your colon and closes the opening in your abdomen.

How Do Doctors Treat Diverticulitis?

If you have diverticulitis with mild symptoms and no other problems, a doctor may recommend that you rest, take oral antibiotics, and follow a liquid diet for a period of time. If your symptoms ease after a few days, the doctor will recommend gradually adding solid foods back into your diet. Severe cases of diverticulitis that come on quickly and cause complications will likely require a hospital stay and involve intravenous (IV) antibiotics. A few days without food or drink will help your colon rest. If the period without food or drink is longer than a few days, your doctor may give you an IV liquid food mixture. The mixture contains:

- Carbohydrates
- Proteins
- Fats
- Vitamins
- Minerals

How Do Doctors Treat Complications of Diverticulitis?

Your doctor may recommend the following to treat complications of diverticulitis:

Abscess

Your doctor may need to drain an abscess if it is large or does not clear up with antibiotics.

Perforation

If you have a perforation, you will likely need surgery to repair the tear or hole. Additional surgery may be needed to remove a small part of your colon if the surgeon cannot repair the perforation.

Peritonitis

Peritonitis requires immediate surgery to clean your abdominal cavity. You may need a colon resection at a later date after a course of antibiotics. You may also need a blood transfusion if you have lost a lot of blood. Without prompt treatment, peritonitis can be fatal.

Fistula

Surgeons can correct a fistula by performing a colon resection and removing the fistula.

Intestinal Obstruction

If your large intestine is completely blocked, you will need emergency surgery, with possible colon resection. Partial blockage is not an emergency, so you can schedule the surgery or other corrective procedures.

What Should I Eat If I Have Diverticulosis or Diverticulitis?

If you have diverticulosis or if you have had diverticulitis in the past, your doctor may recommend eating more foods that are high in fiber. The *Dietary Guidelines for Americans*, 2015–2020, recommends a dietary fiber intake of 14 grams per 1,000 calories consumed. For example, for a 2,000-calorie diet, the fiber recommendation is 28 grams per day.

The amount of fiber in a food is listed on the food's nutrition facts label. Some fiber-rich foods are listed in the table below.

Table 24.1. Grains

Food and Portion Size	Amount of Fiber
⅓–¾ cup high-fiber bran ready-to-eat cereal	9.1 to 14.3 grams
1–1¼ cup of shredded wheat ready-to-eat cereal	5.0 to 9.0 grams
1½ cup whole wheat spaghetti, cooked	3.2 grams
1 small oat bran muffin	3.0 grams

Table 24.2. Fruits

Food and Portion Size	Amount of Fiber
1 medium pear, with skin	5.5 grams
1 medium apple, with skin	4.4 grams
½ cup of raspberries	4.0 grams
½ cup of stewed prunes	3.8 grams

Table 24.3. Vegetables

Food and Portion Size	Amount of Fiber
½ cup of green peas, cooked	3.5 to 4.4 grams
½ cup of mixed vegetables, cooked from frozen	4.0 grams
½ cup of collards, cooked	3.8 grams
1 medium sweet potato, baked in skin	3.8 grams
1 medium potato, baked, with skin	3.6 grams
½ cup of winter squash, cooked	2.9 grams

Table 24.4. Beans

Food and Portion Size	Amount of Fiber
½ cup navy beans, cooked	9.6 grams
½ cup pinto beans, cooked	7.7 grams
½ kidney beans, cooked	5.7 grams

A doctor or dietitian can help you learn how to add more high-fiber foods to your diet.

Should I Avoid Certain Foods If I Have Diverticulosis or Diverticulitis?

Experts now believe you do not need to avoid certain foods if you have diverticulosis or diverticulitis. In the past, doctors might have asked you to avoid nuts; popcorn; and seeds such as sunflower, pumpkin, caraway, and sesame. Research suggests that these foods are not harmful to people with diverticulosis or diverticulitis. The seeds in tomatoes, zucchini, cucumbers, strawberries, and raspberries, as well as poppy seeds, are also fine to eat. Even so, each person is different. You may find that certain types or amounts of foods worsen your symptoms.

Chapter 25

What You Need to Know about Colon Polyps

What Are Colon Polyps?

Colon polyps are growths on the lining of your colon and rectum. You can have more than one colon polyp.

Are Colon Polyps Cancerous?

Colon and rectal cancer—also called colorectal cancer—most often begins as polyps. Most polyps are not cancerous, but some may turn into cancer over time. Removing polyps can help prevent colorectal cancer. Colorectal cancer is the second leading cause of cancer death in the United States.

How Common Are Colon Polyps?

Colon polyps are common in American adults. Anywhere between 15 and 40 percent of adults may have colon polyps. Colon polyps are more common in men and older adults.

This chapter includes text excerpted from "Colon Polyps," National Institute of Diabetes and Digestive and Kidney Diseases (NIDDK), September 2017.

Who Is More Likely to Develop Colon Polyps?

Although anyone can develop colon polyps, you may have a greater chance of developing them if you:

- Are over age 50
- Have someone in your family who has had polyps or colorectal cancer
- Have inflammatory bowel disease (IBD) such as ulcerative colitis (UC) or Crohn disease
- Have obesity
- Smoke cigarettes

When Should I Start Colon Polyp Screening?

Screening is testing for diseases when you have no symptoms. Finding and removing polyps can help prevent colorectal cancer. Your doctor will recommend screening for colorectal cancer starting at age 50 if you don't have health problems or other factors that make you more likely to develop colorectal cancer. If you are at higher risk for colorectal cancer, your doctor may recommend screening at a younger age. You also may need to be tested more often. If you are older than age 75, talk with your doctor about whether you should be screened.

What Are the Symptoms of Colon Polyps?

Most people with colon polyps don't have symptoms. You can't tell that you have polyps because you feel well. When colon polyps do cause symptoms, you may:

- Have bleeding from your rectum. You might notice blood on your underwear or on toilet paper after you've had a bowel movement.
- Have blood in your stool. Blood can make stool look black or can show up as red streaks in your stool.
- Feel tired because you have anemia and not enough iron in your body. Bleeding from colon polyps can lead to anemia and a lack of iron.

Many other health problems can also cause these symptoms. However, if you have bleeding from your rectum or blood in your stool, contact your doctor right away.

What Causes Colon Polyps

Experts aren't sure what causes colon polyps. However, research suggests that certain factors, such as age and family history, can raise your chances of developing colon polyps.

How Do Doctors Diagnose Colon Polyps?

Doctors can find colon polyps only by using certain tests or procedures, such as a colonoscopy or imaging study. Your doctor may first take a medical and family history and perform a physical exam to help decide which test or procedure is best for you. For example, your doctor may ask if you have any symptoms. He or she may also ask if you have a family history of colon polyps or colorectal cancer. After taking a medical and family history, your doctor may perform a physical exam.

Tests and Procedures

- Flexible sigmoidoscopy
- Colonoscopy
- Virtual colonoscopy
- Lower gastrointestinal (GI) series

How Do Doctors Treat Colon Polyps?

Doctors treat colon polyps by removing them. In most cases, doctors use special tools during a colonoscopy or flexible sigmoidoscopy to remove colon polyps. After doctors remove the polyp, they send it for testing to check for cancer. A pathologist will review the test results and send a report to your doctor. Doctors can remove almost all polyps without surgery. If you have colon polyps, your doctor will ask you to get tested regularly in the future because you have a higher chance of developing more polyps.

Seek Care Right Away

Call your doctor right away if you have any of the following symptoms after he or she removes a colon polyp:

- Severe pain in your abdomen
- Fever

- Bloody bowel movements that do not get better
- Bleeding from your anus that does not stop
- Dizziness
- Weakness

How Can I Prevent Colon Polyps?

Researchers don't know a sure way to prevent colon polyps. However, you can take steps to lower your chances of developing colon polyps.

Eating, Diet, and Nutrition

Eating, diet, and nutrition changes—such as eating less red meat and more fruits and vegetables—may lower your chances of developing colon polyps.

Healthy Lifestyle Choices

You can make the following healthy lifestyle choices to help lower your chances of developing colon polyps:

- Get regular physical activity
- Don't smoke cigarettes, and if you do smoke, quit
- Avoid drinking alcohol
- Lose weight if you're overweight

Aspirin

Taking a low dose of aspirin every day for a long period of time may help prevent polyps from developing into colorectal cancer in some people. However, taking aspirin daily may cause side effects such as bleeding in your stomach or intestines. Talk with your doctor before you start taking aspirin daily.

What Type of Eating Plan Is Best to Prevent Colon Polyps?

Research suggests that making the following changes may have health benefits and may lower your chances of developing colon polyps:

- Eating more fruits, vegetables, and other foods with fiber, such as beans and bran cereal.

- Losing weight if you're overweight and not gaining weight if you're already at a healthy weight

Foods to Limit

Research suggests that eating less of the following foods may have health benefits and may lower your chances of developing polyps:

- Fatty foods, such as fried foods

- Red meat, such as beef and pork

- Processed meat, such as bacon, sausage, hot dogs, and lunch meats

Chapter 26

Congenital and Pediatric Disorders of the Lower Gastrointestinal Tract

Chapter Contents

Section 26.1

Gastroschisis

This section includes text excerpted from "Facts about Gastroschisis," Centers for Disease Control and Prevention (CDC), November 21, 2017.

What Is Gastroschisis?

Gastroschisis is a birth defect of the abdominal (belly) wall. The baby's intestines are found outside of the baby's body, exiting through a hole beside the belly button. The hole can be small or large and sometimes other organs, such as the stomach and liver, can also be found outside of the baby's body.

Gastroschisis occurs early during pregnancy when the muscles that make up the baby's abdominal wall do not form correctly. A hole occurs which allows the intestines and other organs to extend outside of the body, usually to the right side of belly button. Because the intestines are not covered in a protective sac and are exposed to the amniotic fluid, the intestines can become irritated, causing them to shorten, twist, or swell.

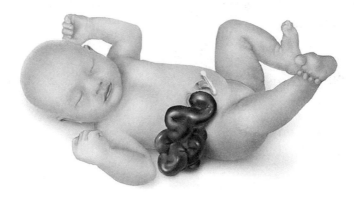

Figure 26.1. *Gastroschisis*

Other Problems

Soon after the baby is born, surgery will be needed to place the abdominal organs inside the baby's body and repair the hole in the abdominal wall. Even after the repair, infants with gastroschisis can have problems with nursing and eating, digestion of food, and absorption of nutrients.

Occurrence

The Centers for Disease Control and Prevention (CDC) estimates that about 1,871 babies are born each year in the United States with gastroschisis, but several studies show that recently this birth defect has become more common, particularly among younger mothers.

What Are the Causes and Risk Factors of Gastroschisis?

The causes of gastroschisis among most infants are unknown. Some babies have gastroschisis because of a change in their genes or chromosomes. Gastroschisis might also be caused by a combination of genes and other factors, such as the things the mother comes in contact with in the environment or what the mother eats or drinks, or certain medicines she uses during pregnancy.

Like many families affected by birth defects, the CDC wants to find out what causes them. Understanding factors that are more common among babies with birth defects will help the CDC learn more about the causes. The CDC funds the Centers for Birth Defects Research and Prevention, which collaborate on large studies such as the National Birth Defects Prevention Study (NBDPS; births 1997–2011) and the Birth Defects Study To Evaluate Pregnancy exposures (BD-STEPS, which began with births in 2014), to understand the causes of and risks for birth defects, like gastroschisis.

CDC researchers have reported important findings about some factors that affect the risk of having a baby with gastroschisis:

- **Younger age**. Teenage mothers were more likely to have a baby with gastroschisis than older mothers.

- **Alcohol and tobacco**. Women who consumed alcohol or were a smoker were more likely to have a baby with gastroschisis.

The CDC continues to study birth defects like gastroschisis in order to learn how to prevent them. If you are pregnant or thinking about getting pregnant, talk with your doctor about ways to increase your chance of having a healthy baby.

What Is the Diagnosis of Gastroschisis?

Gastroschisis can be diagnosed during pregnancy or after the baby is born.

During Pregnancy

During pregnancy, there are screening tests (prenatal tests) to check for birth defects and other conditions. Gastroschisis might result in an abnormal result on a blood or serum screening test or it might be seen during an ultrasound (which creates pictures of the baby's body while inside the womb).

After the Baby Is Born

Gastroschisis is immediately seen at birth.

What Is the Treatment for Gastroschisis?

Soon after the baby is born, surgery will be needed to place the abdominal organs inside the baby's body and repair the defect. If the gastroschisis defect is small (only some of the intestine is outside of the belly), it is usually treated with surgery soon after birth to put the organs back into the belly and close the opening. If the gastroschisis defect is large (many organs outside of the belly), the repair might done slowly, in stages. The exposed organs might be covered with a special material and slowly moved back into the belly. After all of the organs have been put back in the belly, the opening is closed. Babies with gastroschisis often need other treatments as well, including receiving nutrients through an intravenous (IV) line, antibiotics to prevent infection, and careful attention to control their body temperature.

Section 26.2

Hirschsprung Disease

This section includes text excerpted from "Hirschsprung Disease," National Institute of Diabetes and Digestive and Kidney Diseases (NIDDK), September 2015.

What Is Hirschsprung Disease?

Hirschsprung disease is a birth defect in which nerve cells are missing at the end of a child's bowel. Normally, the bowel contains many nerve cells all along its length that control how the bowel works. When the bowel is missing nerve cells, it does not work well. This damage causes blockages in the bowel because the stool does not move through the bowel normally.

Most often, the areas missing the nerve cells are the rectum and the sigmoid colon. However, some children are missing the nerve cells for the entire colon or part of the small intestine.

- In short-segment Hirschsprung disease, nerve cells are missing from the last part of the large intestine.

- In long-segment Hirschsprung disease, nerve cells are missing from most or all of the large intestine and sometimes the last part of the small intestine.

- Rarely, nerve cells are missing in the entire large and small intestine.

In a child with Hirschsprung disease, stool moves through the bowel until it reaches the part lacking nerve cells. At that point, the stool moves slowly or stops.

What Are the Bowel, Large Intestine, Colon, Rectum, and Anus?

The bowel consists of the small and large intestines. The large intestine, which includes the colon and rectum, is the last part of the gastrointestinal (GI) tract. The large intestine's main job is to absorb water and hold stool. The rectum connects the colon to the anus. Stool passes out of the body through the anus. At birth, the large intestine is about two feet long. An adult's large intestine is about five feet long.

What Causes Hirschsprung Disease

During early development of the baby in the mother's womb, nerve cells stop growing toward the end of a child's bowel causing Hirschsprung disease. Most of these cells start at the beginning of the bowel and grow toward the end. Hirschsprung disease occurs when these cells do not reach the end of a child's bowel. Scientists know that genetic defects can increase the chance of a child developing Hirschsprung disease. However, no testing exists that can diagnose a child while the mother is pregnant. Researchers are studying if the mother's health history or lifestyle during pregnancy increases the chance of her baby developing Hirschsprung disease.

Who Gets Hirschsprung Disease?

Hirschsprung disease occurs in approximately one in 5,000 newborns. Children with Down syndrome and other medical problems, such as congenital heart defects, are at much greater risk. For example, about one in 100 children with Down syndrome also has Hirschsprung disease. Hirschsprung disease is congenital, or present at birth; however, symptoms may or may not be obvious at birth. If you have a child with Hirschsprung disease, your chances of having more children with Hirschsprung disease are greater than people who don't have a child with Hirschsprung disease. Also, if a parent has Hirschsprung disease, the chance of their child having Hirschsprung disease is higher. Talk with your doctor to learn more.

What Are the Signs and Symptoms of Hirschsprung Disease?

The main signs and symptoms of Hirschsprung disease are constipation or intestinal obstruction, usually appearing shortly after birth. Many healthy infants and children have difficulty passing stool or infrequent bowel movements. However, unlike healthy children and infants, kids with Hirschsprung disease typically do not respond to constipation medicines given by mouth. Most often, an infant or a child with Hirschsprung disease will have other symptoms, including:

- Growth failure
- Swelling of the abdomen, or belly
- Unexplained fever
- Vomiting

The symptoms can vary; however, how they vary does not depend on how much of the intestine is missing nerve cells. No matter where in the intestine the nerve cells are missing, once the stool reaches this area, the blockage forms and the child develops symptoms.

Symptoms in Newborns

An early symptom in some newborns is a failure to have a first bowel movement within 48 hours after birth. Other symptoms may include:

- Green or brown vomit
- Explosive stools after a doctor inserts a finger into the newborn's rectum
- Swelling of the abdomen
- Diarrhea, often with blood

Symptoms in Toddlers and Older Children

Symptoms of Hirschsprung disease in toddlers and older children may include:

- Not being able to pass stools without enemas or suppositories. An enema involves flushing liquid into the child's anus using a special wash bottle. A suppository is a pill placed into the child's rectum.
- Swelling of the abdomen
- Diarrhea, often with blood
- Slow growth

How Does a Doctor Know If My Child Has Hirschsprung Disease?

A doctor will know if your child has Hirschsprung disease based on:

- A physical exam
- A medical and family history
- Symptoms
- Test results

If your doctor suspects Hirschsprung disease, he or she may refer your child to a pediatric gastroenterologist—a doctor who specializes in digestive diseases in children—for additional evaluation.

Physical Exam

During a physical exam, a doctor usually:

- Reviews your child's height and weight
- Examines your child's abdomen for swelling and examines his or her body for signs of poor nutrition

- Uses a stethoscope to listen to sounds within the abdomen

- Taps on specific areas of your child's body

- Performs a rectal exam—explosive stool after a rectal exam may be a sign of Hirschsprung disease

Medical and Family History

A doctor will ask you to provide your child's medical and family history to help diagnose Hirschsprung disease. The doctor will ask questions about your child's bowel movements. The doctor will also ask about vomiting, swelling of the abdomen, and unexplained fever. The doctor is less likely to diagnose Hirschsprung disease if problems with bowel movements began after one year of age.

Medical Tests

A doctor who suspects Hirschsprung disease will do one or more of the following tests:

- Rectal biopsy

- Abdominal X-ray

- Anorectal manometry

- Lower GI series

How Is Hirschsprung Disease Treated?

Hirschsprung disease is a life-threatening illness, and treatment requires surgery. Children who have surgery for Hirschsprung disease most often feel better after surgery. If growth was slow because of Hirschsprung disease, growth typically improves after surgery. For treatment, a pediatric surgeon will perform a pull-through procedure or an ostomy surgery. During either procedure, the surgeon may remove all or part of the colon, called a colectomy.

Pull-Through Procedure

During a pull-through procedure, a surgeon removes the part of the large intestine that is missing nerve cells and connects the healthy part to the anus. A surgeon most often does a pull-through procedure soon after diagnosis.

Ostomy Surgery

Ostomy surgery is a surgical procedure that reroutes the normal movement of the stool out of the body when a part of the bowel is removed. Creating an ostomy means bringing part of the intestine through the abdominal wall so that stool can leave the body without passing through the anus. The opening in the abdomen through which stool leaves the body is called a stoma. A removable external collection pouch, called an ostomy pouch or ostomy appliance, is attached to the stoma and worn outside the body to collect the stool. The child or caregiver will need to empty the pouch several times each day. Although most children with Hirschsprung disease do not need ostomy surgery, a child sick from Hirschsprung disease may need ostomy surgery to get better before undergoing the pull-through procedure. This gives the inflamed areas of the intestine time to heal. In most cases, an ostomy is temporary and the child will have a second surgery to close the ostomy and reattach the intestine. However, sometimes children with Hirschsprung disease have a permanent ostomy, especially if a long segment of the bowel is missing nerve cells or the child has repeated episodes of bowel inflammation, which healthcare providers call enterocolitis.

Ostomy surgeries include the following:

- Ileostomy surgery is when the surgeon connects the small intestine to the stoma.

- Colostomy surgery is when the surgeon connects part of the large intestine to the stoma.

What Can I Expect as My Child Recovers from Surgery?

After surgery, your child will need time to adjust to the new structure of his or her large intestine.

After the Pull-Through Procedure

Most children feel better after the pull-through procedure. However, some children can have complications or problems after surgery. Problems can include:

- Narrowing of the anus

- Constipation

- Diarrhea

- Leaking stool from the anus
- Delayed toilet training
- Enterocolitis

Typically, these problems improve over time with guidance from your child's doctors. Most children eventually have normal bowel movements.

After Ostomy Surgery

Infants will feel better after ostomy surgery because they will be able to pass gas and stool easily.

Older children will feel better as well, although they must adjust to living with an ostomy. They will need to learn how to take care of the stoma and how to change the ostomy pouch. With a few lifestyle changes, children with ostomies can lead normal lives. However, they may worry about being different from their friends. A special nurse, called an ostomy nurse, can answer questions and show your child how to care for an ostomy.

Enterocolitis

Adults and children with Hirschsprung disease can suffer from enterocolitis before or after surgery. Symptoms of enterocolitis may include:

- A swollen abdomen
- Bleeding from the rectum
- Diarrhea
- Fever
- Lack of energy
- Vomiting

A child with enterocolitis needs to go to the hospital, because enterocolitis can be life threatening. Doctors can treat some children with enterocolitis with a special antibiotic by mouth, often in combination with rectal irrigation at home and in the doctor's office. During rectal irrigation, a doctor inserts a small amount of mild salt water into the child's rectum and allows it to come back out. Doctors will admit children with more severe symptoms of enterocolitis to the hospital for monitoring, rectal irrigation, and intravenous (IV) antibiotics and IV fluid. Doctors give IV antibiotics and fluids through a tube inserted into a vein in the child's arm. In severe or repeated cases of enterocolitis, a child may need a temporary ostomy to let the intestine heal or a revision of the pull-through surgery.

Eating, Diet, and Nutrition

If a surgeon removes the child's colon or bypasses it because of an ostomy, the child will need to drink more liquids to make up for water loss and prevent dehydration. They also need twice as much salt as a healthy child. A doctor can measure the sodium in a child's urine and adjust his or her diet to ensure adequate salt replacement.

Some infants may need tube feedings for a while. A feeding tube is a passageway for the infant to receive infant formula or liquid food directly into his or her stomach or small intestine. The doctor will pass the feeding tube through the nose. In some cases, the doctor will recommend a more permanent feeding tube that he or she puts in place surgically in the child's abdomen.

Section 26.3

Intussusception

This section includes text excerpted from "Questions and Answers about Intussusception and Rotavirus Vaccine," Centers for Disease Control and Prevention (CDC), January 27, 2017.

Most infants who get rotavirus vaccine have no problems. Infants are slightly more likely to be irritable, or to have mild, temporary diarrhea or vomiting after a dose of rotavirus vaccine. There is also a small risk of intussusception from rotavirus vaccination, usually within a week after the first or second dose. This additional risk is estimated to range from about 1 in 20,000 to 1 in 100,000 U.S. infants who get rotavirus vaccine.

What Is Intussusception?

Intussusception is a type of bowel blockage caused when the bowel folds into itself like a telescope. This condition is rare and is most likely to occur during the first year of life. Before rotavirus vaccine was used in the United States, each year about 1,900 infants developed intussusception before the age of one year. With prompt treatment, almost all infants who develop intussusception fully recover.

What Are Known Causes of Intussusception?

Most of the time, the cause is not known. Some cases may be caused by a bowel infection. Some cases may be caused by a polyp or tumor in the bowel—both of these are groups of cells growing in the bowel that are not normal. There is also a small risk of intussusception from rotavirus vaccination.

What Are the Signs of Intussusception in Infants?

For intussusception, look for signs of stomach pain along with severe crying. Early on, these episodes could last just a few minutes and come and go several times in an hour. Babies might pull their legs up to their chest. A baby might also vomit several times or have blood in the stool, or could appear weak or very irritable. These signs would usually happen during the first week after the first or second dose of rotavirus vaccine, but look for them any time after vaccination. If you think it is intussusception, call a doctor right away. If you can't reach your doctor, take your baby to a hospital. Tell them when your baby got the rotavirus vaccine.

How Is Intussusception Treated in the United States?

A radiologist (a specialized doctor in a hospital) usually can unfold the intussusception by using air or fluid to push the folded part of the bowel back into its normal position. In about a third of intussusception cases in infants, surgery is required to unfold the bowel. In a small percentage of infants, the blocked section of bowel must be removed (called resection).

Section 26.4

Necrotizing Enterocolitis

This section includes text excerpted from "Necrotizing
Enterocolitis," Genetic and Rare Diseases Information
Center (GARD), National Center for Advancing Translational
Sciences (NCATS), February 5, 2013. Reviewed September 2018.

Necrotizing enterocolitis (NEC) is a condition characterized by variable injury or damage to the intestinal tract, causing death of intestinal tissue. The condition most often occurs in premature newborns, but it may also occur in term or near-term babies.

Signs and Symptoms

Signs and symptoms may include abdominal distension, bloody stools, vomiting bile-stained fluid, and pneumatosis intestinalis (PI) (gas in the bowel wall) identified on abdominal X-ray. Affected infants occasionally have temperature instability, lethargy, or other findings of sepsis.

Causes

The exact cause of NEC is unknown.

Treatment

Treatment involves stopping feedings, passing a small tube into the stomach to relieve gas, and giving intravenous fluids and antibiotics. Surgery may be needed if there is perforated or necrotic (dead) bowel tissue. About 60–80 percent of affected newborns survive the condition.

Prognosis

The survival of infants with necrotizing enterocolitis (NEC) has steadily improved since the late 20th century. The mortality rate in NEC ranges from 10 percent to more than 50 percent in infants who weigh less than 1500 grams (depending on the severity) compared with a mortality rate of 0–20 percent in babies who weigh more than 2500 grams. Extremely premature infants (1000 grams) are still particularly vulnerable, with reported mortality rates of 40–100 percent.

Of the infants who survive, about 50 percent develop a long-term complication and 10 percent of the infants will have late gastrointestinal problems, but the remaining 50 percent do not have any long-term sequelae. The two most common complications are intestinal stricture and short gut syndrome. Intestinal stricture occurs when an area of the intestine heals with scarring that impinges on the inside of the bowel. It is most common in infants treated without surgery. Short gut syndrome is the most serious postoperative complication in NEC, occurring in as many as 23 percent after resection. It is a malabsorption syndrome resulting from removing excessive or critical portions of the small bowel. The neonatal gut typically grows and adapts over time, but this growth may take up to two years, but it can result in persistent loose stools or frequent bowel movements. Babies who can never successfully tube feed and/or who develop life-threatening liver disease may need organ transplantation.

Most of the babies who have not had extensive intestinal resection have normal gastrointestinal function at 1–10 years of age. Recurrent NEC is an uncommon complication (occurring in about four to six percent), but it can occur after either operative or nonoperative management of NEC. Infants who survive NEC are also at increased risk for neurodevelopmental problems; however, these problems may result from underlying prematurity rather than from NEC.

Section 26.5

Omphalocele

This section includes text excerpted from "Facts about Omphalocele," Centers for Disease Control and Prevention (CDC), November 21, 2017.

What Is Omphalocele?

Omphalocele, also known as exomphalos, is a birth defect of the abdominal (belly) wall. The infant's intestines, liver, or other organs stick outside of the belly through the belly button. The organs are covered in a thin, nearly transparent sac that hardly ever is open or broken.

As the baby develops during weeks six through ten of pregnancy, the intestines get longer and push out from the belly into the umbilical cord. By the eleventh week of pregnancy, the intestines normally go back into the belly. If this does not happen, an omphalocele occurs. The omphalocele can be small, with only some of the intestines outside of the belly, or it can be large, with many organs outside of the belly.

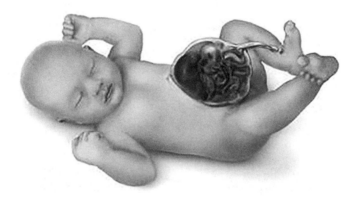

Figure 26.2. *Omphalocele*

Other Problems

Because some or all of the abdominal (belly) organs are outside of the body, babies born with an omphalocele can have other problems. The abdominal cavity, the space in the body that holds these organs, might not grow to its normal size. Also, infection is a concern, especially if the sac around the organs is broken. Sometimes, an organ might become pinched or twisted, and loss of blood flow might damage the organ.

Occurrence

The Centers for Disease Control and Prevention (CDC) estimates that each year about 775 babies in the United States are born with an omphalocele. In other words, about 1 out of every 5,386 babies born in the United States each year is born with an omphalocele. Many babies born with an omphalocele also have other birth defects, such as heart defects, neural tube defects, and chromosomal abnormalities.

Causes and Risk Factors

The causes of omphalocele among most infants are unknown. Some babies have omphalocele because of a change in their genes or chromosomes. Omphalocele might also be caused by a combination of genes and other factors, such as the things the mother comes in contact with in the environment or what the mother eats or drinks, or certain medicines she uses during pregnancy.

Understanding factors that are more common among babies with a birth defect will help the CDC learn more about the causes. CDC funds the Centers for Birth Defects Research and Prevention (CBDRP), which collaborate on large studies such as the National Birth Defects Prevention Study (NBDPS; births 1997–2011), to understand the causes of and risks for birth defects, such as omphalocele.

CDC researchers have reported important findings about some factors that can affect the risk of having a baby with an omphalocele:

- **Alcohol and tobacco**. Women who consumed alcohol or were heavy smokers (more than one pack a day) were more likely to have a baby with omphalocele.

- **Certain medications**. Women who used selective serotonin reuptake inhibitors (SSRIs) during pregnancy were more likely to have a baby with an omphalocele.

- **Obesity**. Women who were obese or overweight before pregnancy were more likely to have a baby with an omphalocele.

The CDC continues to study birth defects such as omphalocele and how to prevent them. If you are pregnant or thinking about getting pregnant, talk with your doctor about ways to increase your chances of having a healthy baby.

Diagnosis

An omphalocele can be diagnosed during pregnancy or after a baby is born.

During Pregnancy

During pregnancy, there are screening tests (prenatal tests) to check for birth defects and other conditions. An omphalocele might result in an abnormal result on a blood or serum screening test or it might be seen during an ultrasound (which creates pictures of the baby).

After a Baby Is Born

In some cases, an omphalocele might not be diagnosed until after a baby is born. An omphalocele is seen immediately at birth.

Treatments

Treatment for infants with an omphalocele depends on a number of factors, including:

- The size of the omphalocele

- The presence of other birth defects or chromosomal abnormalities

- The baby's gestational age

If the omphalocele is small (only some of the intestine is outside of the belly), it usually is treated with surgery soon after birth to put the intestine back into the belly and close the opening. If the omphalocele is large (many organs outside of the belly), the repair might be done in stages. The exposed organs might be covered with a special material, and slowly, over time, the organs will be moved back into the belly. When all the organs have been put back in the belly, the opening is closed.

Chapter 27

Anorectal Disorders

Chapter Contents

Section 27.1

Proctitis

This section includes text excerpted from "Proctitis,"
National Institute of Diabetes and Digestive and Kidney
Diseases (NIDDK), August 2016.

What Is Proctitis?

Proctitis is inflammation of the lining of your rectum. Depending on the cause, proctitis may happen suddenly and last a short time or may be long lasting.

Who Is More Likely to Develop Proctitis?

You are more likely to develop proctitis if you have:

- Engaged in anal sex with a person infected with a sexually transmitted disease (STD)

- Infections such as STDs and foodborne illnesses

- An inflammatory bowel disease (IBD) such as ulcerative colitis (UC) or Crohn disease

- Had radiation therapy to your pelvic area or lower abdomen, due to certain types of cancers

- Injured your anus or rectum

- Taken certain antibiotics

Men are more likely than women to get acute proctitis. Adults are more likely than children to get acute proctitis.

What Are the Complications of Proctitis?

If your proctitis isn't treated or doesn't respond to treatment, you may have complications, including:

- Abscesses—painful, swollen, pus-filled areas caused by infection

- Chronic or severe bleeding that can lead to anemia

- Fistulas—an abnormal passage, or tunnel, between two organs or between an organ and the outside of the body

- Rectal stricture—an abnormal narrowing of your rectum

- Ulcers—sores in the lining of your intestines

What Are the Symptoms of Proctitis?

The most common symptom of proctitis is tenesmus—an uncomfortable, frequent urge to have a bowel movement. Other symptoms of proctitis may include:

- Discharge of mucus or pus from your rectum

- A feeling of fullness in your rectum

- Pain in your anus or rectum

- Pain during bowel movements

- Cramping in your abdomen

- Pain on the left side of your abdomen

- Bleeding from your rectum

- Bloody bowel movements

- Diarrhea

- Constipation

- Swollen lymph nodes in your groin

If you are human immunodeficiency virus (HIV)-positive and have proctitis caused by genital herpes, your symptoms may be worse.

Seek Help Right Away

If you have the following symptoms, you should see a doctor right away:

- Bleeding from your rectum

- Discharge of mucus or pus from your rectum

- Severe pain in your abdomen

What Causes Proctitis
Infections

Sexually transmitted diseases (STDs) can cause proctitis if you have had anal sex with a person infected with an STD. Common STD infections that can cause proctitis include:

- Gonorrhea
- Chlamydia
- Syphilis
- Genital herpes

Infections associated with foodborne illness, such as *Salmonella*, *Shigella*, and *Campylobacter* infections, can also cause proctitis. Children with strep throat may sometimes get proctitis. They may infect the skin around their anus while cleaning the area after using the toilet or by scratching with hands that have strep bacteria from their mouth or nose. The bacteria may cause inflammation of the anus. Strep bacteria that get into the rectum may cause proctitis.

Inflammatory Bowel Disease

Two types of inflammatory bowel disease—ulcerative colitis and Crohn disease—may cause proctitis. Ulcerative colitis causes inflammation and ulcers in the large intestine. Crohn disease causes inflammation and irritation of any part of the digestive tract—most often in the end of the small intestine. However, ulcerative colitis and Crohn disease can also affect the rectum and cause proctitis.

Radiation Therapy

If you have had radiation therapy in your pelvic area or lower abdomen due to certain cancers, you may develop a condition that is similar to proctitis, called radiation proctopathy or radiation proctitis. This condition is different because the intestinal lining does not become inflamed. Up to 75 percent of patients develop radiation proctitis following pelvic radiation therapy.

Injury to the Anus or Rectum

Injury to your anus or rectum from anal sex or from putting objects or substances—including enemas—into your anus or rectum can cause proctitis.

Certain Antibiotics

Use of certain antibiotics can lead to an infection that can cause proctitis in some people. Antibiotics are medicines that kill bacteria. Even though antibiotics are meant to kill infection-causing bacteria, some antibiotics can kill good bacteria that normally live in your digestive tract. The loss of good bacteria may let a harmful bacterium called *Clostridium difficile,* or *C. difficile*, grow in the colon and rectum. *C. difficile* causes proctitis when it infects the lining of the rectum. Antibiotics that can kill good bacteria, leading to *C. difficile* infection, include:

- Clindamycin

- Those, such as cephalosporins, that treat a wide range of bacterial infections

- Any penicillin-based antibiotic such as amoxicillin

How Do Doctors Diagnose Proctitis?

Your doctor diagnoses proctitis based on your medical history, a physical exam, lab tests, and medical procedures.

Medical History

Your doctor will review your symptoms and ask you about your medical history, including:

- Current and past medical conditions

- History of radiation therapy

- Current use of antibiotics

Your doctor will also ask you about your sexual activities, including those that increase your risk of proctitis caused by a sexually transmitted disease (STD).

Physical Exam

Your doctor will perform a physical exam, which will include a digital rectal exam. During a digital rectal exam, your doctor will check for pain, bleeding, and problems such as internal hemorrhoids, polyps, and ulcers.

What Tests and Procedures Do Doctors Use to Diagnose Proctitis?
Lab Tests

Your doctor may perform one or more of the following lab tests to diagnose proctitis.

- Blood test
- Rectal culture
- Stool test

Medical Procedures

Your doctor may perform one or more of the following medical procedures to diagnose proctitis. Your doctor can also diagnose some causes of proctitis, such as Crohn disease and ulcerative colitis, and some complications of proctitis with these procedures.

- Colonoscopy
- Flexible sigmoidoscopy
- Proctoscopy—a procedure to look inside the rectum and anus using a proctoscope

How Do Doctors Treat Proctitis?

Treatment of proctitis depends on its cause and the severity of your symptoms.

Proctitis Caused by Infection

If lab tests confirm that your proctitis is due to an infection, your doctor will prescribe medicine based on the type of infection. A doctor may prescribe:

- Antibiotics to treat bacterial infections such as sexually transmitted diseases and foodborne illnesses
- Antiviral medicines to treat viral infections such as genital herpes

Proctitis Caused by Inflammatory Bowel Disease

When inflammatory bowel disease such as Crohn disease or ulcerative colitis causes proctitis, the goals of treatment are to decrease the inflammation in your intestines, prevent flare-ups of your symptoms, and keep you in remission. Your doctor may prescribe one of the following medicines:

- Aminosalicylates
- Corticosteroids

Proctitis Caused by Radiation Therapy

Doctors treat symptoms caused by radiation therapy in your pelvic area based on the severity of your symptoms. If you have mild symptoms, such as occasional bleeding or tenesmus, your proctitis may heal without treatment. Your doctor may prescribe medicines such as sucralfate (Carafate) or corticosteroid enemas to ease your pain and reduce symptoms.

Proctitis Caused by Injury to Your Anus or Rectum

When injury to your anus or rectum is the cause of your proctitis, you should stop the activity causing the injury. Healing most often occurs in four to six weeks. Your doctor may recommend antidiarrheal medicines and pain relievers.

Proctitis Caused by Certain Antibiotics

When the use of certain antibiotics results in *Clostridium difficile* (*C. difficile*) infection and causes your proctitis, your doctor will stop the antibiotic that triggered the *C. difficile* infection. He or she will prescribe a different antibiotic such as metronidazole (Flagyl), vancomycin (Vancocin), or fidaxomicin (Dificid).

How Can I Prevent Proctitis?

Doctors don't know how to prevent all types of proctitis. To prevent STD-related proctitis you should:

- Use a condom during anal sex.
- Don't have sex with anyone who has any symptoms of an STD, such as pain or a burning sensation during urination or discharge from the penis.
- Reduce your number of sex partners.

If injury to your anus or rectum caused your proctitis, stopping the activity that caused the injury often will stop the inflammation and keep proctitis from coming back.

How Do Doctors Treat the Complications of Proctitis?

If you have continual or severe bleeding, your doctor may use colonoscopy or flexible sigmoidoscopy to perform procedures that destroy rectal tissues to stop the bleeding. These procedures include:

- Thermal therapy, which uses a heat probe, an electric current, or a laser

- Cryoablation, which uses extremely cold temperatures

A surgeon may perform surgery to treat other complications of proctitis, such as abscesses, fistulas, rectal stricture, and ulcers in your intestine. Your doctor may recommend surgery to remove your rectum when other medical treatments fail, the side effects of medicines threaten your health, or your complications are severe.

How Can My Diet Help Reduce Symptoms of Proctitis?

Depending on the cause of your proctitis, changing your diet can help reduce symptoms. Your doctor may recommend that you eat more foods that are high in fiber. Eating foods that are high in fiber can make stools softer and easier to pass and can help prevent constipation. A doctor or dietitian can help you learn how to add more high-fiber foods to your diet.

If your proctitis is caused by ulcerative colitis or Crohn disease, a high-fiber diet may make symptoms worse. If you have ulcerative colitis or Crohn disease, talk with your doctor about what foods are right for you.

If you have diarrhea, you may need to avoid certain foods that can make diarrhea worse:

- Caffeine

- Fructose, a sugar found in fruits, fruit juices, and honey and added to many foods and soft drinks as a sweetener called high-fructose corn syrup

- Lactose, a sugar found in milk and milk products

- Sugar alcohols, sweeteners used in food products that are labeled "sugar-free"

Talk with your doctor before changing your diet.

Your doctor may recommend nutritional supplements or vitamins that can help reduce some proctitis symptoms:

- Omega-3 fatty acids

- Probiotics

- Vitamin C

- Vitamin E

For safety reasons, talk with your doctor before using dietary supplements or any other complementary or alternative medicines or medical practices.

Section 27.2

Rectocele

"Rectocele," © 2017 Omnigraphics.
Reviewed September 2018.

Pelvic organ prolapse, which is the descent of a pelvic organ toward or through the vaginal opening, is a common condition in women. Rectocele, a type of pelvic organ prolapse, involves the bulging (herniation) of the rectum into the vaginal wall as a result of a weakness in the recto-vaginal septum, which is the connective tissue separating the lower part of the rectum and the vagina.

The condition is more common among older women, and may occur in isolation or together with other pelvic floor disorders, such as a prolapsed bladder (cystocele) or prolapsed small intestine (enterocele). Rectocele is also referred to as posterior prolapse.

Causes

While many factors can cause rectocele, it occurs mostly in conjunction with the weakening of the pelvic floor that can occur with pregnancy, childbirth, and age. It may also be caused by pelvic floor weakness associated with hysterectomy (surgical removal of the uterus) or other pelvic surgeries. Other factors that are known to increase the risk of rectocele include chronic constipation, persistent cough, and lifting of heavy weights. These can exert pressure on the pelvic floor and weaken it. According to some studies, assisted delivery using forceps has also been linked to an increased risk of rectocele.

Symptoms

Most cases of posterior prolapse are usually discovered during a routine physical examination and are asymptomatic. Typically, a small pressure or protrusion is felt within the vagina and is accompanied by little or no discomfort. Sometimes, a rectocele may be accompanied by symptoms categorized as either vaginal or rectal. Vaginal symptoms involve the actual protrusion of the prolapsed tissue through the vaginal opening; discomfort or pain during sexual intercourse; and less frequently, vaginal bleeding.

On the other hand, rectal symptoms mostly include difficulty having a bowel movement. Rectal symptoms, particularly in moderate to severe cases of posterior prolapse, are usually accompanied by stool being trapped in the rectocele, which can lead to fecal incontinence and rectal discomfort. Stool trapping can lead to excessive straining and frequent urges to defecate, and most women who experience rectal symptoms may resort to splinting—pressing against the vaginal wall with a wad of tissue or fingers to reduce straining and push stool out during a bowel movement.

Diagnosis

A pelvic examination is the first step in diagnosing a rectocele. The patient may be asked to simulate bowel movement by straining or bearing down so the doctor can examine the size and location of the prolapsed tissue. This may be followed up with imaging tests, such as magnetic resonance imaging (MRI) or a special type of X-ray called defecography, which makes a real time visualization of the patient's defecation. Imaging studies such as those provided by a defecogram are being increasingly used for assessing pelvic floor dysfunction and deciding the line of treatment.

Treatment

Most cases of rectocele can be successfully managed with diet and lifestyle changes. Just as laxatives, increased intake of water and dietary fiber also helps ease bowel movement. In recent years, bio-feedback has emerged as an effective tool in the management of dys-functional defecation associated with pelvic floor disorders such as rectocele. This type of therapy aims to restore normal defecation by improving rectal sensory perception.

Rectocele may also be managed with vaginal pessary, one of the oldest and most effective devices for the nonsurgical management of rectocele. Pessaries are designed to provide mechanical support to the collapsed tissues within the walls of the vagina. Pelvic floor strengthening exercises are also particularly useful in the conservative management of rectocele.

Surgical intervention is considered only when symptoms inter-fere with daily activities and hamper quality of life (QOL). Generally, chronic constipation and obstructed defecation are the most common indications for surgical repair of rectocele.

Surgery

A rectocele repair can be performed by a colorectal surgeon or a gynecologist. There are four main approaches for a rectocele surgery:

1. Transanal (through the anus)

2. Transvaginal (through the vagina)

3. Transperineal (area between anus and vagina)

4. Transabdominal (through an incision in the abdomen)

While transvaginal reconstruction is the most commonly performed rectocele repair, other approaches can be considered based on the size of the rectocele, severity of symptoms, and presence of other health factors. Surgery, by and large, involves removal of redundant tissue followed by stapling of the prolapsed tissue. Sometimes, a mesh or a prosthetic patch is used to reinforce the repair and strengthen the recto-vaginal septum.

Prophylactic Measures

Activities aimed at strengthening the pelvic floor muscles can go a long way in preventing or worsening a posterior prolapse. Commonly recommended prophylactic measures include:

- Correcting constipation or other metabolic disorders that increase intra-abdominal pressure.

- Avoiding strenuous occupational or recreational activity that could exert pressure on the abdomen and cause potential damage to the pelvic floor.

- Maintaining a healthy body weight.

- Quitting smoking.

- Hormone replacement therapy may be recommended for postmenopausal women to reduce the urogenital atrophy associated with estrogen loss and strengthen the vaginal tissue.

References

1. "Posterior Vaginal Prolapse (Rectocele)," Mayo Clinic, July 25, 2017.

2. Beck, David E., Nechol, Allen L. "Rectocele," National Center for Biotechnology Information (NCBI), June 2010.

3. Lefevre, Roger, Davila, Willy G. "Functional Disorders: Rectocele," National Center for Biotechnology Information (NCBI), May 2008.

Section 27.3

Anal Fissure

An anal fissure or anal ulcer is a narrow cut or crack in the lining of the anus that may extend into the anal canal. It usually causes severe pain and bleeding during bowel movements, especially when passing hard stools. These fissures can affect people of all ages and have equal gender distribution. Most anal fissures are acute in nature and heal on their own in a few weeks. However, in chronic cases, the condition can be prolonged for more than eight weeks.

Symptoms

The typical symptoms of an anal fissure are:

- Visible tear in the anal skin
- Small lump on the skin near the anal crack or a skin tag
- Itching and burning sensation around the anal area
- Severe pain during and bowel movements
- Bright red bleeding during bowel movements
- Blood streaks on the surface of the stool

Causes

Trauma in the anus is the major cause of anal fissures. The conditions that induce trauma are:

- Constipation
- Straining during bowel movements
- Passing hard stool
- Repeated diarrhea
- Straining during childbirth
- Tight anal sphincter muscles
- Reduced blood supply to the anus
- Anal sex

Anal fissures are more common among infants and young children, who are more prone to constipation or diarrhea. Some diseases such as inflammatory bowel disease (IBD), anal cancer, tuberculosis, leukemia, and sexually transmitted diseases (STDs) can also cause anal fissure.

Diagnosis

The diagnosis of anal fissures usually involves careful visual examination of the area around the anus. Sometimes, the diagnosis may involve inserting an anoscope or endoscope into the rectum for a better evaluation. This method helps doctors to diagnose other associated conditions such as hemorrhoids.

Treatment

Most acute anal fissures do not require extensive medical treatments. Certain lifestyle changes and home remedies can be helpful to heal such conditions. In order to get rid of acute anal fissures:

- eat fiber-rich vegetables and raw fruits
- drink plenty of water and stay hydrated
- be active and exercise regularly
- keep the anal area dry and clean
- use over-the-counter (OTC) stool softeners
- treat diarrhea immediately
- take warm baths called sitz baths to relax anal muscles

If the condition is chronic, then home remedies may be insufficient and medications may need to be prescribed. The following medicines can be helpful in treating chronic anal fissures:

- Nitroglycerin ointment or a hydrocortisone cream
- Calcium channel blockers
- Botox injections into the anal sphincter to prevent spasms in anus

If the fissures fail to respond to all of the above conservative treatments, then a lateral internal sphincterotomy (LIS) can be considered. LIS is a surgical procedure that involves making a small cut in the anal sphincter muscle. The surgery helps heal the fissure by relieving pain and pressure.

References

1. "Anal Fissure," Healthline, August 29, 2018.
2. "Anal Fissure," Mayo Clinic, January 6, 2018.
3. "Anal Fissure Directory," WebMD, June 14, 2018.

Section 27.4

Anal Abscess (Fistula)

An anal abscess is a medical condition in which a collection of pus develops in a small cavity near the anus or rectum. The abscess occurs when an internal anal gland gets blocked due to infections caused by bacteria or other foreign bodies. When an anal abscess is left untreated, it may lead to a complication called anal fistula. A fistula is a small tunnel-like structure that connects the infected gland inside the anus to the outer surface of the skin. In some cases, fistulas cause persistent drainage of pus from the abscess. The fistulas are classified as: intersphincteric, transsphincteric, suprasphincteric, and extrasphincteric.

Symptoms

The most common symptoms of anal abscess and fistula are:

- Pain and swelling around the anal area
- Pain during bowel movements
- Constipation
- Bleeding
- Fatigue
- Fever and chills
- Discharge of foul-smelling pus
- Skin irritation and redness around the anus
- Painful urination

Causes

The major cause of an anal fistula is an anal abscess. But an anal abscess may have many different causes and risk factors:

- Constipation
- Diarrhea
- Diabetes

- Sexually transmitted diseases (STDs)
- Inflammatory bowel diseases (IBDs) such as Crohn disease
- Diverticulitis
- Use of steroids such as prednisone
- Recent chemotherapy treatment
- Anal sex

Diagnosis

Anal abscess and fistula are usually diagnosed through physical examination. In the case of an anal abscess, the doctor looks for redness and swelling around the anal area and a swollen lump or nodule along the rim of the anus. If there are no such visible signs, then an endoscope is used to obtain a better view. In cases in which the patient is suspected of having a fistula, the doctor looks for an external opening in the anal skin. Special instruments such as ultrasound or magnetic resonance imaging (MRI) are used to track the path of the fistula.

Treatment

The common treatment for anal abscess and fistula is to remove the pus from the infected area through surgery. Most of these surgeries are performed on an outpatient basis with local anesthesia. However, critical cases may require a short-term hospitalization. Sometimes, catheters are used to drain the pus completely. If the opening on the outer surface of the skin heals with the tunnel or fistula still under the skin, then there may be a recurrence of abscess. Therefore, it is important to eliminate the fistula completely. In order to do that, the skin and muscle over the fistula are cut into a groove, which allows the fistula to heal from the inside out.

After the surgery, it is recommended that patients soak the affected area in a warm bath regularly in order to speed up the healing.

References

1. "Anal/Rectal Abscess," Healthline, December 11, 2017.

2. Ratini, Melinda. "Anal Abscess," WebMD, September 11, 2017.

3. "Anal Fistula," Cleveland Clinic, January 16, 2015.

4. "Abscess and Fistula Expanded Information," American Society of Colon and Rectal Surgeons (ASCRS), November 6, 2012.

Chapter 28

Hemorrhoids

What Are Hemorrhoids?

Hemorrhoids, also called piles, are swollen and inflamed veins around your anus or in your lower rectum.

The two types of hemorrhoids are:

- External hemorrhoids, which form under the skin around the anus

- Internal hemorrhoids, which form in the lining of the anus and lower rectum

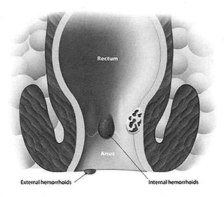

Figure 28.1. *Hemorrhoids*

This chapter includes text excerpted from "Hemorrhoids," National Institute of Diabetes and Digestive and Kidney Diseases (NIDDK), October 2016.

How Common Are Hemorrhoids?

Hemorrhoids are common in both men and women and affect about 1 in 20 Americans. About half of adults older than age 50 have hemorrhoids.

Who Is More Likely to Get Hemorrhoids?

You are more likely to get hemorrhoids if you:

- Strain during bowel movements
- Sit on the toilet for long periods of time
- Have chronic constipation or diarrhea
- Eat foods that are low in fiber
- Are older than age 50
- Are pregnant
- Often lift heavy objects

What Are the Complications of Hemorrhoids?

Complications of hemorrhoids can include the following:

- Blood clots in an external hemorrhoid
- Skin tags—extra skin left behind when a blood clot in external hemorrhoid dissolves
- Infection of a sore on an external hemorrhoid
- Strangulated hemorrhoid—when the muscles around your anus cut off the blood supply to an internal hemorrhoid that has fallen through your anal opening
- Anemia

What Are the Symptoms of Hemorrhoids?

The symptoms of hemorrhoids depend on the type you have. If you have external hemorrhoids, you may have:

- Anal itching
- One or more hard, tender lumps near your anus
- Anal ache or pain, especially when sitting

Too much straining, rubbing, or cleaning around your anus may make your symptoms worse. For many people, the symptoms of external hemorrhoids go away within a few days.

If you have internal hemorrhoids, you may have:

- Bleeding from your rectum—bright red blood on stool, on toilet paper, or in the toilet bowl after a bowel movement

- A hemorrhoid that has fallen through your anal opening, called prolapse

Internal hemorrhoids that are not prolapsed most often are not painful. Prolapsed internal hemorrhoids may cause pain and discomfort. Although hemorrhoids are the most common cause of anal symptoms, not every anal symptom is caused by a hemorrhoid. Some hemorrhoid symptoms are similar to those of other digestive tract problems. For example, bleeding from your rectum may be a sign of bowel diseases such as Crohn disease, ulcerative colitis (UC), or cancer of the colon or rectum.

When Should I Seek a Doctor's Help?

You should seek a doctor's help if you:

- Still have symptoms after one week of at-home treatment
- Have bleeding from your rectum

What Causes Hemorrhoids

The causes of hemorrhoids include:

- Straining during bowel movements
- Sitting on the toilet for long periods of time
- Chronic constipation or diarrhea
- A low-fiber diet
- Weakening of the supporting tissues in your anus and rectum that happens with aging
- Pregnancy
- Often lifting heavy objects

How Are Hemorrhoids Diagnosed?

Your doctor can often diagnose hemorrhoids based on your medical history and a physical exam. He or she can diagnose external hemorrhoids by checking the area around your anus. To diagnose internal hemorrhoids, your doctor will perform a digital rectal exam and may perform procedures to look inside your anus and rectum.

Medical History

Your doctor will ask you to provide your medical history and describe your symptoms. He or she will ask you about your eating habits, toilet habits, enema and laxative use, and current medical conditions.

Physical Exam

Your doctor will check the area around your anus for:

- Lumps or swelling
- Internal hemorrhoids that have fallen through your anal opening, called prolapse
- External hemorrhoids with a blood clot in a vein
- Leakage of stool or mucus
- Skin irritation
- Skin tags—extra skin that is left behind when a blood clot in external hemorrhoid dissolves
- Anal fissures—a small tear in the anus that may cause itching, pain, or bleeding

Your doctor will perform a digital rectal exam to:

- Check the tone of the muscles in your anus
- Check for tenderness, blood, internal hemorrhoids, and lumps or masses

Procedures

Your doctor may use the following procedures to diagnose internal hemorrhoids:

- Anoscopy
- Rigid proctosigmoidoscopy

Your doctor may diagnose internal hemorrhoids while performing procedures for other digestive tract problems or during a routine examination of your rectum and colon. These procedures include colonoscopy and flexible sigmoidoscopy.

How Can I Treat My Hemorrhoids?

You can most often treat your hemorrhoids at home by:

- Eating foods that are high in fiber
- Taking a stool softener or a fiber supplement such as psyllium (Metamucil) or methylcellulose (Citrucel)
- Drinking water or other nonalcoholic liquids each day as recommended by your healthcare professional
- Not straining during bowel movements
- Not sitting on the toilet for long periods of time
- Taking over-the-counter (OTC) pain relievers such as acetaminophen, ibuprofen, naproxen, or aspirin
- Sitting in a tub of warm water, called a sitz bath, several times a day to help relieve pain

Applying OTC hemorrhoid creams or ointments or using suppositories—a medicine you insert into your rectum—may relieve mild pain, swelling, and itching of external hemorrhoids. Most often, doctors recommend using OTC products for one week. You should follow up with your doctor if the products:

- Do not relieve your symptoms after one week
- Cause side effects such dry skin around your anus or a rash

Most prolapsed internal hemorrhoids go away without at-home treatment. However, severely prolapsed or bleeding internal hemorrhoids may need medical treatment.

How Do Doctors Treat Hemorrhoids?

Doctors treat hemorrhoids with procedures during an office visit or in an outpatient center or a hospital. Office treatments include the following:

- **Rubber band ligation.** Rubber band ligation is a procedure that doctors use to treat bleeding or prolapsing internal hemorrhoids. A doctor places a special rubber band around the base of the hemorrhoid. The band cuts off the blood supply. The banded part of the hemorrhoid shrivels and falls off, most often within a week. Scar tissue forms in the remaining part of the hemorrhoid, often shrinking the hemorrhoid. Only a doctor should perform this procedure—you should never try this treatment yourself.

- **Sclerotherapy.** A doctor injects a solution into an internal hemorrhoid, which causes scar tissue to form. The scar tissue cuts off the blood supply, often shrinking the hemorrhoid.

- **Infrared photocoagulation.** A doctor uses a tool that directs infrared light at an internal hemorrhoid. Heat created by the infrared light causes scar tissue to form, which cuts off the blood supply, often shrinking the hemorrhoid.

- **Electrocoagulation.** A doctor uses a tool that sends an electric current into an internal hemorrhoid. The electric current causes scar tissue to form, which cuts off the blood supply, often shrinking the hemorrhoid.

Outpatient center or hospital treatments include the following:

- **Hemorrhoidectomy.** A doctor, most often a surgeon, may perform a hemorrhoidectomy to remove large external hemorrhoids and prolapsing internal hemorrhoids that do not respond to other treatments. Your doctor will give you anesthesia for this treatment.

- **Hemorrhoid stapling.** A doctor, most often a surgeon, may use a special stapling tool to remove internal hemorrhoid tissue and pull a prolapsing internal hemorrhoid back into the anus. Your doctor will give you anesthesia for this treatment.

- Sometimes complications of hemorrhoids also require treatment.

How Can I Prevent Hemorrhoids?

You can help prevent hemorrhoids by:

- Eating foods that are high in fiber

- Drinking water or other nonalcoholic liquids each day as recommended by your healthcare professional

- Not straining during bowel movements

- Not sitting on the toilet for long periods of time
- Avoiding regular heavy lifting

What Should I Eat If I Have Hemorrhoids?

Your doctor may recommend that you eat more foods that are high in fiber. Eating foods that are high in fiber can make stools softer and easier to pass and can help treat and prevent hemorrhoids. Drinking water and other liquids, such as fruit juices and clear soups, can help the fiber in your diet work better. Ask your doctor about how much you should drink each day based on your health and activity level and where you live.

The *2015–2020 Dietary Guidelines for Americans* recommends a dietary fiber intake of 14 grams per 1,000 calories consumed. For example, for a 2,000-calorie diet, the fiber recommendation is 28 grams per day.

The amount of fiber in a food is listed on the food's nutrition facts label. Some fiber-rich foods are listed in the table below.

Table 28.1. Fiber-Rich Foods

Food and Portion Size	Amount of Fiber
Grains	
⅓–¾ cup high-fiber bran, ready-to-eat cereal	9.1 to 14.3 grams
1–1¼ cups of shredded wheat, ready-to-eat cereal	5.0 to 9.0 grams
1½ cups whole-wheat spaghetti, cooked	3.2 grams
One small oat bran muffin	3.0 grams
Fruits	
One medium pear, with skin	5.5 grams
One medium apple, with skin	4.4 grams
½ cup of raspberries	4.0 grams
½ cup of stewed prunes	3.8 grams
Vegetables	
½ cup of green peas, cooked	3.5–4.4 grams
½ cup of mixed vegetables, cooked from frozen	4.0 grams
½ cup of collards, cooked	3.8 grams
One medium sweet potato, baked in skin	3.8 grams
One medium potato, baked, with skin	3.6 grams
½ cup of winter squash, cooked	2.9 grams

Table 28.1. Continued

Food and Portion Size	Amount of Fiber
Beans	
½ cup navy beans, cooked	9.6 grams
½ cup pinto beans, cooked	7.7 grams
½ cup kidney beans, cooked	5.7 grams

A doctor or dietitian can help you learn how to add more high-fiber foods to your diet.

What Should I Avoid Eating If I Have Hemorrhoids?

If your hemorrhoids are caused by chronic constipation, try not to eat too many foods with little or no fiber, such as:

- Cheese
- Chips
- Fast food
- Ice cream
- Meat
- Prepared foods, such as some frozen and snack foods
- Processed foods, such as hot dogs and some microwavable dinners

Chapter 29

Structural Defects of the Lower GI Tract

What Are Anatomic Problems of the Lower GI Tract?

- Anatomic problems of the lower gastrointestinal (GI) tract are structural defects. Anatomic problems that develop before birth are known as congenital abnormalities. Other anatomic problems may occur any time after birth—from infancy into adulthood.

- The GI tract is a series of hollow organs joined in a long, twisting tube from the mouth to the anus. The movement of muscles in the GI tract, along with the release of hormones and enzymes, allows for the digestion of food. Organs that make up the GI tract are the mouth, esophagus, stomach, small intestine, large intestine—which includes the appendix, cecum, colon, and rectum—and anus. The intestines are sometimes called the bowel. The last part of the GI tract—called the lower GI tract—consists of the large intestine and anus.

- The large intestine is about five feet long in adults and absorbs water and any remaining nutrients from partially digested

This chapter includes text excerpted from "Anatomic Problems of the Lower GI Tract," National Institute of Diabetes and Digestive and Kidney Diseases (NIDDK), July 2013. Reviewed September 2018.

food passed from the small intestine. The large intestine then changes waste from liquid to a solid matter called stool. Stool passes from the colon to the rectum. The rectum is six to eight inches long in adults and is located between the last part of the colon—called the sigmoid colon—and the anus. The rectum stores stool prior to a bowel movement. During a bowel movement, the muscles of the rectal wall contract to move stool from the rectum to the anus, a one-inch-long opening through which stool leaves the body.

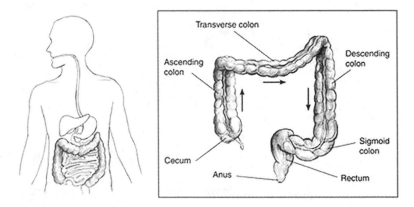

Figure 29.1. *Lower GI Tract*

- Anatomic problems of the lower GI tract may involve parts of organs being in the wrong place, shaped abnormally, or incorrectly connected to other organs. Anatomic problems that affect the large intestine or anus include:

  - Malrotation

  - Volvulus

  - Intussusception

  - Fistula

  - Imperforate anus

  - Colonic atresia

How Does the Lower GI Tract Develop?

About four weeks into gestation—the nine-month period from conception to birth—the intestines of the developing baby, or fetus, consist of a thin, straight tube that connects the stomach and the rectum. Over the next two weeks, the rapidly developing intestines outgrow the baby's abdomen and move into the umbilical cord, which connects the baby to the mother. During gestational weeks 10–12, the baby's abdomen has grown large enough to hold the intestines, which return to the abdomen, rotating counterclockwise to their final position. The intestines are held in place by tissue called mesentery.

What Is Malrotation?

Malrotation is when the intestines do not rotate completely or correctly during gestation. Malrotation can cause serious medical problems in some infants and children, while others may never develop problems. Surgeons estimate that problems with malrotation occur in a small percentage of cases and are usually diagnosed in the first month of life. Boys are more likely than girls to be diagnosed with malrotation during infancy, but problems identified later in childhood are equally likely in boys and girls. Malrotation rarely occurs in adults.

Malrotation can prevent the cecum—the beginning of the large intestine—from moving to its normal position in the lower right area of the abdomen. If this happens, bands of mesentery can block the small intestine, creating an intestinal obstruction—also called bowel obstruction—a life-threatening event and a medical emergency. Malrotation may also leave the mesentery only narrowly attached to the back of the abdomen. This incomplete attachment may result in the intestine twisting—a serious condition called volvulus.

Symptoms of Malrotation

Infants who have serious problems resulting from malrotation experience pain that can be severe, and they often vomit bile—a greenish-yellow fluid. Other symptoms may include:

- Abdominal tenderness, swelling, or bloating
- Bloody or dark-red stools
- Constipation—a condition in which a child has fewer than two bowel movements a week
- Dehydration, or abnormal loss of body fluids—decreased tears and little or no urine or dark-yellow urine may be observed
- Signs of shock—paleness, sweating, confusion, and rapid pulse
- Weight loss

Older children with problems from malrotation may have the above symptoms as well as nausea, abdominal pain, diarrhea, or an abnormal growth rate, as compared with their peers. Infants or children with any of the above symptoms should be evaluated immediately by a healthcare provider.

Diagnosis and Treatment of Malrotation

Doctors use X-rays of the abdomen and imaging studies to diagnose intestinal problems related to malrotation.

- Computerized tomography (CT) scan
- Upper GI series
- Lower GI series

The above tests are all performed at a hospital or outpatient center by an X-ray technician, and the images are interpreted by a radiologist—a doctor who specializes in medical imaging. Surgery is almost always required to correct problems resulting from malrotation. A surgeon performs the procedure in a hospital and the child is given general anesthesia. With early diagnosis and treatment, surgery is usually successful and may involve:

- Repositioning the large and small intestines
- Dividing the bands of mesentery blocking the small intestine
- Removing the appendix, a four-inch pouch attached to the cecum
- Untwisting the large intestine if volvulus has occurred

What Is Volvulus?

Volvulus occurs when the intestine twists around itself and the mesentery that supports it, creating an obstruction. The area of intestine above the obstruction continues to function and fills with food, fluid, and gas. The mesentery may become so tightly twisted that blood flow to the affected part of the intestine is cut off. This situation can lead to death of the blood-starved tissue and tearing of the intestinal wall—a life-threatening event and a medical emergency.

Volvulus can be caused by malrotation or by other medical conditions such as:

- An enlarged colon
- Hirschsprung disease, a disease of the large intestine that causes severe constipation or intestinal obstruction

- Abdominal adhesions, or bands of scar tissue that form as part of the healing process following abdominal injury, infection, or surgery

Sigmoid volvulus—twisting of the sigmoid colon—accounts for the majority of cases, with cecal volvulus—twisting of the cecum and ascending colon—occurring less frequently.

Sigmoid Volvulus

Anatomic problems that increase a person's risk of developing sigmoid volvulus include:

- An elongated or movable sigmoid colon that is not attached to the left wall of the abdomen

- A narrow mesentery connection at the base of the sigmoid colon

- Malrotation that presents with problems in infancy

Sigmoid volvulus that occurs after infancy is more commonly seen in people who:

- Are male

- Are older than age 60

- Live in a nursing or psychiatric facility

- Have a history of mental-health conditions

Symptoms of Sigmoid Volvulus

Sigmoid volvulus symptoms can be severe and occur suddenly. Symptoms may include:

- Abdominal cramping

- Bloody stools

- Constipation

- Nausea

- Signs of shock

- Vomiting

People with any of these symptoms should be evaluated immediately by a healthcare provider. Other symptoms may develop more slowly but worsen with time, such as constipation, inability to pass gas, and abdominal swelling. People with these symptoms should also contact a healthcare provider.

Diagnosis and Treatment of Sigmoid Volvulus

Prompt diagnosis and appropriate treatment of sigmoid volvulus generally lead to a successful outcome. Doctors use X-rays, upper or lower GI series, computed tomography (CT) scans, and flexible sigmoidoscopy—another common diagnostic test—to help diagnose sigmoid volvulus.

If volvulus is found, the doctor may use the sigmoidoscope to untwist the colon. However, if the colon is twisted tightly or if the blood flow has been cut off, immediate surgery will be needed. Surgery involves restoring the blood supply, if possible, to the affected part of the sigmoid colon. Sometimes the affected part of the colon must be removed and the healthy ends reattached, a procedure called an intestinal resection. Resection prevents volvulus from recurring; untwisting the volvulus with the sigmoidoscope may not prevent recurrence.

Cecal volvulus

Cecal volvulus is twisting of the cecum and ascending colon. Normally, the cecum and ascending colon are fixed to the abdominal wall. If improperly attached, they can move and become twisted.

Symptoms of Cecal Volvulus

More commonly seen in people ages 30–60, cecal volvulus may be caused by abdominal adhesions, severe coughing, or pregnancy. People with cecal volvulus often have intermittent chronic symptoms—those that come and go over a longer period of time—including:

- Abdominal cramping or swelling

- Nausea

- Vomiting

People with any of the above symptoms should be evaluated immediately by a healthcare provider. Other symptoms may develop more slowly but worsen with time, such as constipation, inability to pass gas, and abdominal swelling. People with these symptoms should also contact a healthcare provider.

Diagnosis and Treatment of Cecal Volvulus

Doctors use X-rays, upper or lower GI series, and CT scans to diagnose cecal volvulus. Imaging shows whether the cecum is out of place and inflated with trapped air. Imaging may also show that the appendix, which is attached to the cecum, is filled with air. To treat cecal volvulus, surgeons use a procedure called cecopexy to reposition the cecum and attach it to the abdominal wall. If the cecum is seriously damaged by volvulus, the surgeon will perform intestinal resection surgery. Cecopexy and intestinal resection surgery have high rates of success and usually prevent the recurrence of cecal volvulus.

What Is Imperforate Anus?

Imperforate anus occurs during gestation and involves abnormal development of the rectum and anus. This condition results in a blocked or missing anus, which allows little or no stool to pass from the rectum. Imperforate anus is uncommon and occurs slightly more often in boys than in girls. Types of imperforate anus include:

- An anus that is narrow or blocked by a thin membrane—this condition is also called anal atresia

- An anus that is missing or incorrectly placed

- A rectum that is not connected to the anus

- A rectum that is connected to the urinary tract or genitals by a fistula

Although most girls with imperforate anus have a less severe form of the condition, such as anal atresia, some are born with a more severe form of imperforate anus called cloaca—a common opening for the rectum, bladder, and vagina.

Symptoms of Imperforate Anus

Imperforate anus is observed when a newborn is first examined after birth. In addition to visible indications such as an incorrectly placed anus, imperforate anus may be associated with symptoms that include abdominal swelling and the absence of bowel movements.

Diagnosis and Treatment of Imperforate Anus

The severity of imperforate anus depends on where the blockage is situated—low, intermediate, or high—in relation to the set of muscles that support the rectum and other organs within the pelvic region. X-rays of the abdomen and CT scans can help determine the severity of the condition. The doctor may perform other tests to look for abnormalities in the urinary tract.

Correcting the imperforate anus almost always requires surgery, and the type of procedure depends on the location and severity of the defect. For example, a low imperforate anus may only require gently widening the anus. Sometimes anoplasty—a surgery to rebuild or move the anus—is needed within the first days after birth. Intermediate or high imperforate anus may require multiple surgeries done in stages. Girls with cloaca may require multiple extensive and complicated surgeries.

The outcome of surgery is measured by the child's ability to eventually control bowel movements. Most children treated for imperforate anus develop voluntary bowel movements at the usual age of toilet training. However, some children may not achieve good bowel control after surgery because the anal muscles do not develop properly. Factors affecting the outcome of surgery include:

- Location of the defect—treatment of low imperforate anus has a more successful long-term outcome than intermediate or high imperforate anus

- The child's sex—girls tend to have a low imperforate anus, which can be corrected more easily and has more successful long-term results

- Age at the time of surgery—the younger the child when surgery is done, the more successful the outcome

What Is Colonic Atresia?

Colonic atresia (CA) is an extremely rare congenital anomaly that occurs when a section of the colon closes before birth. Symptoms appear in infants soon after birth and include vomiting, abdominal swelling, and the absence of bowel movements. Intestinal resection surgery is performed immediately after diagnosis.

Eating, Diet, and Nutrition

Eating, diet, and nutrition have not been shown to play a role in causing or preventing anatomic problems of the lower GI tract.

Chapter 30

Other Disorders of the Lower Gastrointestinal Tract

Chapter Contents

Section 30.1

Abdominal Adhesions

This section includes text excerpted from "Abdominal Adhesions," National Institute of Diabetes and Digestive and Kidney Diseases (NIDDK), September 2013. Reviewed September 2018.

What Are Abdominal Adhesions?

Abdominal adhesions are bands of fibrous tissue that can form between abdominal tissues and organs. Normally, internal tissues and organs have slippery surfaces, preventing them from sticking together as the body moves. However, abdominal adhesions cause tissues and organs in the abdominal cavity to stick together.

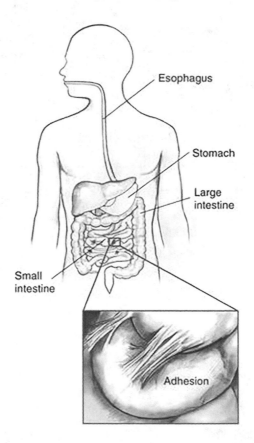

Figure 30.1. *Abdominal Adhesions*

What Is the Abdominal Cavity?

The abdominal cavity is the internal area of the body between the chest and hips that contains the lower part of the esophagus, stomach, small intestine, and large intestine. The esophagus carries food and liquids from the mouth to the stomach, which slowly pumps them into the small and large intestines. Abdominal adhesions can kink, twist, or pull the small and large intestines out of place, causing an intestinal obstruction. Intestinal obstruction, also called a bowel obstruction, results in the partial or complete blockage of movement of food or stool through the intestines.

What Causes Abdominal Adhesions

Abdominal surgery is the most frequent cause of abdominal adhesions. Surgery-related causes include:

- Cuts involving internal organs

- Handling of internal organs

- Drying out of internal organs and tissues

- Contact of internal tissues with foreign materials, such as gauze, surgical gloves, and stitches

- Blood or blood clots that were not rinsed away during surgery

Abdominal adhesions can also result from inflammation not related to surgery, including:

- Appendix rupture

- Radiation treatment

- Gynecological infections

- Abdominal infections

Rarely, abdominal adhesions form without apparent cause.

How Common Are Abdominal Adhesions and Who Is at Risk?

Of patients who undergo abdominal surgery, 93 percent develop abdominal adhesions. Surgery in the lower abdomen and pelvis, including bowel and gynecological operations, carries an even greater chance of abdominal adhesions. Abdominal adhesions can become larger and tighter as time passes, sometimes causing problems years after surgery.

What Are the Symptoms of Abdominal Adhesions?

In most cases, abdominal adhesions do not cause symptoms. When symptoms are present, chronic abdominal pain is the most common.

What Are the Complications of Abdominal Adhesions?

Abdominal adhesions can cause intestinal obstruction and female infertility—the inability to become pregnant after a year of trying. Abdominal adhesions can lead to female infertility by preventing fertilized eggs from reaching the uterus, where fetal development takes place. Women with abdominal adhesions in or around their fallopian tubes have an increased chance of ectopic pregnancy—a fertilized egg growing outside the uterus. Abdominal adhesions inside the uterus may result in repeated miscarriages—a pregnancy failure before 20 weeks.

How Are Abdominal Adhesions and Intestinal Obstructions Diagnosed?

Abdominal adhesions cannot be detected by tests or seen through imaging techniques such as X-rays or ultrasound. Most abdominal adhesions are found during surgery performed to examine the abdomen. However, abdominal X-rays, a lower gastrointestinal (GI) series, and computerized tomography (CT) scans can diagnose intestinal obstructions.

How Are Abdominal Adhesions and Intestinal Obstructions Treated?

Abdominal adhesions that do not cause symptoms generally do not require treatment. Surgery is the only way to treat abdominal adhesions that cause pain, intestinal obstruction, or fertility problems. More surgery, however, carries the risk of additional abdominal adhesions. People should speak with their healthcare provider about the best way to treat their abdominal adhesions. Complete intestinal obstructions usually require immediate surgery to clear the blockage. Most partial intestinal obstructions can be managed without surgery.

How Can Abdominal Adhesions Be Prevented?

Abdominal adhesions are difficult to prevent; however, certain surgical techniques can minimize abdominal adhesions. Laparoscopic surgery decreases the potential for abdominal adhesions because several tiny incisions are made in the lower abdomen instead of one large incision. The surgeon inserts a laparoscope—a thin tube with a tiny video camera attached—into one of the small incisions. The camera sends a magnified image from inside the body to a video monitor. Patients will usually receive general anesthesia during this surgery.

If laparoscopic surgery is not possible and a large abdominal incision is required, at the end of surgery a special film-like material can be inserted between organs or between the organs and the abdominal incision. The film-like material, which looks similar to wax paper and is absorbed by the body in about a week, hydrates organs to help prevent abdominal adhesions.

Other steps taken during surgery to reduce abdominal adhesions include:

- Using starch- and latex-free gloves
- Handling tissues and organs gently
- Shortening surgery time
- Using moistened drapes and swabs
- Occasionally applying saline solution

Eating, Diet, and Nutrition

Researchers have not found that eating, diet, and nutrition play a role in causing or preventing abdominal adhesions. A person with a partial intestinal obstruction may relieve symptoms with a liquid or low-fiber diet, which is more easily broken down into smaller particles by the digestive system.

Section 30.2

Intestinal Pseudo-Obstruction

This section includes text excerpted from "Intestinal Pseudo-Obstruction," National Institute of Diabetes and Digestive and Kidney Diseases (NIDDK), February 2014. Reviewed September 2018.

What Is Intestinal Pseudo-Obstruction?

Intestinal pseudo-obstruction is a rare condition with symptoms that resemble those caused by a blockage, or obstruction, of the intestines, also called the bowel. However, when a healthcare provider examines the intestines, no blockage exists. Instead, the symptoms are due to nerve or muscle problems that affect the movement of food, fluid, and air through the intestines.

The intestines are part of the gastrointestinal (GI) tract and include the small intestine and the large intestine. The small intestine is the organ where most digestion occurs. The small intestine measures about 20 feet and includes the:

- Duodenum, the first part of the small intestine

- Jejunum, the middle section of the small intestine

- Ileum, the lower end of the small intestine

The large intestine absorbs water from stool and changes it from a liquid to a solid form, which passes out of the body during a bowel movement. The large intestine measures about five feet and includes the:

- Cecum, the first part of the large intestine, which is connected to the ileum

- Colon, the part of the large intestine extending from the cecum to the rectum

- Rectum, the lower end of the large intestine leading to the anus

Who Is More Likely to Have Intestinal Pseudo-Obstruction?

This condition can occur in people of any age. Some infants are born with congenital intestinal pseudo-obstruction, and some people develop this condition as adults. Intestinal pseudo-obstruction may be acute, occurring suddenly and lasting a short time, or it may be chronic, or long lasting. Acute colonic pseudo-obstruction (ACPO), also called Ogilvie syndrome or acute colonic ileus, mostly affects older adults. In this condition, the colon becomes distended or enlarged, after:

- Surgery, such as operations to open the abdomen or replace a hip or knee

- Injury, such as a hip fracture

- Illness, such as a serious infection

Acute colonic pseudo-obstruction can lead to serious complications. However, people with the condition usually get better with treatment.

What Causes Intestinal Pseudo-Obstruction

Problems with nerves, muscles, or interstitial cells of Cajal cause intestinal pseudo-obstruction. Interstitial cells of Cajal are called "pacemaker" cells because they set the pace of intestinal contractions. These cells convey messages from nerves to muscles.

Problems with nerves, muscles, or interstitial cells of Cajal prevent normal contractions of the intestines and cause problems with the movement of food, fluid, and air through the intestines.

Primary or idiopathic intestinal pseudo-obstruction is intestinal pseudo-obstruction that occurs by itself. In some people with primary intestinal pseudo-obstruction, mutations, or changes, in genes—traits passed from parent to child—cause the condition. However, health-care providers do not typically order genetic testing for an intestinal pseudo-obstruction, as they don't commonly recognize gene mutations as a cause.

Some people have duplications or deletions of genetic material in the *Filamin A, alpha (FLNA)* gene. Researchers believe that these genetic changes may impair the function of a protein, causing problems with the nerve cells in the intestines. As a result, the nerves cannot work with the intestinal muscles to produce normal contractions that move food, fluid, and air through the digestive tract. Also, these genetic changes may account for some of the other signs and symptoms that can occur with intestinal pseudo-obstruction, such as bladder symptoms and muscle weakness.

A condition called mitochondrial neurogastrointestinal encephalopathy (MNGIE) may also cause primary intestinal pseudo-obstruction. In people with this condition, mitochondria—structures in cells that

411

produce energy—do not function normally. Mitochondrial neurogas-trointestinal encephalopathy can also cause other symptoms, such as problems with nerves in the limbs and changes in the brain.

Secondary intestinal pseudo-obstruction develops as a complication of another medical condition. Causes of secondary intestinal pseu-do-obstruction include:

- Abdominal or pelvic surgery
- Diseases that affect muscles and nerves, such as lupus erythematosus, scleroderma, and Parkinson disease
- Infections
- Medications, such as opiates and antidepressants, that affect muscles and nerves
- Radiation to the abdomen
- Certain cancers, including lung cancer

What Are the Symptoms of Intestinal Pseudo-Obstruction?

Intestinal pseudo-obstruction symptoms may include:

- Abdominal swelling or bloating, also called distension
- Abdominal pain
- Nausea
- Vomiting
- Constipation
- Diarrhea

Over time, the condition can cause malnutrition, bacterial over-growth in the intestines, and weight loss. Malnutrition is a condition that develops when the body does not get the right amount of the vitamins, minerals, and other nutrients it needs to maintain healthy tissues and organ function. Some people develop problems with their esophagus, stomach, or bladder.

How Is Intestinal Pseudo-Obstruction Diagnosed?

To diagnose intestinal pseudo-obstruction, a healthcare provider may suggest the person consult a gastroenterologist—a doctor who specializes in digestive diseases. A healthcare provider will perform a physical exam; take a complete medical history, imaging studies, and a biopsy; and perform blood tests. A healthcare provider may order other tests to confirm the diagnosis. The healthcare provider also will look for the cause of the condition, such as an underlying illness.

Intestinal pseudo-obstruction can be difficult to diagnose, especially primary intestinal pseudo-obstruction. As a result, a correct diagnosis may take a long time.

Physical Exam

A physical exam is one of the first things a healthcare provider may do to help diagnose intestinal pseudo-obstruction. During a physical exam, a healthcare provider usually:

- Examines a person's body
- Uses a stethoscope to listen to bodily sounds
- Taps on specific areas of the person's body

Medical History

The healthcare provider will ask a person to provide a medical and family history to help diagnose intestinal pseudo-obstruction.

Imaging Studies

A healthcare provider may order the following imaging studies:
- Abdominal X-ray
- Upper GI series
- Lower GI series
- Computerized tomography (CT) scan
- Upper GI endoscopy

Biopsy

A gastroenterologist can obtain a biopsy of the intestinal wall during endoscopy or during surgery, if the person has surgery for intestinal pseudo-obstruction and the cause is unknown. If the healthcare provider needs to examine the nerves in the intestinal wall, a deeper biopsy, which a gastroenterologist can typically obtain only during surgery, is necessary.

413

A biopsy is a procedure that involves taking a piece of the intestinal wall tissue for examination with a microscope. A healthcare provider performs the biopsy in a hospital and uses light sedation and local anesthetic; the healthcare provider uses general anesthesia if performing the biopsy during surgery. A pathologist—a doctor who specializes in diagnosing diseases—examines the intestinal tissue in a lab. Diagnosing problems in the nerve pathways of the intestinal tissue requires special techniques that are not widely available.

A healthcare provider can also use a biopsy obtained during endoscopy to rule out celiac disease. Celiac disease is an autoimmune disorder in which people cannot tolerate gluten because it damages the lining of their small intestine and prevents absorption of nutrients. Gluten is a protein found in wheat, rye, and barley and in products such as vitamin and nutrient supplements, lip balms, and certain medications.

Blood Tests

A blood test involves drawing blood at a healthcare provider's office or a commercial facility and sending the sample to a lab for analysis. The blood test can show the presence of other diseases or conditions that may be causing a person's symptoms. The blood test also can show levels of essential vitamins and minerals to help detect malnutrition.

Manometry

Manometry is a test that measures muscle pressure and movements in the GI tract, such as how well the smooth muscles of the stomach and small intestine contract and relax. A gastroenterologist performs the test at a hospital or an outpatient center. While the person is under sedation, a healthcare provider places a thin tube, or manometry tube, into the stomach and moves it down into the small intestine. A gastroenterologist may use an endoscope to place this tube. A healthcare provider will move the person to a manometry room and connect the manometry tube to a computer. When the person wakes up from sedation, the computer records the pressure inside the intestine while the person is fasting and after the person has eaten a meal. Manometry can confirm the diagnosis of intestinal pseudo-obstruction and show the extent of the condition.

Gastric Emptying Tests

Gastric emptying tests can show if a disorder called gastroparesis is causing a person's symptoms. People with gastroparesis, which literally refers to a paralyzed stomach, have severely delayed gastric emptying, or the delayed movement of food from the stomach to the small intestine. Some patients with intestinal pseudo-obstruction also have gastroparesis.

Types of gastric emptying tests include the following:

- Gastric emptying scintigraphy
- Breath test
- SmartPill

How Is Intestinal Pseudo-Obstruction Treated?

A healthcare provider will treat intestinal pseudo-obstruction with nutritional support, medications, and, in some cases, decompression. Rarely, a person will need surgery. If an illness, a medication, or both cause intestinal pseudo-obstruction, a healthcare provider will treat the underlying illness, stop the medication, or do both.

Nutritional Support

People with intestinal pseudo-obstruction often need nutritional support to prevent malnutrition and weight loss. Enteral nutrition provides liquid food through a feeding tube inserted through the nose into the stomach or placed directly into the stomach or small intestine. A healthcare provider inserts the feeding tube, sometimes using X-ray or endoscopy for guidance, and teaches the person how to care for the tube after returning home. Enteral nutrition is sufficient for most people with intestinal pseudo-obstruction. In a severe case, a person may need intravenous (IV) feeding, also called parenteral nutrition, which provides liquid food through a tube placed in a vein.

Enteral nutrition is possible because the intestinal lining is normal in most people with intestinal pseudo-obstruction. Enteral nutrition is preferred over parenteral nutrition because it has a much lower risk of complications.

Medications

A healthcare provider prescribes medications to treat the different symptoms and complications of intestinal pseudo-obstruction, such as:

- Antibiotics to treat bacterial infections
- Pain medication, which should be used sparingly, if at all, because most pain medications delay intestinal transit

- Medication to make intestinal muscles contract
- Antinausea medications
- Antidiarrheal medications
- Laxatives

Decompression

A person with acute colonic pseudo-obstruction and a greatly enlarged colon who does not respond to medications may need a procedure, called decompression, to remove gas from the colon. A gastroenterologist can perform the procedure in a hospital or an outpatient center. The gastroenterologist may choose to decompress the colon by using colonoscopy. During colonoscopy, the gastroenterologist inserts a flexible tube into the colon through the anus. A healthcare provider gives the person a light sedative, and possibly pain medication, to relax. If the person requires long-term decompression, the gastroenterologist also can decompress the colon through a surgical opening in the cecum. In this case, the healthcare provider gives the person local anesthesia.

Surgery

In severe cases of intestinal pseudo-obstruction, a person may need surgery to remove part of the intestine. However, surgery should be performed rarely, if at all, because intestinal pseudo-obstruction is a generalized disorder that typically affects the entire intestine. Removing part of the intestine cannot cure the disease.

A surgeon will perform the surgery at a hospital; a person will need general anesthesia. A few highly specialized treatment centers offer small intestine transplantation. A healthcare provider may recommend small intestine transplantation when all other treatments have failed.

Eating, Diet, and Nutrition

Researchers have not found that eating, diet, and nutrition play a role in causing or preventing intestinal pseudo-obstruction. Following special diets usually does not help improve the disorder. However, eating frequent, small meals with pureed foods or liquids may ease digestion. Vitamin and trace mineral supplements may help a person who is malnourished.

Section 30.3

Inguinal Hernia

This section includes text excerpted from "Inguinal Hernia,"
National Institute of Diabetes and Digestive and Kidney
Diseases (NIDDK), June 2014. Reviewed September 2018.

What Is an Inguinal Hernia?

An inguinal hernia happens when contents of the abdomen—usually fat or part of the small intestine—bulge through a weak area in
the lower abdominal wall. The abdomen is the area between the chest
and the hips. The area of the lower abdominal wall is also called the
inguinal or groin region.

Two types of inguinal hernias are:

- Indirect inguinal hernias, which are caused by a defect in the
  abdominal wall that is congenital, or present at birth

- Direct inguinal hernias, which usually occur only in male adults
  and are caused by a weakness in the muscles of the abdominal
  wall that develops over time

Inguinal hernias occur at the inguinal canal in the groin region.

What Is the Inguinal Canal?

The inguinal canal is a passage through the lower abdominal wall.
People have two inguinal canals—one on each side of the lower abdomen. In males, the spermatic cords pass through the inguinal canals
and connect to the testicles in the scrotum—the sac around the testicles. The spermatic cords contain blood vessels, nerves, and a duct,
called the spermatic duct, that carries sperm from the testicles to the
penis. In females, the round ligaments, which support the uterus, pass
through the inguinal canals.

What Causes Inguinal Hernias

The cause of inguinal hernias depends on the type of inguinal
hernia.

Indirect inguinal hernias. A defect in the abdominal wall that
is present at birth causes an indirect inguinal hernia.

417

During the development of the fetus in the womb, the lining of the abdominal cavity forms and extends into the inguinal canal. In males, the spermatic cord and testicles descend out from inside the abdomen and through the abdominal lining to the scrotum through the inguinal canal. Next, the abdominal lining usually closes off the entrance to the inguinal canal a few weeks before or after birth. In females, the ovaries do not descend out from inside the abdomen, and the abdominal lining usually closes a couple of months before birth.

Sometimes the lining of the abdomen does not close as it should, leaving an opening in the abdominal wall at the upper part of the inguinal canal. Fat or part of the small intestine may slide into the

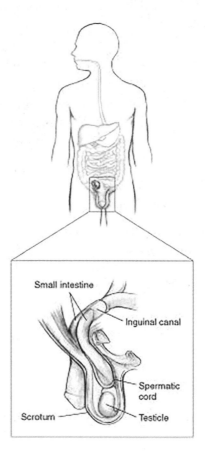

Figure 30.2. *Inguinal Hernia*

Indirect inguinal hernia in a male

inguinal canal through this opening, causing a hernia. In females, the ovaries may also slide into the inguinal canal and cause a hernia.

Indirect hernias are the most common type of inguinal hernia. Indirect inguinal hernias may appear in two to three percent of male children; however, they are much less common in female children, occurring in less than one percent.

Direct inguinal hernias. Direct inguinal hernias usually occur only in male adults as aging and stress or strain weaken the abdominal muscles around the inguinal canal. Previous surgery in the lower abdomen can also weaken the abdominal muscles. Females rarely form this type of inguinal hernia. In females, the broad ligament of the uterus acts as an additional barrier behind the muscle layer of the lower abdominal wall. The broad ligament of the uterus is a sheet of tissue that supports the uterus and other reproductive organs.

Who Is More Likely to Develop an Inguinal Hernia?

Males are much more likely to develop inguinal hernias than females. About 25 percent of males and about two percent of females will develop an inguinal hernia in their lifetimes. Some people who have an inguinal hernia on one side will have or will develop a hernia on the other side. People of any age can develop inguinal hernias. Indirect hernias can appear before age one and often appear before age 30; however, they may appear later in life. Premature infants have a higher chance of developing an indirect inguinal hernia. Direct hernias, which usually only occur in male adults, are much more common in men older than age 40 because the muscles of the abdominal wall weaken with age. People with a family history of inguinal hernias are more likely to develop inguinal hernias. Studies also suggest that people who smoke have an increased risk of inguinal hernias.

What Are the Signs and Symptoms of an Inguinal Hernia?

The first sign of an inguinal hernia is a small bulge on one or, rarely, on both sides of the groin—the area just above the groin crease between the lower abdomen and the thigh. The bulge may increase in size over time and usually disappears when lying down.

Other signs and symptoms can include:

- Discomfort or pain in the groin—especially when straining, lifting, coughing, or exercising—that improves when resting

- Feelings such as weakness, heaviness, burning, or aching in the groin

- A swollen or an enlarged scrotum in men or boys

Indirect and direct inguinal hernias may slide in and out of the abdomen into the inguinal canal. A healthcare provider can often move them back into the abdomen with gentle massage.

What Are the Complications of Inguinal Hernias?

Inguinal hernias can cause the following complications:

- **Incarceration.** An incarcerated hernia happens when part of the fat or small intestine from inside the abdomen becomes stuck in the groin or scrotum and cannot go back into the abdomen. A healthcare provider is unable to massage the hernia back into the abdomen.

- **Strangulation.** When an incarcerated hernia is not treated, the blood supply to the small intestine may become obstructed, causing "strangulation" of the small intestine. This lack of blood supply is an emergency situation and can cause the section of the intestine to die.

How Are Inguinal Hernias Diagnosed?

A healthcare provider diagnoses an inguinal hernia with:

- A medical and family history

- A physical exam

- Imaging tests, including X-rays

Medical and family history. Taking a medical and family history may help a healthcare provider diagnose an inguinal hernia. Often the symptoms that the patient describes will be signs of an inguinal hernia.

Physical exam. A physical exam may help diagnose an inguinal hernia. During a physical exam, a healthcare provider usually examines the patient's body. The healthcare provider may ask the patient to stand and cough or strain so the healthcare provider can feel for a bulge caused by the hernia as it moves into the groin or scrotum. The healthcare provider may gently try to massage the hernia back into its proper position in the abdomen.

Imaging tests. A healthcare provider does not usually use imaging tests, including X-rays, to diagnose an inguinal hernia unless he or she:

- Is trying to diagnose a strangulation or an incarceration
- Cannot feel the inguinal hernia during a physical exam, especially in patients who are overweight
- Is uncertain if the hernia or another condition is causing the swelling in the groin or other symptoms

Specially trained technicians perform imaging tests at a healthcare provider's office, an outpatient center, or a hospital.

A radiologist—a doctor who specializes in medical imaging—interprets the images. A patient does not usually need anesthesia.

Tests may include the following:

- Abdominal X-ray
- Computerized tomography (CT) scan
- Abdominal ultrasound

How Are Inguinal Hernias Treated?

Repair of an inguinal hernia via surgery is the only treatment for inguinal hernias and can prevent incarceration and strangulation. Healthcare providers recommend surgery for most people with inguinal hernias and especially for people with hernias that cause symptoms. Research suggests that men with hernias that cause few or no symptoms may be able to safely delay surgery until their symptoms increase. Men who delay surgery should watch for symptoms and see a healthcare provider regularly. Healthcare providers usually recommend surgery for infants and children to prevent incarceration. Emergent, or immediate, surgery is necessary for incarcerated or strangulated hernias.

A general surgeon—a doctor who specializes in abdominal surgery—performs hernia surgery at a hospital or surgery center, usually on an outpatient basis. Recovery time varies depending on the size of the hernia, the technique used, and the age and health of the person.

Hernia surgery is also called herniorrhaphy. The two main types of surgery for hernias are:

- **Open hernia repair.** During an open hernia repair, a healthcare provider usually gives a patient local anesthesia in the abdomen with sedation; however, some patients may have:

  - Sedation with a spinal block, in which a healthcare provider injects anesthetics around the nerves in the spine, making the body numb from the waist down

  - General anesthesia

- The surgeon makes an incision in the groin, moves the hernia back into the abdomen, and reinforces the abdominal wall with stitches. Usually, the surgeon also reinforces the weak area with a synthetic mesh or "screen" to provide additional support.

- **Laparoscopic hernia repair.** A surgeon performs laparoscopic hernia repair with the patient under general anesthesia. The surgeon makes several small, half-inch incisions in the lower abdomen and inserts a laparoscope—a thin tube with a tiny video camera attached. The camera sends a magnified image from inside the body to a video monitor, giving the surgeon a close-up view of the hernia and surrounding tissue. While watching the monitor, the surgeon repairs the hernia using synthetic mesh or "screen."

People who undergo laparoscopic hernia repair generally experience a shorter recovery time than those who have an open hernia repair. However, the surgeon may determine that laparoscopy is not the best option if the hernia is large or if the person has had previous pelvic surgery.

Most adults experience discomfort and require pain medication after either an open hernia repair or a laparoscopic hernia repair. Intense activity and heavy lifting are restricted for several weeks. The surgeon will discuss when a person may safely return to work. Infants and children also experience some discomfort; however, they usually resume normal activities after several days.

Surgery to repair an inguinal hernia is quite safe, and complications are uncommon. People should contact their healthcare provider if any of the following symptoms appear:

- Redness around or drainage from the incision
- Fever

- Bleeding from the incision
- Pain that is not relieved by medication or pain that suddenly worsens

Possible long-term complications include:

- Long-lasting pain in the groin
- Recurrence of the hernia, requiring a second surgery
- Damage to nerves near the hernia

How Can Inguinal Hernias Be Prevented?

People cannot prevent the weakness in the abdominal wall that causes indirect inguinal hernias. However, people may be able to prevent direct inguinal hernias by maintaining a healthy weight and not smoking.

People can keep inguinal hernias from getting worse or keep inguinal hernias from recurring after surgery by:

- Avoiding heavy lifting
- Using the legs, not the back, when lifting objects
- Preventing constipation and straining during bowel movements
- Maintaining a healthy weight
- Not smoking

Eating, Diet, and Nutrition

Researchers have not found that eating, diet, and nutrition play a role in causing inguinal hernias. A person with an inguinal hernia may be able to prevent symptoms by eating high-fiber foods. Fresh fruits, vegetables, and whole grains are high in fiber and may help prevent constipation and straining that cause some of the painful symptoms of a hernia. The surgeon will provide instructions on eating, diet, and nutrition after inguinal hernia surgery. Most people drink liquids and eat a light diet the day of the operation and then resume their usual diet the next day.

Section 30.4

Short Bowel Syndrome

This section includes text excerpted from "Short Bowel
Syndrome," National Institute of Diabetes and
Digestive and Kidney Diseases (NIDDK), July 2015.

What Is Short Bowel Syndrome?

Short bowel syndrome is a group of problems related to poor absorption of nutrients. Short bowel syndrome typically occurs in people who have:

- Had at least half of their small intestine removed and sometimes all or part of their large intestine removed
- Significant damage of the small intestine
- Poor motility, or movement, inside the intestines

Short bowel syndrome may be mild, moderate, or severe, depending on how well the small intestine is working. People with short bowel syndrome cannot absorb enough water, vitamins, minerals, protein, fat, calories, and other nutrients from food. What nutrients the small intestine has trouble absorbing depends on which section of the small intestine has been damaged or removed.

What Is the Small Intestine?

The small intestine is the tube-shaped organ between the stomach and large intestine. Most food digestion and nutrient absorption take place in the small intestine. The small intestine is about 20 feet long and includes the duodenum, jejunum, and ileum:

- Duodenum—the first part of the small intestine, where iron and other minerals are absorbed
- Jejunum—the middle section of the small intestine, where carbohydrates, proteins, fat, and most vitamins are absorbed
- Ileum—the lower end of the small intestine, where bile acids and vitamin B_{12} are absorbed

What Is the Large Intestine?

The large intestine is about five feet long in adults and absorbs water and any remaining nutrients from partially digested food passed from the small intestine. The large intestine then changes waste from liquid to a solid matter called stool.

What Causes Short Bowel Syndrome

The main cause of short bowel syndrome is surgery to remove a portion of the small intestine. This surgery can treat intestinal diseases, injuries, or birth defects.

Some children are born with an abnormally short small intestine or with part of their bowel missing, which can cause short bowel syndrome. In infants, short bowel syndrome most commonly occurs following surgery to treat necrotizing enterocolitis, a condition in which part of the tissue in the intestines is destroyed.

Short bowel syndrome may also occur following surgery to treat conditions such as:

- Cancer and damage to the intestines caused by cancer treatment

- Crohn disease, a disorder that causes inflammation, or swelling, and irritation of any part of the digestive tract

- Gastroschisis, which occurs when the intestines stick out of the body through one side of the umbilical cord

- Internal hernia, which occurs when the small intestine is displaced into pockets in the abdominal lining

- Intestinal atresia, which occurs when a part of the intestines doesn't form completely

- Intestinal injury from loss of blood flow due to a blocked blood vessel

- Intestinal injury from trauma

- Intussusception, in which one section of either the large or small intestine folds into itself, much like a collapsible telescope

- Meconium ileus, which occurs when the meconium, a newborn's first stool, is thicker and stickier than normal and blocks the ileum

- Midgut volvulus, which occurs when blood supply to the middle of the small intestine is completely cut off

- Omphalocele, which occurs when the intestines, liver, or other organs stick out through the navel, or belly button

Even if a person does not have surgery, disease or injury can damage the small intestine.

How Common Is Short Bowel Syndrome?

Short bowel syndrome is a rare condition. Each year, short bowel syndrome affects about three out of every million people.

What Are the Signs and Symptoms of Short Bowel Syndrome?

The main symptom of short bowel syndrome is diarrhea—loose, watery stools. Diarrhea can lead to dehydration, malnutrition, and weight loss. Dehydration means the body lacks enough fluid and electrolytes—chemicals in salts, including sodium, potassium, and chloride—to work properly. Malnutrition is a condition that develops when the body does not get the right amount of vitamins, minerals, and nutrients it needs to maintain healthy tissues and organ function. Loose stools contain more fluid and electrolytes than solid stools. These problems can be severe and can be life threatening without proper treatment.

Other signs and symptoms may include:

- Bloating
- Cramping
- Fatigue, or feeling tired
- Foul-smelling stool
- Heartburn
- Too much gas
- Vomiting
- Weakness

People with short bowel syndrome are also more likely to develop food allergies and sensitivities, such as lactose intolerance. Lactose intolerance is a condition in which people have digestive symptoms—such as bloating, diarrhea, and gas—after eating or drinking milk or milk products.

What Are the Complications of Short Bowel Syndrome?

The complications of short bowel syndrome may include:

- Malnutrition

- Peptic ulcers—sores on the lining of the stomach or duodenum caused by too much gastric acid

- Kidney stones—solid pieces of material that form in the kidneys

- Small intestinal bacterial overgrowth—a condition in which abnormally large numbers of bacteria grow in the small intestine

How Is Short Bowel Syndrome Diagnosed?

A healthcare provider diagnoses short bowel syndrome based on:

- A medical and family history

- A physical exam

- Blood tests

- Fecal fat tests

- An X-ray of the small and large intestines

- Upper gastrointestinal (GI) series

- Computerized tomography (CT) scan

Medical and Family History

Taking a medical and family history may help a healthcare provider diagnose short bowel syndrome. He or she will ask the patient about symptoms and may request a history of past operations.

Physical Exam

A physical exam may help diagnose short bowel syndrome. During a physical exam, a healthcare provider usually:

- Examines a patient's body, looking for muscle wasting or weight loss and signs of vitamin and mineral deficiencies

- Uses a stethoscope to listen to sounds in the abdomen

- Taps on specific areas of the patient's body

Blood Tests

A blood test involves drawing a patient's blood at a healthcare provider's office or a commercial facility and sending the sample to a lab for analysis. Blood tests can show mineral and vitamin levels and measure complete blood count.

Fecal Fat Tests

A fecal fat test measures the body's ability to break down and absorb fat. For this test, a patient provides a stool sample at a healthcare provider's office. The patient may also use a take-home test kit. The patient collects stool in plastic wrap that he or she lays over the toilet seat and places a sample into a container. A patient can also use a special tissue provided by the healthcare provider's office to collect the sample and place the tissue into the container. For children wearing diapers, the parent or caretaker can line the diaper with plastic to collect the stool. The healthcare provider will send the sample to a lab for analysis. A fecal fat test can show how well the small intestine is working.

X-Ray

An X-ray is a picture created by using radiation and recorded on film or on a computer. The amount of radiation used is small. An X-ray technician performs the X-ray at a hospital or an outpatient center, and a radiologist—a doctor who specializes in medical imaging—interprets the images. An X-ray of the small intestine can show that the last segment of the large intestine is narrower than normal. Blocked stool causes the part of the intestine just before this narrow segment to stretch and bulge.

Upper Gastrointestinal Series

Upper GI series, also called a barium swallow, uses X-rays and fluoroscopy to help diagnose problems of the upper GI tract. A patient may experience bloating and nausea for a short time after the test. For several days afterward, barium liquid in the GI tract causes white or light-colored stools. A healthcare provider will give the patient specific instructions about eating and drinking after the test. Upper GI series can show narrowing and widening of the small and large intestines.

Computerized Tomography Scan

Computerized tomography scans use a combination of X-rays and computer technology to create images. For a CT scan, a healthcare provider may give the patient a solution to drink and an injection of a special dye, called a contrast medium. The patient does not need anesthesia. CT scans can show bowel obstruction and changes in the intestines.

How Is Short Bowel Syndrome Treated?

A healthcare provider will recommend treatment for short bowel syndrome based on a patient's nutritional needs. Treatment may include:

- Nutritional support
- Medications
- Surgery
- Intestinal transplant

Nutritional Support

The main treatment for short bowel syndrome is nutritional support, which may include the following:

- Oral rehydration
- Parenteral nutrition
- Enteral nutrition
- Vitamin and mineral supplements
- Special diet

Medications

A healthcare provider may prescribe medications to treat short bowel syndrome, including:

- Antibiotics to prevent bacterial overgrowth
- H2 blockers to treat too much gastric acid secretion
- Proton pump inhibitors (PPIs) to treat too much gastric acid secretion
- Choleretic agents to improve bile flow and prevent liver disease
- Bile-salt binders to decrease diarrhea
- Anti-secretin agents to reduce gastric acid in the intestine

- Hypomotility agents to increase the time it takes food to travel through the intestines, leading to Increased nutrient absorption

- Growth hormones to improve intestinal absorption

- Teduglutide to improve intestinal absorption

Surgery

The goal of surgery is to increase the small intestine's ability to absorb nutrients. Approximately half of the patients with short bowel syndrome need surgery. Surgery used to treat short bowel syndrome includes procedures that:

- Prevent blockage and preserve the length of the small intestine

- Narrow any dilated segment of the small intestine

- Slow the time it takes for food to travel through the small intestine

- Lengthen the small intestine

Long-term treatment and recovery, which for some may take years, depend in part on:

- What sections of the small intestine were removed

- How much of the intestine is damaged

- How well the muscles of the intestine work

- How well the remaining small intestine adapts over time

Intestinal Transplant

An intestinal transplant is surgery to remove a diseased or an injured small intestine and replace it with a healthy small intestine from a person who has just died, called a donor. Sometimes a living donor can provide a segment of his or her small intestine.

A healthcare provider will tailor treatment to the severity of the patient's disease:

- Treatment for mild short bowel syndrome involves eating small, frequent meals; drinking fluid; taking nutritional supplements; and using medications to treat diarrhea.

- Treatment for moderate short bowel syndrome is similar to that for mild short bowel syndrome, with the addition of parenteral nutrition as needed.

- Treatment for severe short bowel syndrome involves the use of parenteral nutrition and oral rehydration solutions. Patients may receive enteral nutrition or continue normal eating, even though most of the nutrients are not absorbed. Both enteral nutrition and normal eating stimulate the remaining intestine to work better and may allow patients to discontinue parenteral nutrition. Some patients with severe short bowel syndrome require parenteral nutrition indefinitely or surgery.

Can Short Bowel Syndrome Be Prevented?

People can ask their healthcare providers about surgical techniques that minimize scar tissue. Scientists have not yet found a way to prevent short bowel syndrome that is present at birth, as its cause is unknown.

Eating, Diet, and Nutrition

Researchers have not found that eating, diet, and nutrition play a role in causing or preventing short bowel syndrome.

Part Five

Disorders of the Digestive System's Solid Organs: The Liver and Pancreas

Chapter 31

Viral Hepatitis

What Is the Liver?

The liver is the body's largest internal organ. The liver is called the body's metabolic factory because of the important role it plays in metabolism—the way cells change food into energy after food is digested and absorbed into the blood. The liver has many important functions, including:

- Taking up, storing, and processing nutrients from food— including fat, sugar, and protein—and delivering them to the rest of the body when needed

- Making new proteins, such as clotting factors and immune factors

- Producing bile. In addition to carrying toxins and waste products out of the body, bile helps the body digest fats and the fat-soluble vitamins A, D, E, and K

- Removing waste products the kidneys cannot remove, such as fats, cholesterol, toxins, and medications

This chapter contains text excerpted from the following sources: Text under the heading "What Is Liver?" is excerpted from "Wilson Disease," National Institute of Diabetes and Digestive and Kidney Diseases (NIDDK), July 2014. Reviewed September 2018; Text beginning with the heading "What Is Viral Hepatitis?" is excerpted from "Viral Hepatitis," Office on Women's Health (OWH), U.S. Department of Health and Human Services (HHS), July 2, 2018.

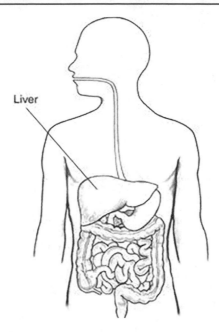

Figure 31.1. *Liver*

A healthy liver is necessary for survival. The liver can regenerate most of its, cells when they become damaged. However, if injury to the liver is too severe or long lasting, regeneration is incomplete and the liver creates scar tissue.

What Is Viral Hepatitis?

Viral hepatitis is inflammation of the liver caused by the hepatitis virus. Inflammation happens when your immune system senses a danger, like a virus, and sends white blood cells to surround the area to protect your body. This causes redness, swelling, and sometimes pain.

Hepatitis damages the liver and can cause scarring of the liver, called cirrhosis. Cirrhosis can cause liver cancer, liver failure, and death. Your liver changes the food you eat into energy. It also cleans alcohol and other toxins from your blood, helps your stomach and intestines digest food, and makes proteins that your body needs to control and stop bleeding.

What Are the Different Types of Viral Hepatitis?

The most common types of viral hepatitis in the United States are:

- Hepatitis A

- Hepatitis B
- Hepatitis C

Does Viral Hepatitis Affect Women Differently Than Men?

Yes, certain types of viral hepatitis affect women differently than men.

Hepatitis A affects women and men in similar ways.

Hepatitis B affects women differently than men:

- **Birth control.** Women with severe liver damage may not be able to use birth control. This is because a damaged liver may have problems breaking down estrogen.

- **Pregnancy.** The risk of passing hepatitis B to your baby during pregnancy is high. Hepatitis B raises your risk for pregnancy complications. Talk to your doctor about taking hepatitis B medicine to lower the risk of passing hepatitis B to your baby. Certain hepatitis B medicines are safe to take during pregnancy but are not recommended for everyone.

Hepatitis C affects women differently than men:

- **Younger women.** Research shows that acute (short-term) hepatitis C goes away on its own more often for younger women than men. Also, in women with chronic hepatitis C, liver damage usually happens more slowly than it does for men. Researchers think the hormone estrogen may help protect the liver from damage.

- **Menstrual cycles.** You may miss menstrual periods or have shorter periods. This can happen as a side effect of hepatitis medicines. Since hepatitis C is spread through blood, the risk of passing hepatitis C to a partner is higher during your menstrual period.

- **Birth control.** Women with severe liver damage may not be able to use birth control that contains estrogen. This is because a damaged liver may have problems breaking down estrogen.

- **Pregnancy.** Experts think the risk of passing hepatitis C to your baby during pregnancy is low. But hepatitis C raises your risk for pregnancy complications such as premature birth and gestational diabetes. Some hepatitis C medicines can also cause serious harm to your baby if taken during pregnancy.

- **Menopause.** Liver damage happens more quickly for women after menopause. Hepatitis C medicines also may not work as well for women after menopause as they do for men.

Who Gets Viral Hepatitis?

Viral hepatitis is common in the United States and affects women and men. Hepatitis B and C are more common than hepatitis A.

- In 2015, hepatitis A affected an estimated 2,500 Americans. The percentage of people with hepatitis A has gone down by 95 percent since the hepatitis A vaccine became available in 1995.

- Chronic hepatitis B may affect more than 1 million Americans. Asian-Americans and Pacific Islanders have the highest rates of hepatitis B infection. About 50 percent of the people living with Hepatitis B are Asian-Americans and Pacific Islanders.

- Within this high-risk group, hepatitis B is usually passed from a mother to her baby during pregnancy. Babies born with hepatitis B are likely to have it their entire lives and are at higher risk of liver damage and liver cancer.

- Hepatitis C is the most common type of viral hepatitis infection in the United States. An estimated 3.5 million Americans have chronic hepatitis C. The Centers for Disease Control and Prevention (CDC) recommends that everyone born between 1945 and 1965 (also called baby boomers) get tested at least once for hepatitis C because it is so common in this age group.

How Do You Get Hepatitis A?

Hepatitis A is found in an infected person's stool (poop). Hepatitis A is spread through:

- Eating or drinking contaminated food or water

  - You can get hepatitis A by eating food prepared by a person with the virus who didn't wash his or her hands after using the bathroom and then touched the food.

  - You can get hepatitis A by eating raw or undercooked shellfish that came from sewage-contaminated water.

- Vaginal, oral, or anal sex. Hepatitis A can be spread even if the infected person has no symptoms.

- Touching unclean diaper changing areas or toilets. If an infant or toddler had hepatitis A and soiled the changing area, others who come into contact with the stool could become infected.

You are more likely to get hepatitis A if you travel out of the country to a developing country with poor sanitation or without access to clean water and have not gotten vaccinated for hepatitis A. Ask your doctor if you need a hepatitis A vaccination.

How Do You Get Hepatitis B?

Hepatitis B is found in an infected person's blood and other body fluids, such as semen and vaginal fluid.
Hepatitis B is usually spread through:

- Vaginal, oral, or anal sex. This is the most common way hepatitis B is spread. Hepatitis B can be spread even if the infected person has no symptoms.

- Birth to a mother who has hepatitis B

- Sharing or reusing needles, syringes, and drug preparation equipment such as cookers and cotton when injecting drugs. Hands or drug preparation equipment that have even tiny amounts of blood on them can spread hepatitis B.

- Accidental needle stick or other sharp instrument injury (higher risk for healthcare workers)

A less common way to spread hepatitis B is through prechewed food to a baby from a mother who has hepatitis B. However, hepatitis B cannot be spread through breastfeeding.

How Do You Get Hepatitis C?

Hepatitis C is found in an infected person's blood and other body fluids.
Hepatitis C is usually spread through:

- Sharing or reusing needles, syringes, and drug preparation equipment such as cookers and cotton when injecting drugs. This is the most common way hepatitis C is spread in the United States. Hands or drug preparation equipment that have even tiny amounts of blood on them can also spread hepatitis C.

- Accidental needle stick or other sharp instrument injury (higher risk for healthcare workers)

Less common ways to spread hepatitis C:

- Vaginal, oral, or anal sex
- Birth to a mother who has hepatitis, though this is rare
- Sharing personal items like razors and toothbrushes
- Tattoos or body piercings
- Blood transfusions done in the United States before the 1990s (when hepatitis C testing began) or in other parts of the world where hepatitis C testing is less common

What Are the Symptoms of Viral Hepatitis?

The symptoms of viral hepatitis are similar for all types of hepatitis. They include:

- Low-grade fever (a temperature between 99.5°F and 101°F)
- Fatigue (tiredness)
- Loss of appetite
- Upset stomach
- Vomiting
- Stomach pain
- Dark urine
- Clay-colored bowel movements
- Joint pain
- Jaundice, which is when the skin and whites of the eyes turn yellow

People who are newly infected are most likely to have one or more of these symptoms, but some people with viral hepatitis do not have any symptoms. New hepatitis A infections usually cause symptoms, but as many as half the people with new hepatitis B and hepatitis C infections do not have symptoms.

Certain blood tests can show if you have hepatitis, even if you do not have symptoms. People with chronic hepatitis B or C often develop symptoms when their liver becomes damaged.

Why Do All Baby Boomers Need to Be Tested for Viral Hepatitis?

The CDC recommends that all Americans born between 1945 and 1965 (called baby boomers) get a one-time test for hepatitis C. This is because three in four adults with hepatitis C are baby boomers, and most baby boomers do not know they have it.

It's likely that many baby boomers with hepatitis C were infected many years ago before the blood supply was tested for hepatitis C.

How Is Viral Hepatitis Diagnosed?

Talk to your doctor if you have symptoms of viral hepatitis. Your doctor will:

- Ask questions about your health history
- Do a physical exam
- Order blood tests that look for parts of the virus or antibodies that your body makes in response to the virus. Other tests may measure the amount of the virus in your blood.

How Do I Know If I Have Acute or Chronic Viral Hepatitis?

Hepatitis A, B, and C all start out as an acute (short-term) infection. Some acute infections can develop into lifelong, chronic infections. Your doctor may do a blood test to see if the infection is acute or chronic.

- Hepatitis A causes acute infection only. Most people recover with no lasting health problems.
- Hepatitis B and C can cause both acute and chronic infections. Some people recover from the acute infection and cannot spread the infection to others. For other people, the infection develops into a chronic infection and can be spread to others.

How Is Acute (Short-Term) Viral Hepatitis Treated?

Acute viral hepatitis usually goes away on its own. Hepatitis A causes only acute infection, but hepatitis B and C often cause chronic or lifelong infection. If you have acute hepatitis A, B, or C, you may feel sick for a few months before you get better.

Your doctor may recommend rest and making sure you get enough fluids. Avoid alcohol and certain medicines, like the pain reliever acetaminophen, because they can damage the liver during this time. Some people with acute viral hepatitis need to be hospitalized to manage the symptoms.

If you think you have hepatitis, go to the doctor right away.

How Is Chronic (Long-Term) Viral Hepatitis Treated?

If you have chronic viral hepatitis, your treatment depends on the type of hepatitis you have:

- **Hepatitis B.** You will probably meet with your doctor regularly, every 6–12 months, to watch for signs of liver disease and liver cancer. If you plan to become pregnant in the future, talk to your doctor first. You may need antiviral medicines to treat hepatitis B, but many people do not need medicine.

- **Hepatitis C.** If you have hepatitis C, talk with your doctor about whether you need medicine. Certain approved antiviral medicines treat and may cure hepatitis C in adults. If you have health insurance, ask about your copay or coinsurance and which medicines are covered under your plan.

What Can Happen If Viral Hepatitis Is Not Treated?

Most people recover from hepatitis A with no treatment or long-lasting health problems.

Chronic hepatitis B and C can lead to serious health problems, such as:

- Cirrhosis or scarring of the liver

- Liver cancer

- Liver failure

People with liver failure may need a liver transplant to survive. In the United States, cirrhosis caused by chronic hepatitis C is currently the most common reason for needing a liver transplant. Viral hepatitis is also the most common cause of liver cancer.

What Should I Do If I Think I Have Been Exposed to Viral Hepatitis?

Call your doctor or your local or state health department if you think you may have been exposed.

- If you may have been exposed to hepatitis A or B, your doctor may recommend getting a vaccine (shot) to keep you from getting the infection.

- The CDC recommends that people who are exposed to hepatitis C, such as a healthcare worker after an accidental needle stick, get tested for hepatitis C infection. New antiviral medicines for hepatitis C cure most of the people who take them. If you have health insurance, ask about your copay and coinsurance and which medicines are covered under your plan.

How Can I Prevent Viral Hepatitis?

You can lower your risk of getting viral hepatitis with the following steps. The steps work best when used together. No single step can protect you from every kind of viral hepatitis.

Steps to lower your risk of viral hepatitis:

- Get vaccinated. Getting vaccinated is the best way to prevent hepatitis A and B. There is no vaccine for hepatitis C. The hepatitis A and hepatitis B vaccines are recommended for anyone who wants protection from the viruses and for people with certain risk factors and health problems. Ask your doctor if you need the vaccines.

- Wash your hands after using the bathroom and changing diapers and before preparing or eating food.

- If you have sex, use condoms. Condoms lower your risk of getting or passing sexually transmitted infections (STIs), including viral hepatitis. Viral hepatitis can be passed through menstrual blood, vaginal fluid, and semen (cum). Make sure to put the condom on before the penis touches your vagina, mouth, or anus. Other methods of birth control like birth control pills, shots, implants, or diaphragms, will not protect you from viral hepatitis.

- Limit your number of sex partners. Your risk of getting viral hepatitis goes up with the number of lifetime sex partners you have.

- If you use needles or syringes for any reason, do not share them with others.

- Do not share personal items that could have blood on them, such as razors, nail clippers, toothbrushes, or glucose monitors.

- Do not get tattoos or body piercings from an unlicensed person or facility.

- Wear protective gloves if you have to touch another person's blood.

- If you are a healthcare or public safety worker, get vaccinated for hepatitis A and B, and always follow recommended standard precautions and infection-control principles, including safe injection practices.

Do I Need the Viral Hepatitis Vaccines?

Maybe. The hepatitis A and B vaccines can protect you from getting infected. Talk to your doctor or nurse about getting the recommended vaccines.

There is no vaccine yet to prevent hepatitis C. But you can take other steps to lower your risk of getting hepatitis C.

Who Should Get the Hepatitis A Vaccine?

The hepatitis A vaccine is given in two doses, 6–18 months apart. Two doses are needed for lasting protection.

The vaccine is recommended for:

- All children, starting at 1 year (12–23 months old)

- Men who have sex with men

- People who travel or work in a part of the world where hepatitis A is common, such as certain parts of Central or South America, Asia, Africa, and eastern Europe.

- People who use illegal drugs

- People who are treated with clotting factor concentrates, such as people with hemophilia

- People with chronic liver disease (CLD)

- People who work with hepatitis A in a laboratory or with hepatitis A–infected primates

- Members of households planning to adopt a child, or care for a newly arriving adopted child, from a country where hepatitis A is common.

Who Should Get the Hepatitis B Vaccine?

The hepatitis B vaccine is usually given in three doses over six months. The vaccine is recommended for:

- All children at birth
- All children and teens younger than 19 who have not been vaccinated
- Men who have sex with men
- People who live with or have sex with someone who is infected with hepatitis B
- People with more than one sex partner
- People who share equipment to inject drugs
- People with chronic liver or kidney disease
- People with HIV
- People younger than 60 with diabetes
- People whose jobs expose them to human blood or other body fluids
- Residents and staff of facilities for people with developmental disabilities
- People who travel to parts of the world where hepatitis B is common, such as Southeast Asia, sub-Saharan Africa, the Amazon Basin in South America, the Pacific Islands, parts of Eastern Europe, and parts of the Middle East

How Long Do the Hepatitis A and B Vaccines Protect You?

During your lifetime, you need:

- One series of the hepatitis A vaccine (two shots given at least six months apart)
- One series of the hepatitis B vaccine (three or four shots given over a six-month period)

Most people don't need a booster dose of either vaccine. But if you have had dialysis, a medical procedure to clean your blood, or have a weakened immune system, your doctor might recommend additional doses of the hepatitis B vaccine.

How Can I Get Free or Low-Cost Hepatitis A and B Vaccines?

The hepatitis A and hepatitis B vaccines are covered under most insurance plans.

- If you have insurance, check with your insurance provider to find out what's included in your plan.

- Medicare Part B covers hepatitis B vaccines for people at risk.

- If you have Medicaid, the benefits covered are different in each state.

Chapter 32

Cirrhosis of the Liver

What Is Cirrhosis?

Cirrhosis is a condition in which your liver is scarred and permanently damaged. Scar tissue replaces healthy liver tissue and prevents your liver from working normally. Scar tissue also partly blocks the flow of blood through your liver. As cirrhosis gets worse, your liver begins to fail.

Many people are not aware that they have cirrhosis, since they may not have signs or symptoms until their liver is badly damaged.

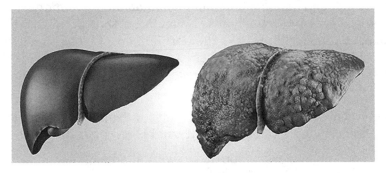

Figure 32.1. *Healthy Liver and Liver with Cirrhosis*

This chapter includes text excerpted from "Cirrhosis," National Institute of Diabetes and Digestive and Kidney Diseases (NIDDK), March 2018.

How Common Is Cirrhosis?

Researchers estimate that about 1 in 400 adults in the United States has cirrhosis. Cirrhosis is more common in adults ages 45–54. About 1 in 200 adults ages 45–54 in the United States has cirrhosis. Researchers believe the actual numbers may be higher because many people with cirrhosis are not diagnosed.

Who Is More Likely to Get Cirrhosis?

People are more likely to get cirrhosis if they have certain health conditions. People are also more likely to get cirrhosis if they:

- Have abused alcohol for a long time
- Have type 2 diabetes
- Are men
- Are older than age 50

What Are the Complications of Cirrhosis?

As the liver fails, complications may develop. In some people, complications may be the first sign of the disease. Complications of cirrhosis may include the following.

Portal Hypertension

Portal hypertension is the most common serious complication of cirrhosis. Portal hypertension is a condition that occurs when scar tissue partly blocks and slows the normal flow of blood through your liver, which causes high blood pressure in the portal vein. Portal hypertension and its treatments may lead to other complications, including:

- Enlarged veins—called varices—in your esophagus, stomach, or intestines, which can lead to internal bleeding if the veins burst
- Swelling in your legs, ankles, or feet, called edema
- Buildup of fluid in your abdomen—called ascites—which can lead to a serious infection in the space that surrounds your liver and intestines
- Confusion or difficulties thinking caused by the buildup of toxins in your brain, called hepatic encephalopathy (HE)

Infections

Cirrhosis increases your chance of getting bacterial infections, such as urinary tract infections and pneumonia.

Liver Cancer

Cirrhosis increases your chance of getting liver cancer. Most people who develop liver cancer already have cirrhosis.

Liver Failure

Cirrhosis may eventually lead to liver failure. With liver failure, your liver is badly damaged and stops working. Liver failure is also called end-stage liver disease. This may require a liver transplant.

Other Complications

Other complications of cirrhosis may include:

- Bone diseases, such as osteoporosis
- Gallstones
- Problems with the bile ducts—the tubes that carry bile out of the liver
- Malabsorption and malnutrition
- Bruising and bleeding easily
- Sensitivity to medicines
- Insulin resistance and type 2 diabetes

What Are the Symptoms of Cirrhosis?

You may have no signs or symptoms of cirrhosis until your liver is badly damaged.

Early symptoms of cirrhosis may include:

- Feeling tired or weak
- Poor appetite
- Losing weight without trying
- Nausea and vomiting
- Mild pain or discomfort in the upper right side of your abdomen

As liver function gets worse, you may have other symptoms, including:

- Bruising and bleeding easily
- Confusion, difficulties thinking, memory loss, personality changes, or sleep disorders
- Swelling in your lower legs, ankles, or feet, called edema
- Bloating from buildup of fluid in your abdomen, called ascites
- Severe itchy skin
- Darkening of the color of your urine
- Yellowish tint to the whites of your eyes and skin called jaundice

What Causes Cirrhosis

Cirrhosis has different causes. Some people with cirrhosis have more than one cause of liver damage.

Most Common Causes

The most common causes of cirrhosis are:

- Alcoholic liver disease (ALD)—damage to the liver and its function due to alcohol abuse
- Nonalcoholic fatty liver disease (NAFLD)
- Chronic hepatitis C
- Chronic hepatitis B

Less Common Causes

Some of the less common causes of cirrhosis include:

- Autoimmune hepatitis
- Diseases that damage, destroy, or block bile ducts, such as primary biliary cholangitis (PBC) and primary sclerosing cholangitis (PSC)
- Inherited liver diseases—diseases passed from parents to children through genes—that affect how the liver works, such as Wilson disease, hemochromatosis, and alpha-1-antitrypsin deficiency (A1AD)

- Long-term use of certain medicines
- Chronic heart failure with liver congestion, a condition in which blood flow out of the liver is slowed

How Do Doctors Diagnose Cirrhosis?

Doctors diagnose cirrhosis based on your medical history, a physical exam, and the results of tests.

Medical History

Your doctor will ask about your symptoms. He or she will also ask if you have a history of health conditions that make you more likely to develop cirrhosis. Your doctor will ask about your use of alcohol and over-the-counter (OTC) and prescription medicines.

Physical Exam

Your doctor will examine your body, use a stethoscope to listen to sounds in your abdomen, and tap or press on specific areas of your abdomen. He or she will check to see if your liver is larger than it should be. Your doctor will also check for tenderness or pain in your abdomen.

What Tests Do Doctors Use to Diagnose Cirrhosis?
Blood Tests

Your doctor may recommend the following blood tests:

- Liver tests that can show abnormal liver enzyme levels, which may be a sign of liver damage. Your doctor may suspect cirrhosis if you have:

  - Increased levels of the liver enzymes alanine transaminase (ALT), aspartate transaminase (AST), and alkaline phosphatase (ALP)

  - Increased levels of bilirubin

  - Decreased levels of blood proteins

- Complete blood count, which can show signs of infection and anemia that may be caused by internal bleeding

- Tests for viral infections to see if you have hepatitis B or hepatitis C

- Blood tests for autoimmune liver conditions, which include the antinuclear antibody (ANA), anti-smooth muscle antibody (SMA), and antimitochondrial antibody (AMA) tests

Based on the blood test results, your doctor may be able to diagnose certain causes of cirrhosis.

Your doctor can use blood tests to tell how serious your cirrhosis is.

Imaging Tests

Imaging tests can show the size, shape, texture, and stiffness of your liver. Measuring the stiffness of the liver can show scarring. Your doctor can use stiffness measures to see if the scarring is getting better or worse. Imaging tests can also show how much fat is in the liver. Your doctor may use one or more of the following imaging tests:

- Magnetic resonance imaging (MRI)

- Ultrasound

- X-rays such as computerized tomography (CT) scans

- Transient elastography (TE), a special ultrasound that measures the stiffness of your liver and can measure liver fat

Liver Biopsy

Your doctor may perform a liver biopsy to see how much scarring in is your liver. A liver biopsy can diagnose cirrhosis when the results of other tests are uncertain. The biopsy may show the cause of cirrhosis. Sometimes your doctor may find that something other than cirrhosis has caused your liver to become damaged or enlarged. Your doctor can also diagnose liver cancer based on liver biopsy results.

How Do Doctors Treat Cirrhosis?

Doctors do not have specific treatments that can cure cirrhosis. However, they can treat many of the diseases that cause cirrhosis. Some of the diseases that cause cirrhosis can be cured. Treating the underlying causes of cirrhosis may keep your cirrhosis from getting worse and help prevent liver failure. Successful treatment may slowly improve some of your liver scarring.

How Do Doctors Treat the Causes of Cirrhosis?

Doctors most often treat the causes of cirrhosis with medicines. Your doctor will recommend that you stop activities such as drinking alcohol and taking certain medicines that may have caused cirrhosis or may make cirrhosis worse.

Alcoholic Liver Disease (ALD)

If you have alcoholic liver disease (ALD), your doctor will recommend that you completely stop drinking alcohol. He or she may refer you for alcohol treatment.

Nonalcoholic Fatty Liver Disease (NAFLD)

If you have nonalcoholic fatty liver disease (NAFLD), your doctor may recommend losing weight. Weight loss through healthy eating and regular physical activity can reduce fat in the liver, inflammation, and scarring.

Chronic Hepatitis C

If you have chronic hepatitis C, your doctor may prescribe one or more medicines that have been approved to treat hepatitis C since 2013. Studies have shown that these medicines can cure chronic hepatitis C in 80–95 percent of people with this disease.

Chronic Hepatitis B

For chronic hepatitis B, your doctor may prescribe antiviral medicines that slow or stop the virus from further damaging your liver.

Autoimmune Hepatitis

Doctors treat autoimmune hepatitis with medicines that suppress, or decrease the activity of, your immune system.

Diseases That Damage, Destroy, or Block Bile Ducts

Doctors usually treat diseases that damage, destroy, or block bile ducts with medicines such as ursodiol (Actigall, Urso). Doctors may use surgical procedures to open bile ducts that are narrowed or blocked. Diseases that damage, destroy, or block bile ducts include primary biliary cholangitis (PBC) and primary sclerosing cholangitis (PSC).

Inherited Liver Diseases

Treatment of inherited liver diseases depends on the disease. Treatment most often focuses on managing symptoms and complications.

Long-Term Use of Certain Medicines

The only specific treatment for most cases of cirrhosis caused by certain medicines is to stop taking the medicine that caused the problem. Talk with your doctor before you stop taking any medicines.

How Do Doctors Treat the Complications of Cirrhosis?

Treatments for the complications of cirrhosis include the following.

Portal Hypertension

Doctors treat portal hypertension with medicines to lower high blood pressure in the portal vein. Treatments for the complications of portal hypertension include:

- Enlarged veins in your esophagus or stomach, called varices. Your doctor may prescribe medicines to lower the pressure in the veins of your esophagus or stomach. This lowers the chance that the veins become enlarged and burst, causing internal bleeding. If you vomit blood or have black or bloody stools go to a hospital right away. Doctors may perform procedures during upper GI endoscopy or use surgical procedures to stop the internal bleeding.

- Swelling in your legs, ankles, or feet, called edema. Your doctor may prescribe medicines that remove fluid from your body. Your doctor will recommend limiting the amount of salt in your diet.

- Buildup of fluid in your abdomen, called ascites. Your doctor may prescribe medicines that remove fluid from your body. Your doctor will recommend limiting the amount of salt in your diet. If you have large amounts of fluid in your abdomen, your doctor may use a needle or tube to drain the fluid. He or she will check the fluid for signs of infection. Your doctor may prescribe medicines to treat infection or prevent infection.

- Confusion, difficulties thinking, memory loss, personality changes, or sleep disorders, called hepatic encephalopathy. Your doctor may prescribe medicines that help lower the levels of toxins in your brain and improve brain function.

Infections

If you have a bacterial infection, your doctor will prescribe an antibiotic.

Liver Cancer

Your doctor may treat liver cancer with the medical procedures that remove or destroy cancer cells, such as surgery, radiation therapy, and chemotherapy. Doctors also treat liver cancer with a liver transplant.

Liver Failure

Liver failure, also called end-stage liver disease, happens when the liver stops working. The only treatment for liver failure is a liver transplant.

Other Complications

Your doctor may treat other complications through changes in medicines, diet, or physical activity. Your doctor may also recommend surgery.

What Can I Do to Help Keep My Cirrhosis from Getting Worse?

To help keep your cirrhosis from getting worse, you can do the following:

- Do not drink alcohol or use illegal drugs.
- Talk with your doctor before taking:
  - Prescription medicines
  - Prescription and over-the-counter (OTC) sleep aids
  - OTC medicines, including nonsteroidal anti-inflammatory drugs (NSAIDS) and acetaminophen
  - Dietary supplements, including herbal supplements
- Take your medicines as directed.
- Get a vaccine for hepatitis A, hepatitis B, flu, pneumonia caused by certain bacteria, and shingles.
- Get a screening blood test for hepatitis C.
- Eat a healthy, well-balanced diet.
- Avoid raw or undercooked shellfish, fish, and meat.
- Try to keep a healthy body weight.

Talk with your doctor about your risk for getting liver cancer and how often you should be checked.

When Do Doctors Consider a Liver Transplant for Cirrhosis?

Your doctor will consider a liver transplant when cirrhosis leads to liver failure. Doctors consider liver transplants only after they have ruled out all other treatment options. Talk with your doctor about whether a liver transplant is right for you.

What Should I Eat If I Have Cirrhosis?

If you have cirrhosis, you should eat a healthy, well-balanced diet. Talk with your doctor, a dietitian, or a nutritionist about healthy eating.

What Should I Avoid Eating and Drinking If I Have Cirrhosis?

- You should avoid eating raw or undercooked shellfish, fish, and meat. Bacteria or viruses from these foods may cause severe infections in people with cirrhosis.

- Your doctor may recommend limiting salt in your diet and limiting your intake of fats or protein.

- You should completely stop drinking alcohol because it can cause more liver damage.

Chapter 33

Primary Sclerosing Cholangitis

What Is Primary Sclerosing Cholangitis?

Primary sclerosing cholangitis (PSC) is a chronic disease in which the bile ducts inside and outside the liver become inflamed and scarred, and are eventually narrowed or blocked. When the bile ducts are narrowed or blocked, bile builds up in the liver and causes liver damage. This damage can lead to cirrhosis and eventually liver failure. Medical experts believe that PSC is an autoimmune disease, which means that the immune system is overactive and attacks normal, healthy bile duct cells.

How Common Is Primary Sclerosing Cholangitis?

Researchers estimate that about 6–16 people out of 100,000 have PSC. However, this estimate may be low because not all people who have PSC are diagnosed with the disease.

This chapter includes text excerpted from "Primary Sclerosing Cholangitis," National Institute of Diabetes and Digestive and Kidney Diseases (NIDDK), January 2018.

Who Is More Likely to Get Primary Sclerosing Cholangitis?

You are more likely to get PSC if you:

- Are between the ages of 30 and 50

- Are a man

- Have inflammatory bowel disease (IBD), most commonly ulcerative colitis (UC)

- Have a family member who has PSC

What Other Health Problems Do People with Primary Sclerosing Cholangitis Have?

People with PSC may have other health problems, including:

- Inflammatory bowel disease (IBD)

- Gallstones

- Autoimmune diseases, such type 1 diabetes, celiac disease, and thyroid diseases

About 7 out of 10 people who have PSC also have IBD.

What Are the Complications of Primary Sclerosing Cholangitis?

Complications of PSC include:

- Low levels of fat-soluble vitamins

- Bile duct infection

- Cirrhosis

- Liver failure

- Bile duct cancer

- Gallbladder cancer

People with PSC and IBD have a greater chance of getting colorectal cancer.

What Are the Symptoms of Primary Sclerosing Cholangitis?

The main symptoms of PSC are:

- Feeling tired or weak
- Itchy skin

Other symptoms may include:

- Losing weight without trying
- Poor appetite
- Fever
- Pain in the abdomen

As the disease gets worse, you may get symptoms of cirrhosis and liver failure, such as:

- Bloating
- Bruising and bleeding easily
- Confusion, difficulty thinking, or memory loss
- Redness in the palms of your hands
- Swelling in your legs, ankles, or feet
- Yellowish eyes and skin called jaundice

Because PSC gets worse slowly, you can have the disease for years before you have any symptoms. Many people have no symptoms when they are first diagnosed with PSC.

What Causes Primary Sclerosing Cholangitis

The cause of PSC is not known. However, one or more of the following may play a role in causing the disease:

- Genes
- Immune system problems
- Changes in the bacteria in your gastrointestinal (GI) tract, also called gut flora or gut microbiome
- Bile duct injury caused by bile acids

How Do Doctors Diagnose Primary Sclerosing Cholangitis?

Doctors diagnose PSC based on your medical and family history, a physical exam, and the results of medical tests.

Your doctor will ask you about your symptoms. He or she may also ask whether:

- You have a history of inflammatory bowel disease (IBD), particularly ulcerative colitis (UC)

- One of your parents or siblings has PSC

- You have a history of autoimmune disease, such type 1 diabetes, celiac disease, and thyroid diseases

During a physical exam, your doctor may:

- Use a stethoscope to listen to sounds in your abdomen

- Tap or press on specific areas of your abdomen

- Look for symptoms of cirrhosis and liver failure

- Check to see if your liver and spleen are larger than they should be

- Check for tenderness or pain in your abdomen

Your doctor may also check for and ask about symptoms of a bile duct infection, which may include:

- Fever

- Chills

- Nausea

- Vomiting

- Yellowish eyes and skin called jaundice

What Medical Tests Do Doctors Use to Diagnose Primary Sclerosing Cholangitis?
Blood Tests

Liver function tests can show abnormal liver enzyme levels in your blood. Abnormal levels of certain liver enzymes may be a sign of damage to your liver or bile ducts. Blood tests can also show higher-than-normal levels of certain antibodies in the blood, which may be a sign of PSC. Another blood test, called a white blood cell (WBC) count, measures the number of WBCs in your blood. A high WBC count may be a sign of a bile duct infection.

Imaging Tests

Your doctor may perform one or more of the following imaging tests of your liver and bile ducts:

- Ultrasound

- Computed tomography (CT) scans

- Magnetic resonance imaging (MRI) scans

- Magnetic resonance cholangiopancreatography (MRCP)

- Endoscopic retrograde cholangiopancreatography (ERCP)

- Percutaneous transhepatic cholangiography (PTC). PTC is an X-ray of the bile ducts. A special dye injected into the bile ducts lets a doctor see the bile ducts on the X-ray. PTC can show narrowing or blockage in the bile ducts.

- Transient elastography, a special ultrasound that measures the stiffness of your liver

Imaging tests may help diagnose PSC by ruling out other causes of bile duct damage, such as autoimmune hepatitis and tumors.

Liver Biopsy

In some cases, your doctor may perform a liver biopsy to

- Confirm the diagnosis of PSC

- See whether the disease is advanced, as shown by the amount of liver scarring or cirrhosis

- Rule out other diseases that may be causing your symptoms

How Do Doctors Treat Primary Sclerosing Cholangitis?

Doctors can't cure primary sclerosing cholangitis (PSC) or keep the disease from getting worse. However, they can treat narrowed or blocked bile ducts and the symptoms and complications of PSC.

Narrowed or Blocked Bile Ducts

If your bile ducts are narrowed or blocked, your doctor may use medical procedures, such as endoscopic retrograde cholangiopancreatography (ERCP) and percutaneous transhepatic cholangiography, to open them and help keep them open.

Itchy Skin

Your doctor may recommend over-the-counter (OTC) products and medicines or prescribe medicines to treat itchy skin. OTC products and medicines include

- Skin creams and lotions that contain camphor, menthol, pramoxine, or capsaicin

- Antihistamines such as fexofenadine

For mild itchy skin, your doctor may prescribe hydroxyzine. For severe itchy skin, your doctor may prescribe cholestyramine.

Low Levels of Fat-Soluble Vitamins in Your Body

If you have low levels of fat-soluble vitamins in your body, your doctor may recommend dietary supplements of vitamins A, D, E, and K. Follow your doctor's instructions on the type and amount of vitamins you should take.

Bile Duct Infection

Your doctor may prescribe an antibiotic to treat a bile duct infection.

Cirrhosis

If your PSC has caused cirrhosis, your doctor may treat the health problems related to cirrhosis with medicines, surgery, and other medical procedures. If cirrhosis leads to liver failure, you may need a liver transplant.

When Do Doctors Consider a Liver Transplant for Primary Sclerosing Cholangitis?

Your doctor may consider a liver transplant if your PSC has caused liver failure. Doctors consider liver transplants only after all other treatment options have failed.

What Can I Do to Prevent Further Liver Damage?

To help prevent further liver damage, you can do the following:

- Carefully follow your doctor's instructions.

- Take your medicines and vitamins as directed.

- If you smoke, quit smoking.

- Do not drink any alcohol or use illegal drugs.

- Have regular checkups, as recommended by your doctor.

- Talk with your doctor before taking:

  - Prescription medicines

  - Over-the-counter (OTC) medicines

  - Dietary supplements

  - Complementary and alternative medicines (CAM)

- Try to keep a healthy body weight.

What Should I Eat If I Have Primary Sclerosing Cholangitis?

You should eat well-balanced meals that give you enough calories and nutrients. If you have low levels of fat-soluble vitamins in your body, your doctor may recommend eating foods that are high in vitamins A, D, E, and K. A healthcare professional such as a dietitian or nutritionist can help you plan meals that are good sources of these vitamins.

What Should I Avoid Eating If I Have Primary Sclerosing Cholangitis?

You should avoid eating raw shellfish such as oysters, which can have bacteria that may cause severe infections in people with liver disease. Your doctor may recommend that you avoid foods that are high in salt, fat, and carbohydrates, especially those with added sugars.

Your doctor will recommend that you stop drinking alcohol, or at least limit your intake to no more than one or two drinks per week. If you have PSC and cirrhosis, your doctor will recommend that you don't drink any alcohol at all.

Chapter 34

Other Liver Disorders

Chapter Contents

Section 34.1

Porphyria

This section includes text excerpted from "Porphyria,"
National Institute of Diabetes and Digestive and Kidney
Diseases (NIDDK), February 2014. Reviewed September 2018.

What Are Porphyrias?

Porphyrias are rare disorders that affect mainly the skin or nervous
system and may cause abdominal pain. These disorders are usually
inherited, meaning they are caused by abnormalities in genes passed
from parents to children. When a person has a porphyria, cells fail to
change body chemicals called porphyrins and porphyrin precursors
into heme, the substance that gives blood its red color. The body makes
heme mainly in the bone marrow and liver. Bone marrow is the soft,
sponge-like tissue inside the bones; it makes stem cells that develop
into one of the three types of blood cells—red blood cells (RBCs), white
blood cells (WBCs), and platelets.

The process of making heme is called the heme biosynthetic pathway. One of the eight enzymes controls each step of the process. The
body has a problem making heme if any one of the enzymes is at a low
level, also called a deficiency. Porphyrins and porphyrin precursors of
heme then build up in the body and cause illness.

What Is Heme and What Does It Do?

Heme is a red pigment composed of iron linked to a chemical called
protoporphyrin. Heme has important functions in the body. The largest
amounts of heme are in the form of hemoglobin, found in RBCs and bone
marrow. Hemoglobin carries oxygen from the lungs to all parts of the
body. In the liver, heme is a component of proteins that break down hormones, medications, and other chemicals and keep liver cells functioning
normally. Heme is an important part of nearly every cell in the body.

What Are the Types of Porphyria?

Each of the eight types of porphyria corresponds to low levels of
a specific enzyme in the heme biosynthetic pathway. Experts often
classify porphyrias as acute or cutaneous based on the symptoms a
person experiences:

- Acute porphyrias affect the nervous system. They occur rapidly and last only a short time.

- Cutaneous porphyrias affect the skin.

Two types of acute porphyrias, hereditary coproporphyria (HCP) and variegate porphyria (VP), can also have cutaneous symptoms. Experts also classify porphyrias as erythropoietic or hepatic:

- In erythropoietic porphyrias, the body overproduces porphyrins, mainly in the bone marrow.

- In hepatic porphyrias, the body overproduces porphyrins and porphyrin precursors, mainly in the liver.

The below table lists each type of porphyria, the deficient enzyme responsible for the disorder, and the main location of porphyrin buildup.

Table 34.1. Types of Porphyria

Type of Porphyria	Deficient Enzyme
Delta-aminolevulinate-dehydratase deficiency porphyria	Delta-aminolevulinic acid dehydratase (ALAD)
Acute intermittent porphyria (AIP)	Porphobilinogen deaminase (PBGD)
Hereditary coproporphyria (HCP)	Coproporphyrinogen oxidase (CPOX)
Variegate porphyria (VP)	Protoporphyrinogen oxidase (PPOX)
Congenital erythropoietic porphyria (CEP)	Uroporphyrinogen III cosynthase
Porphyria cutanea tarda (PCT)	Uroporphyrinogen decarboxylase (UROD) (~75% deficiency)
Hepatoerythropoietic porphyria (HEP)	Uroporphyrinogen decarboxylase (~90% deficiency)
Erythropoietic protoporphyria (EPP)*	Ferrochelatase (FECH) (~75% deficiency)

* *Protoporphyria XLPP (X-linked protoporphyria) is a variant of erythropoietic protoporphyria.*

How Common Is Porphyria?

The exact rates of porphyria are unknown and vary around the world. For example, PCT is most common in the United States, and variegate porphyria (VP) is most common in South America.

467

What Causes Porphyria

Most porphyrias are inherited disorders. Scientists have identified genes for all eight enzymes in the heme biosynthetic pathway. Most porphyrias result from inheriting an abnormal gene, also called a gene mutation, from one parent. Some porphyrias, such as congenital erythropoietic porphyria (CEP), hepatoerythropoietic porphyria (HEP), and erythropoietic protoporphyria (EPP), occur when a person inherits two abnormal genes, one from each parent. The likeliness of a person passing the abnormal gene or genes to the next generation depends on the type of porphyria.

Porphyria cutanea tarda (PCT) is usually an acquired disorder, meaning factors other than genes cause the enzyme deficiency. This type of porphyria can be triggered by:

- Too much iron

- Use of alcohol or estrogen

- Smoking

- Chronic hepatitis C—a long-lasting liver disease that causes inflammation, or swelling, of the liver

- Human immunodeficiency virus (HIV)—the virus that causes acquired immunodeficiency syndrome (AIDS)

- Abnormal genes associated with hemochromatosis—the most common form of iron overload disease, which causes the body to absorb too much iron

For all types of porphyria, symptoms can be triggered by:
- Use of alcohol
- Smoking
- Use of certain medications or hormones
- Exposure to sunlight
- Stress
- Dieting and fasting

What Are the Symptoms of Porphyria?

Some people with porphyria-causing gene mutations have latent porphyria, meaning they have no symptoms of the disorder. Symptoms of cutaneous porphyrias include:

- Oversensitivity to sunlight

- Blisters on exposed areas of the skin

- Itching and swelling on exposed areas of the skin

Symptoms of acute porphyrias include:

- Pain in the abdomen—the area between the chest and hips

- Pain in the chest, limbs, or back

- Nausea and vomiting

- Constipation—a condition in which an adult has fewer than three bowel movements a week or a child has fewer than two bowel movements a week, depending on the person

- Urinary retention—the inability to empty the bladder completely

- Confusion

- Hallucinations

- Seizures and muscle weakness

Symptoms of acute porphyrias can develop over hours or days and last for days or weeks. These symptoms can come and go over time, while symptoms of cutaneous porphyrias tend to be more continuous. Porphyria symptoms can vary widely in severity.

How Is Porphyria Diagnosed?

A healthcare provider diagnoses porphyria with blood, urine, and stool tests. These tests take place at a healthcare provider's office or a commercial facility. A blood test involves drawing blood and sending the sample to a lab for analysis. For urine and stool tests, the patient collects a sample of urine or stool in a special container. A healthcare provider tests the samples in the office or sends them to a lab for analysis. High levels of porphyrins or porphyrin precursors in blood, urine, or stool indicate porphyria. A healthcare provider may also recommend deoxyribonucleic acid (DNA) testing of a blood sample to look for known gene mutations that cause porphyrias.

How Is Porphyria Treated?

Treatment for porphyria depends on the type of porphyria the person has and the severity of the symptoms.

Acute Porphyrias

A healthcare provider treats acute porphyrias with heme or glucose loading to decrease the liver's production of porphyrins and porphyrin precursors. A patient receives heme intravenously once a day for four days. Glucose loading involves giving a patient a glucose solution by mouth or intravenously. Heme is usually more effective and is the treatment of choice unless symptoms are mild. In rare instances, if symptoms are severe, a healthcare provider will recommend liver transplantation to treat acute porphyria. In liver transplantation, a surgeon removes a diseased or an injured liver and replaces it with a healthy, whole liver or a segment of a liver from another person, called a donor. A patient has liver transplantation surgery in a hospital under general anesthesia. Liver transplantation can cure liver failure.

Cutaneous Porphyrias

The most important step a person can take to treat a cutaneous porphyria is to avoid sunlight as much as possible. Other cutaneous porphyrias are treated as follows:

- **Porphyria cutanea tarda (PCT).** A healthcare provider treats PCT by removing factors that tend to activate the disease and by performing repeated therapeutic phlebotomies to reduce iron in the liver. Therapeutic phlebotomy is the removal of about a pint of blood from a vein in the arm. A technician performs the procedure at a blood donation center, such as a hospital, clinic, or bloodmobile. A patient does not require anesthesia. Another treatment approach is low-dose hydroxychloroquine tablets to reduce porphyrins in the liver.

- **Erythropoietic protoporphyria (EPP).** People with EPP may be given beta-carotene or cysteine to improve sunlight tolerance, though these medications do not lower porphyrin levels. Experts recommend hepatitis A and hepatitis B vaccines and avoiding alcohol to prevent protoporphyria liver failure. A healthcare provider may use liver transplantation or a combination of medications to treat people who develop liver failure. Unfortunately, liver transplantation does not correct the primary defect, which is the continuous overproduction of protoporphyria by bone marrow. Successful bone marrow transplantations may successfully cure EPP. A healthcare provider only considers bone marrow transplantation if the disease is severe and leading to secondary liver disease.

- **Congenital erythropoietic porphyria (CEP) and hepatoerythropoietic porphyria (HEP).** People with CEP or HEP may need surgery to remove the spleen or blood transfusions to treat anemia. A surgeon removes the spleen in a hospital, and a patient receives general anesthesia. With a blood transfusion, a patient receives blood through an intravenous (IV) line inserted into a vein. A technician performs the procedure at a blood donation center, and a patient does not need anesthesia.

Secondary Porphyrinurias

Conditions called secondary porphyrinuria, such as disorders of the liver and bone marrow, as well as a number of drugs, chemicals, and toxins are often mistaken for porphyria because they lead to mild or moderate increases in porphyrin levels in the urine. Only high—not mild or moderate—levels of porphyrin or porphyrin precursors lead to a diagnosis of porphyria.

Eating, Diet, and Nutrition

People with an acute porphyria should eat a diet with an average-to-high level of carbohydrates. The recommended dietary allowance for carbohydrates is 130 grams per day for adults and children 1 year of age or older; pregnant and breastfeeding women need higher intakes. People should avoid limiting intake of carbohydrates and calories, even for short periods of time, as this type of dieting or fasting can trigger symptoms. People with an acute porphyria who want to lose weight should talk with their healthcare providers about diets they can follow to lose weight gradually. People undergoing therapeutic phlebotomies should drink plenty of milk, water, or juice before and after each procedure. A healthcare provider may recommend vitamin and mineral supplements for people with a cutaneous porphyria.

Section 34.2

Type I Glycogen Storage Disease

This section includes text excerpted from "Glycogen Storage
Disease Type I," Genetics Home Reference (GHR), National
Institutes of Health (NIH), September 18, 2018.

What Is Type I Glycogen Storage Disease?

Glycogen storage disease type I (also known as GSDI or von Gierke
disease) is an inherited disorder caused by the buildup of a complex
sugar called glycogen in the body's cells. The accumulation of glycogen
in certain organs and tissues, especially the liver, kidneys, and small
intestines, impairs their ability to function normally.

What Are the Signs and Symptoms of Type I Glycogen Storage Disease?

Signs and symptoms of this condition typically appear around
the age of three or four months, when babies start to sleep through
the night and do not eat as frequently as newborns. Affected infants
may have low blood sugar (hypoglycemia), which can lead to seizures. They can also have a buildup of lactic acid in the body (lactic acidosis), high blood levels of a waste product called uric acid
(hyperuricemia), and excess amounts of fats in the blood (hyperlip-
idemia). As they get older, children with GSDI have thin arms and
legs and short stature. An enlarged liver may give the appearance of
a protruding abdomen. The kidneys may also be enlarged. Affected
individuals may also have diarrhea and deposits of cholesterol in
the skin (xanthomas).

People with GSDI may experience delayed puberty. Beginning in
young to mid-adulthood, affected individuals may have thinning of
the bones (osteoporosis), a form of arthritis resulting from uric acid
crystals in the joints (gout), kidney disease, and high blood pressure
in the blood vessels that supply the lungs (pulmonary hypertension).
Females with this condition may also have abnormal development of
the ovaries (polycystic ovaries). In affected teens and adults, tumors
called adenomas may form in the liver. Adenomas are usually noncancerous (benign), but occasionally these tumors can become cancerous
(malignant).

What Are the Types?

Researchers have described two types of GSDI, which differ in their signs and symptoms and genetic cause. These types are known as glycogen storage disease type Ia (GSDIa) and glycogen storage disease type Ib (GSDIb). Two other forms of GSDI have been described, and they were originally named types Ic and Id. However, these types are now known to be variations of GSDIb; for this reason, GSDIb is sometimes called GSD type I non-a.

Many people with GSDIb have a shortage of white blood cells (neutropenia), which can make them prone to recurrent bacterial infections. Neutropenia is usually apparent by age one. Many affected individuals also have inflammation of the intestinal walls (inflammatory bowel disease (IBD)). People with GSDIb may have oral problems including cavities, inflammation of the gums (gingivitis), chronic gum (periodontal) disease, abnormal tooth development, and open sores (ulcers) in the mouth. The neutropenia and oral problems are specific to people with GSDIb and are typically not seen in people with GSDIa.

How Common Is Type I Glycogen Storage Disease?

The overall incidence of GSDI is 1 in 100,000 individuals. GSDIa is more common than GSDIb, accounting for 80 percent of all GSDI cases.

What Causes Type I Glycogen Storage Disease

Mutations in two genes, *G6PC* and *SLC37A4*, cause GSDI. *G6PC* gene mutations cause GSDIa, and *SLC37A4* gene mutations cause GSDIb. The proteins produced from the *G6PC* and *SLC37A4* genes work together to break down a type of sugar molecule called glucose 6-phosphate. The breakdown of this molecule produces the simple sugar glucose, which is the primary energy source for most cells in the body.

Mutations in the *G6PC* and *SLC37A4* genes prevent the effective breakdown of glucose 6-phosphate. Glucose 6-phosphate that is not broken down to glucose is converted to glycogen and fat so it can be stored within cells. Too much glycogen and fat stored within a cell can be toxic. This buildup damages organs and tissues throughout the body, particularly the liver and kidneys, leading to the signs and symptoms of GSDI.

473

Inheritance Pattern

This condition is inherited in an autosomal recessive pattern, which means both copies of the gene in each cell have mutations. The parents of an individual with an autosomal recessive condition each carry one copy of the mutated gene, but they typically do not show signs and symptoms of the condition.

What Are the Other Names of Type I Glycogen Storage Disease?

- Glucose-6-phosphate deficiency
- Glucose-6-phosphate transport defect
- GSD I
- GSD type I
- Hepatorenal form of glycogen storage disease
- Hepatorenal glycogenosis
- Von Gierke disease

Section 34.3

Hemochromatosis

This section includes text excerpted from "Hemochromatosis,"
National Institute of Diabetes and Digestive and Kidney
Diseases (NIDDK), March 2014. Reviewed September 2018.

What Is Hemochromatosis?

Hemochromatosis is the most common form of iron overload disease. Too much iron in the body causes hemochromatosis. Iron is important because it is part of hemoglobin, a molecule in the blood that transports oxygen from the lungs to all body tissues. However, too much iron in the body leads to iron overload—a buildup of extra iron that, without treatment, can damage organs such as the liver, heart, and pancreas;

endocrine glands; and joints. The three types of hemochromatosis are primary hemochromatosis, also called hereditary hemochromatosis; secondary hemochromatosis; and neonatal hemochromatosis.

What Causes Hemochromatosis
Primary Hemochromatosis

Inherited genetic defects cause primary hemochromatosis, and mutations in the *HFE* gene are associated with up to 90 percent of cases. The *HFE* gene helps regulate the amount of iron absorbed from food. The two known mutations of *HFE* are *C282Y* and *H63D*. *C282Y* defects are the most common cause of primary hemochromatosis.

People inherit two copies of the *HFE* gene—one copy from each parent. Most people who inherit two copies of the *HFE* gene with the *C282Y* defect will have higher-than-average iron absorption. However, not all of these people will develop health problems associated with hemochromatosis. One study found that 31 percent of people with two copies of the *C282Y* defect developed health problems by their early fifties. Men who develop health problems from *HFE* defects typically develop them after age 40. Women who develop health problems from *HFE* defects typically develop them after menopause.

People who inherit two *H63D* defects or one *C282Y* and one *H63D* defect may have higher-than-average iron absorption. However, they are unlikely to develop iron overload and organ damage.

Rare defects in other genes may also cause primary hemochromatosis. Mutations in the hemojuvelin or hepcidin genes cause juvenile hemochromatosis, a type of primary hemochromatosis. People with juvenile hemochromatosis typically develop severe iron overload and liver and heart damage between ages 15 and 30.

Secondary Hemochromatosis

Hemochromatosis that is not inherited is called secondary hemochromatosis. The most common cause of secondary hemochromatosis is frequent blood transfusions in people with severe anemia. Anemia is a condition in which red blood cells are fewer or smaller than normal, which means they carry less oxygen to the body's cells. Types of anemia that may require frequent blood transfusions include:

- Congenital, or inherited, anemias such as sickle cell disease (SCD), thalassemia, and Fanconi syndrome (FS)

- Severe acquired anemias, which are not inherited, such as aplastic anemia and autoimmune hemolytic anemia

Liver diseases—such as alcoholic liver disease, nonalcoholic steatohepatitis (NASH), and chronic hepatitis C infection—may cause mild iron overload. However, this iron overload causes much less liver damage than the underlying liver disease causes.

Neonatal Hemochromatosis

Neonatal hemochromatosis is a rare disease characterized by liver failure and death in fetuses and newborns. Researchers are studying the causes of neonatal hemochromatosis and believe more than one factor may lead to the disease.

Experts previously considered neonatal hemochromatosis a type of primary hemochromatosis. However, studies suggest genetic defects that increase iron absorption do not cause this disease. Instead, the mother's immune system may produce antibodies—proteins made by the immune system to protect the body from foreign substances such as bacteria or viruses—that damage the liver of the fetus. Women who have had one child with neonatal hemochromatosis are at risk for having more children with the disease. Treating these women during pregnancy with intravenous (IV) immunoglobulin—a solution of antibodies from healthy people—can prevent fetal liver damage.

Researchers supported by the National Institute of Diabetes and Digestive and Kidney Diseases (NIDDK) recently found that a combination of exchange transfusion—removing blood and replacing it with donor blood—and IV immunoglobulin is an effective treatment for babies born with neonatal hemochromatosis.

Who Is More Likely to Develop Hemochromatosis?

Primary hemochromatosis mainly affects Caucasians of Northern European descent. This disease is one of the most common genetic disorders in the United States. About four to five out of every 1,000 Caucasians carry two copies of the *C282Y* mutation of the *HFE* gene and are susceptible to developing hemochromatosis. About one out of every 10 Caucasians carries one copy of *C282Y*.

Hemochromatosis is extremely rare in African Americans, Asian Americans, Hispanics/Latinos, and American Indians. *HFE* mutations are usually not the cause of hemochromatosis in these populations.

Both men and women can inherit the gene defects for hemochromatosis; however, not all will develop the symptoms of hemochromatosis. Men usually develop symptoms at a younger age than women. Women lose blood—which contains iron—regularly during menstruation; therefore, women with the gene defects that cause hemochromatosis may not develop iron overload and related symptoms and complications until after menopause.

What Are the Symptoms of Hemochromatosis?

A person with hemochromatosis may notice one or more of the following symptoms:

- Joint pain
- Fatigue, or feeling tired
- Unexplained weight loss
- Abnormal bronze or gray skin color
- Abdominal pain
- Loss of sex drive

Not everyone with hemochromatosis will develop these symptoms.

What Are the Complications of Hemochromatosis?

Without treatment, iron may build up in the organs and cause complications, including:

- Cirrhosis, or scarring of liver tissue
- Diabetes
- Irregular heart rhythms or weakening of the heart muscle
- Arthritis
- Erectile dysfunction (ED)

The complication most often associated with hemochromatosis is liver damage. Iron buildup in the liver causes cirrhosis, which increases the chance of developing liver cancer. For some people, complications may be the first sign of hemochromatosis. However, not everyone with hemochromatosis will develop complications.

How Is Hemochromatosis Diagnosed?

Healthcare providers use medical and family history, a physical exam, and routine blood tests to diagnose hemochromatosis or other conditions that could cause the same symptoms or complications.

- **Medical and family history.** Taking a medical and family history is one of the first things a healthcare provider may do to help diagnose hemochromatosis. The healthcare provider will look for clues that may indicate hemochromatosis, such as a family history of arthritis or unexplained liver disease.

- **Physical exam.** After taking a medical history, a healthcare provider will perform a physical exam, which may help diagnose hemochromatosis. During a physical exam, a healthcare provider usually:

  - Examines a patient's body

  - Uses a stethoscope to listen to bodily sounds

  - Taps on specific areas of the patient's body

- **Blood tests.** A blood test involves drawing blood at a healthcare provider's office or a commercial facility and sending the sample to a lab for analysis. Blood tests can determine whether the amount of iron stored in the body is higher than normal:

  - The transferrin saturation test shows how much iron is bound to the protein that carries iron in the blood. Transferrin saturation values above or equal to 45 percent are considered abnormal.

  - The serum ferritin test detects the amount of ferritin—a protein that stores iron—in the blood. Levels above 300 μg/L in men and 200 μg/L in women are considered abnormal. Levels above 1,000 μg/L in men or women indicate a high chance of iron overload and organ damage.

If either test shows higher-than-average levels of iron in the body, healthcare providers can order a special blood test that can detect two copies of the C282Y mutation to confirm the diagnosis. If the mutation is not present, healthcare providers will look for other causes.

- **Liver biopsy.** Healthcare providers may perform a liver biopsy, a procedure that involves taking a piece of liver tissue for examination with a microscope for signs of damage or disease.

The healthcare provider may ask the patient to temporarily stop taking certain medications before the liver biopsy. The healthcare provider may ask the patient to fast for eight hours before the procedure.

During the procedure, the patient lies on a table, right hand resting above the head. The healthcare provider applies a local anesthetic to the area where he or she will insert the biopsy needle. If needed, a healthcare provider will also give sedatives and pain medication. The healthcare provider uses a needle to take a small piece of liver tissue. He or she may use ultrasound, computerized tomography scans, or other imaging techniques to guide the needle. After the biopsy, the patient must lie on the right side for up to two hours and is monitored an additional two to four hours before being sent home.

A healthcare provider performs a liver biopsy at a hospital or an outpatient center. The healthcare provider sends the liver sample to a pathology lab where the pathologist—a doctor who specializes in diagnosing disease—looks at the tissue with a microscope and sends a report to the patient's healthcare provider. The biopsy shows how much iron has accumulated in the liver and whether the patient has liver damage.

Hemochromatosis is rare, and healthcare providers may not think to test for this disease. Thus, the disease is often not diagnosed or treated. The initial symptoms can be diverse, vague, and similar to the symptoms of many other diseases. Healthcare providers may focus on the symptoms and complications caused by hemochromatosis rather than on the underlying iron overload. However, if a healthcare provider diagnoses and treats the iron overload caused by hemochromatosis before organ damage has occurred, a person can live a normal, healthy life.

Who Should Be Tested for Hemochromatosis?

Experts recommend testing for hemochromatosis in people who have symptoms, complications, or a family history of the disease. Some researchers have suggested widespread screening for the *C282Y* mutation in the general population. However, screening is not cost effective. Although the *C282Y* mutation occurs quite frequently, the disease caused by the mutation is rare, and many people with two copies of the mutation never develop iron overload or organ damage.

Researchers and public health officials suggest the following:

- Siblings of people who have hemochromatosis should have their blood tested to see if they have the *C282Y* mutation.

- Parents, children, and other close relatives of people who have hemochromatosis should consider being tested.

- Healthcare providers should consider testing people who have severe and continuing fatigue, unexplained cirrhosis, joint pain or arthritis, heart problems, erectile dysfunction (ED), or diabetes because these health issues may result from hemochromatosis.

How Is Hemochromatosis Treated?

Healthcare providers treat hemochromatosis by drawing blood. This process is called phlebotomy. Phlebotomy rids the body of extra iron. This treatment is simple, inexpensive, and safe.

Based on the severity of the iron overload, a patient will have phlebotomy to remove a pint of blood once or twice a week for several months to a year, and occasionally longer. Healthcare providers will test serum ferritin levels periodically to monitor iron levels. The goal is to bring serum ferritin levels to the low end of the average range and keep them there. Depending on the lab, the level is 25–50 μg/L.

After phlebotomy reduces serum ferritin levels to the desired level, patients may need maintenance phlebotomy treatment every few months. Some patients may need phlebotomies more often. Serum ferritin tests every six months or once a year will help determine how often a patient should have blood drawn. Many blood donation centers provide free phlebotomy treatment for people with hemochromatosis.

Treating hemochromatosis before organs are damaged can prevent complications such as cirrhosis, heart problems, arthritis, and diabetes. Treatment cannot cure these conditions in patients who already have them at diagnosis. However, treatment will help most of these conditions improve. The treatment's effectiveness depends on the degree of organ damage. For example, treating hemochromatosis can stop the progression of liver damage in its early stages and lead to a normal life expectancy. However, if a patient develops cirrhosis, his or her chance of developing liver cancer increases, even with phlebotomy treatment. Arthritis usually does not improve even after phlebotomy removes extra iron.

Eating, Diet, and Nutrition

Iron is an essential nutrient found in many foods. People with hemochromatosis absorb much more iron from the food they eat compared with healthy people. People with hemochromatosis can help prevent iron overload by:

- eating only moderate amounts of iron-rich foods, such as red meat and organ meat
- avoiding supplements that contain iron
- avoiding supplements that contain vitamin C, which increases iron absorption

People with hemochromatosis can take steps to help prevent liver damage, including:

- Limiting the amount of alcoholic beverages they drink because alcohol increases their chance of cirrhosis and liver cancer
- Avoiding alcoholic beverages entirely if they already have cirrhosis

Section 34.4

Wilson Disease

This section includes text excerpted from "Wilson Disease," National Institute of Diabetes and Digestive and Kidney Diseases (NIDDK), July 2014. Reviewed September 2018.

What Is Wilson Disease?

Wilson disease is a genetic disease that prevents the body from removing extra copper. The body needs a small amount of copper from food to stay healthy; however, too much copper is poisonous. Normally, the liver filters extra copper and releases it into bile. Bile is a fluid made by the liver that carries toxins and wastes out of the body through the gastrointestinal tract. In Wilson disease, the liver does not filter copper correctly and copper builds up in the liver, brain, eyes, and other organs. Over time, high copper levels can cause life-threatening organ damage.

What Causes Wilson Disease

Wilson disease is caused by an inherited autosomal recessive mutation, or change, in the *ATP7B* gene. In an autosomal recessive disease, the child has to inherit the gene mutation from both parents to have an increased likelihood for the disease. The chance of a child inheriting autosomal recessive mutations from both parents with a gene mutation is 25 percent, or one in four. If only one parent carries the mutated gene, the child will not get the disease, although the child may inherit one copy of the gene mutation. The child is called a "carrier" of the disease and can pass the gene mutation to the next generation. Genetic testing is a procedure that identifies changes in a patient's genes and can show whether a parent or child is a carrier of a mutated gene. Autosomal recessive diseases are typically not seen in every generation of an affected family.

The following chart shows the chance of inheriting an autosomal recessive mutation from parents who both carry the mutated gene.

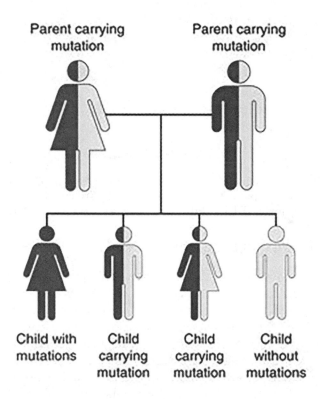

Figure 34.1. *Autosomal Recessive Mutation*

Who Is More Likely to Develop Wilson Disease?

Men and women develop Wilson disease at equal rates. About one in 30,000 people have Wilson disease. Symptoms usually appear between ages 5 and 35; however, new cases have been reported in people ages 3–72.

A person's risk of being a carrier or having Wilson disease increases when his or her family has a known history of Wilson disease. Some people may not know about a family history of the condition because the mutation is often passed to a child by a parent who is a carrier. A person's chances of having Wilson disease increase if a healthcare provider has diagnosed one or both parents with the condition.

What Are the Signs and Symptoms of Wilson Disease?

The signs and symptoms of Wilson disease vary, depending on what organs of the body are affected. Wilson disease is present at birth; however, the signs and symptoms of the disease do not appear until the copper builds up in the liver, the brain, or other organs.

When people have signs and symptoms, they usually affect the liver, the central nervous system (CNS), or both. The CNS includes the brain, the spinal cord, and nerves throughout the body. Sometimes a person does not have symptoms and a healthcare provider discovers the disease during a routine physical exam or blood test, or during an illness. Children can have Wilson disease for several years before any signs and symptoms occur. People with Wilson disease may have:

- Liver-related signs and symptoms

- CNS-related signs and symptoms

- Mental health-related signs and symptoms

- Other signs and symptoms

Liver-Related Signs and Symptoms

People with Wilson disease may develop signs and symptoms of chronic, or long lasting, liver disease:

- Weakness

- Fatigue, or feeling tired

- Loss of appetite

483

- Nausea

- Vomiting

- Weight loss

- Pain and bloating from fluid accumulating in the abdomen

- Edema—swelling, usually in the legs, feet, or ankles and less often in the hands or face

- Itching

- Spiderlike blood vessels, called spider angiomas, near the surface of the skin

- Muscle cramps

- Jaundice, a condition that causes the skin and whites of the eyes to turn yellow

Some people with Wilson disease may not develop signs or symptoms of liver disease until they develop acute liver failure—a condition that develops suddenly.

Central Nervous System (CNS)-Related Signs and Symptoms

Central nervous system (CNS)-related symptoms usually appear in people after the liver has retained a lot of copper; however, signs and symptoms of liver disease may not be present. CNS-related symptoms occur most often in adults and sometimes occur in children. Signs and symptoms include:

- Tremors or uncontrolled movements

- Muscle stiffness

- Problems with speech, swallowing, or physical coordination

A healthcare provider may refer people with these symptoms to a neurologist—a doctor who specializes in nervous system diseases.

Mental Health-Related Signs and Symptoms

Some people will have mental health-related signs and symptoms when copper builds up in the central nervous system. Signs and symptoms may include:

- Personality changes

- Depression

- Feeling anxious, or nervous, about most things

- Psychosis—when a person loses contact with reality

Other Signs and Symptoms

Other signs and symptoms of Wilson disease may include:

- Anemia, a condition in which red blood cells (RBCs) are fewer or smaller than normal, which prevents the body's cells from getting enough oxygen

- Arthritis, a condition in which a person has pain and swelling in one or more joints

- High levels of amino acids, protein, uric acid, and carbohydrates in urine

- Low platelet or white blood cell (WBC) count

- Osteoporosis, a condition in which the bones become less dense and more likely to fracture

Kayser-Fleischer (KF) Rings

Kayser-Fleischer (KF) rings result from a buildup of copper in the eyes and are the most unique sign of Wilson disease. During an eye exam, a healthcare provider will see a rusty-brown ring around the edge of the iris and in the rim of the cornea. The iris is the colored part of the eye surrounding the pupil. The cornea is the transparent outer membrane or layer that covers the eye.

People with Wilson disease who show signs of nervous system damage usually have Kayser-Fleischer rings. However, the rings are present in only 40–66 percent of people with signs of liver damage alone.

What Are the Complications of Wilson Disease?

People who have Wilson disease that is not treated or diagnosed early can have serious complications, such as:

- Cirrhosis—scarring of the liver

- Kidney damage—as liver function decreases, the kidneys may be damaged

- Persistent nervous system problems when nervous system symptoms do not resolve

- Liver cancer—hepatocellular carcinoma is a type of liver cancer that can occur in people with cirrhosis

- Liver failure—a condition in which the liver stops working properly

- Death, if left untreated

How Is Wilson Disease Diagnosed?

Healthcare providers typically see the same symptoms of Wilson disease in other conditions, and the symptoms of Wilson disease do not occur together often, making the disease difficult to diagnose.

A healthcare provider may use several tests and exams to diagnose Wilson disease, including the following:

Medical and Family History

A healthcare provider may take a medical and family history to help diagnose Wilson disease.

Physical Exam

A physical exam may help diagnose Wilson disease. During a physical exam, a healthcare provider usually:

- examines a patient's body

- uses a stethoscope to listen to sounds related to the abdomen

A healthcare provider will use a special light called a slit lamp to look for Kayser-Fleischer rings in the eyes.

Blood Tests

A nurse or technician will draw blood samples at a healthcare provider's office or a commercial facility and send the samples to a lab for analysis. A healthcare provider may:

- Perform liver enzyme or function tests—blood tests that may indicate liver abnormalities

- Check copper levels in the blood. Since the copper is deposited into the organs and is not circulating in the blood, most people with Wilson disease have a lower-than-normal level of copper in the blood. In cases of acute liver failure caused by Wilson disease, the level of blood copper is often higher than normal

- Check the level of ceruloplasmin—a protein that carries copper in the bloodstream. Most people with Wilson disease have a lower-than-normal ceruloplasmin level

- Conduct genetic testing. A healthcare provider may recommend genetic testing in cases of a known family history of Wilson disease

Urine Tests

24-hour urine collection. A patient will collect urine at home in a special container provided by a healthcare provider's office or a commercial facility. A healthcare provider sends the sample to a lab for analysis. A 24-hour urine collection will show increased copper in the urine in most patients who have symptoms due to Wilson disease.

Liver Biopsy

A liver biopsy is a procedure that involves taking a small piece of liver tissue for examination with a microscope for signs of damage or disease. The healthcare provider may ask the patient to stop taking certain medications temporarily before the liver biopsy. He or she may also ask the patient to fast—eat or drink nothing—for eight hours before the procedure.

During the procedure, the patient lies on a table, right hand resting above the head. The healthcare provider applies a local anesthetic to the area where he or she will insert the biopsy needle. If needed, a healthcare provider will also give sedatives and pain medication. The healthcare provider uses the needle to take a small piece of liver tissue. He or she may use ultrasound, computerized tomography scans, or other imaging techniques to guide the needle. After the biopsy, the patient must lie on the right side for up to two hours and is monitored an additional two to four hours before being sent home.

A pathologist—a doctor who specializes in diagnosing diseases—examines the liver tissue in a lab. The test can show cirrhosis of the liver. Sometimes the liver biopsy will show copper buildup in the liver cells; however, the results can vary because the copper does not always deposit evenly into the liver. Therefore, healthcare providers often find it more useful to analyze a piece of liver tissue for copper content. Most patients with Wilson disease have high levels of copper in the liver tissue when compared with carriers or with people who do not have Wilson disease.

Imaging Tests

A healthcare provider may order imaging tests to evaluate brain abnormalities in patients who have nervous system symptoms often seen with Wilson disease, or in patients diagnosed with Wilson disease. Healthcare providers do not use brain imaging tests to diagnose Wilson disease, though certain findings may suggest the patient has the disease.

Magnetic resonance imaging (MRI). An MRI is a test that takes pictures of the body's internal organs and soft tissues without using X-rays. A specially trained technician performs the procedure in an outpatient center or a hospital, and a radiologist—a doctor who specializes in medical imaging—interprets the images. The patient does not need anesthesia, though people with a fear of confined spaces may receive light sedation, taken by mouth. An MRI may include the injection of a special dye, called contrast medium. With most MRI machines, the patient will lie on a table that slides into a tunnel-shaped device that may be open ended or closed at one end. Some machines allow the patient to lie in a more open space. The technician will take a sequence of images from different angles to create a detailed picture of the brain. During sequencing, the patient will hear loud mechanical knocking and humming noises. MRI can show if other diseases or conditions are causing the patient's neurological symptoms.

Computerized tomography (CT) scan. A CT scan uses a combination of X-rays and computer technology to create images. For a CT scan, a healthcare provider may give the patient a solution to drink and an injection of contrast medium. CT scans require the patient to lie on a table that slides into a tunnel-shaped device where a technician takes the X-rays. An X-ray technician performs the procedure in an outpatient center or a hospital. A radiologist interprets the images. The patient does not need anesthesia. A CT scan can show if other diseases or conditions are causing the patient's neurological symptoms.

How Is Wilson Disease Treated?

A healthcare provider will treat Wilson disease with a lifelong effort to reduce and control the amount of copper in the body. Treatment may include:

- Medications

- Changes in eating, diet, and nutrition

- A liver transplant

Medications

A healthcare provider will prescribe medications to treat Wilson disease. The medications have different actions that healthcare providers use during different phases of the treatment.

Chelating agents. Chelating agents are medications that remove extra copper from the body by releasing it from organs into the bloodstream. Once the copper is in the bloodstream, the kidneys then filter the copper and pass it into the urine. A healthcare provider usually recommends chelating agents at the beginning of treatment. A potential side effect of chelating agents is that nervous system symptoms may become worse during treatment. The two medications available for this type of treatment include:

- trientine (Syprine)—the risk for side effects and worsening nervous system symptoms appears to be lower with trientine than d-penicillamine. Researchers are still studying the side effects; however, some healthcare providers prefer to prescribe trientine as the first treatment of choice because it appears to be safer.

- d-penicillamine—people taking d-penicillamine may have other reactions or side effects, such as:

  - Fever

  - A rash

  - Kidney problems

  - Bone marrow problems

A healthcare provider will prescribe a lower dose of a chelating agent to women who are pregnant to reduce the risk of birth defects. A healthcare provider should consider future screening on any newborn whose parent has Wilson disease.

Zinc. A healthcare provider will prescribe zinc for patients who do not have symptoms, or after a person has completed successful treatment using a chelating agent and symptoms begin to improve. Zinc, taken by mouth as zinc salts such as zinc acetate (Galzin), blocks the digestive tract's absorption of copper from food. Although most people taking zinc usually do not experience side effects, some people may experience stomach upset. A healthcare provider may prescribe zinc for children with Wilson disease who show no symptoms. Women may take the full dosage of zinc safely during pregnancy.

Maintenance, or long term, treatment begins when symptoms improve and tests show that copper is at a safe level. Maintenance treatment typically includes taking zinc or a lower dose of a chelating agent. A healthcare provider closely monitors the person and reviews regular blood and urine tests to ensure maintenance treatment controls the copper level in the body.

Treatment for people with Wilson disease who have no symptoms may include a chelating agent or zinc in order to prevent symptoms from developing and stop or slow disease progression.

People with Wilson disease will take medications for the rest of their lives. Follow up and adherence to the healthcare provider's treatment plan is necessary to manage symptoms and prevent organ damage.

Changes in Eating, Diet, and Nutrition

People with Wilson disease should reduce their dietary copper intake by avoiding foods that are high in copper, such as:

- Shellfish
- Liver
- Mushrooms
- Nuts
- Chocolate

People should not eat these foods during the initial treatment and talk with the healthcare provider to discuss if they are safe to eat in moderation during maintenance treatment.

People with Wilson disease whose tap water runs through copper pipes or comes from a well should check the copper levels in the tap water. Water that sits in copper pipes may pick up copper residue, but running water lowers the level to within acceptable limits. People with Wilson disease should not use copper containers or cookware to store or prepare food or drinks.

To help ensure coordinated and safe care, people should discuss their use of complementary and alternative medical practices, including their use of vitamins and dietary supplements, with their healthcare provider. If the healthcare provider recommends taking any type of supplement or vitamin, a pharmacist can recommend types that do not contain copper.

People should talk with a healthcare provider about diet changes to reduce copper intake.

Liver Transplant

A liver transplant may be necessary for people when:

- Cirrhosis leads to liver failure

- Acute liver failure happens suddenly

- Treatment is not effective

A liver transplant is an operation to remove a diseased or an injured liver and replace it with a healthy one from another person, called a donor. A successful transplant is a life-saving treatment for people with liver failure.

Most liver transplants are successful. About 85 percent of transplanted livers are functioning after 1 year. Liver transplant surgery provides a cure for Wilson disease in most cases.

How Can Wilson Disease Be Prevented?

A person cannot prevent Wilson disease; however, people with a family history of Wilson disease, especially those with an affected sibling or parent, should talk with a healthcare provider about testing. A healthcare provider may be able to diagnose Wilson disease before symptoms appear. Early diagnosis and treatment of Wilson disease can reduce or even prevent organ damage.

People with a family history of the disease may also benefit from genetic testing that can identify one or more gene mutations. A healthcare provider may refer a person with a family history of Wilson disease to a geneticist—a doctor who specializes in genetic diseases.

Section 34.5

Sarcoidosis

This section includes text excerpted from "Sarcoidosis,"
National Heart, Lung, and Blood Institute (NHLBI), March 29, 2018.

Sarcoidosis is a rare condition in which groups of immune cells form lumps, called granulomas, in various organs in the body. Inflammation, which may be triggered by infection or exposure to certain substances, is thought to play a role in the formation of granulomas.

Sarcoidosis can affect any organ. Most often it affects the lungs and lymph nodes in the chest. You may experience fatigue, which is extreme tiredness, or fever, but you may also experience other signs and symptoms depending on the organ that is affected. Your doctor will diagnose sarcoidosis in part by ruling out other diseases that have similar symptoms.

Determining whether treatment is needed and what type depends on your signs and symptoms, which organs are affected, and how well those organs are working. Medicines used to treat sarcoidosis help reduce inflammation or suppress the immune system. Many people recover with few or no long-term problems. Sometimes the disease causes permanent scarring in the affected organs. When scarring happens in the lungs, this is called pulmonary fibrosis.

What Causes Sarcoidosis?

Sarcoidosis is a condition in which immune cells form lumps, called granulomas, in your organs. Inflammation is thought to cause granulomas to form and may lead to temporary or permanent scarring at the site of the granulomas. Your inherited genes or certain environmental factors may trigger the inflammation that leads to granulomas.

Genetics

Studies suggest that people get sarcoidosis because of genes that make you susceptible to the disease. Some of the genes that are related to sarcoidosis are associated with the immune system.

Environmental Factors

Environmental factors, such as infection or exposure to certain substances, can trigger changes in the immune system and lead to sarcoidosis. Studies suggest that these triggers may cause sarcoidosis only in people with genes that make them susceptible to the disease.

What Are the Risk Factors of Sarcoidosis?
Age

You can be diagnosed with sarcoidosis at any age, but sarcoidosis is most commonly diagnosed in people age 55 and older.

Environment or Occupation

Your risk for sarcoidosis may be higher if you have repeated exposure to environmental substances that cause inflammation, such as insecticides or mold, or if you work in healthcare or as a firefighter. Working in these occupations may expose you to substances that trigger the formation of granulomas.

Family History and Genetics

You have a higher risk of sarcoidosis if you have a close relative with sarcoidosis.

Other Medical Conditions

Sarcoidosis sometimes occurs after lymphoma, a type of blood cancer.

Race or Ethnicity

People of any race can get sarcoidosis, but it is more common in people of African or Scandinavian descent.

Sex

Both men and women can develop sarcoidosis, but it is more common in women.

Screening and Prevention

Currently, there are no screening methods to determine who will develop sarcoidosis. If you are at risk for sarcoidosis, your doctor may recommend you try to avoid insecticides, mold, or other environmental sources of substances known to trigger the formation of granulomas.

Signs, Symptoms, and Complications

Many people who have sarcoidosis have no signs or symptoms. Some people experience general signs and symptoms of sarcoidosis such as fever and weight loss. Others will experience signs and symptoms that will depend on which organs are affected. If inflammation continues, some people may develop permanent scarring, which can lead to life-threatening serious heart or lung complications.

Signs and Symptoms

Many people have general signs and symptoms, such as:

- Depression

- Fatigue

- Fever

- Malaise, or a feeling of discomfort or illness

- Pain and swelling in the joints

- Weight loss

Sarcoidosis most often affects the lungs and the lymph nodes in the chest. Some people with sarcoidosis in the lungs may wheeze, cough, feel short of breath, or have chest pain. However, people with sarcoidosis in the lungs do not always have lung-related symptoms.

If sarcoidosis affects other organs or parts of your body, you may have other symptoms related to those organs:

- Abdominal pain

- A larger than normal spleen

- Anemia

- Burning, itchy, or dry eyes

- Fainting

- Heart palpitations

- Joint pain

- Muscle weakness

- Problems with a liver that is larger than normal, including itching, vomiting, nausea, jaundice, or abdominal pain.

- Problems with the nervous system, including headache, dizziness, vision problems, seizures, mood swings, disturbed behavior, hallucinations, delusions, back pain, or pain associated with particular nerves.

- Skin changes, including erythema nodosum or lupus pernio, a condition that causes skin sores that usually affect the face, especially the nose, cheeks, lips, and ears. The sores associated with lupus pernio tend to last a long time. Lupus pernio occurs mostly in African Americans and can return after sarcoidosis treatment is over.

- Swelling of the salivary glands

- Swollen or tender lymph nodes in other areas of the body besides the chest, such as in your neck, chin, armpits, or groin.

Complications

If sarcoidosis is untreated or if the treatment does not work, inflammation can continue and scarring may develop. Sarcoidosis can cause serious and life-threatening damage to the organs it affects, including:

- Blindness

- Blood and bone marrow problems, including lower-than-usual numbers of red or white blood cells (WBCs)

- Endocrine conditions, including hypercalcemia, diabetes insipidus, and amenorrhea

- Heart complications, including arrhythmia, heart failure, sudden cardiac arrest, cardiomyopathy

- Kidney conditions, such as kidney stones or kidney failure

- Cirrhosis

- Lung diseases, such as pulmonary hypertension and pulmonary fibrosis

- Problems with the nervous system, including brain tumors, meningitis, hydrocephalus, psychiatric problems, and nerve pain

How Is Sarcoidosis Diagnosed?

Your doctor will diagnose sarcoidosis based on your symptoms, a physical exam, imaging tests, or a biopsy of an affected organ. The doctor will also perform tests to rule out other diseases that have similar signs and symptoms.

Diagnostic Tests and Procedures

To diagnose sarcoidosis and determine which organs are affected, your doctor may have you undergo some of the following tests and procedures:

- Biopsy of the lungs, liver, skin, or other affected organs to check for granulomas

- Blood tests, including complete blood counts, to check hormone levels and to test for other conditions that may cause sarcoidosis

- Bronchoscopy, which may include rinsing an area of the lung to get cells or using a needle to take cells from the lymph nodes in the chest

- Chest X-ray to look for granulomas in the lungs and heart and determine the stage of the disease. Often, sarcoidosis is found because a chest X-ray is performed for another reason

- Neurological tests, such as electromyography, evoked potentials, spinal taps, or nerve conduction tests, to detect problems with the nervous system caused by sarcoidosis

- Eye exam to look for eye damage, which can occur without symptoms in a person with sarcoidosis

- Gallium scan, which uses a radioactive material called gallium to look for inflammation, usually in the eyes or lymph nodes

- High-resolution computed tomography (HRCT) scan to look for granulomas

- Magnetic resonance imaging (MRI) to help find granulomas

- Positron emission tomography (PET) scan, a type of imaging that can help find granulomas

- Pulmonary function tests to check whether you have breathing problems

- Ultrasound to look for granulomas

Tests for Other Medical Conditions

To help diagnose sarcoidosis, your doctor may need to perform tests or ask questions to rule out other medical conditions that have similar signs and symptoms as sarcoidosis.

- Blood tests to help the doctor distinguish between sarcoidosis and cancer or infections

- A bronchoscopy to find signs that may suggest an infection or cancer

- Questions about environmental exposure to help determine whether the granulomas are related to sarcoidosis or another condition. Exposure to beryllium, for example, can cause granulomas similar to sarcoidosis even though they are actually associated with chronic beryllium disease (CBD).

- A urinalysis to help the doctor rule out other conditions that resemble sarcoidosis

Stages of Sarcoidosis

Doctors use stages to describe the various imaging findings of sarcoidosis of the lung or lymph nodes of the chest. There are four stages of sarcoidosis, and they indicate where the granulomas are located. In each of the first three stages, sarcoidosis can range from mild to severe. Stage IV is the most severe and indicates permanent scarring in the lungs.

- Stage I: Granulomas are located only in the lymph nodes.

- Stage II: Granulomas are located in the lungs and lymph nodes.

- Stage III: Granulomas are located in the lungs only.

- Stage IV: Pulmonary fibrosis

What Are the Treatments for Sarcoidosis?

The goal of treatment is remission, a state in which the condition is not causing problems. Not everyone who is diagnosed with sarcoidosis needs treatment. Sometimes the condition goes away on its own. Whether you need treatment—and what type you need—will depend on your signs and symptoms, which organs are affected, and whether those organs are working well. Some people do not respond to treatment.

Medicines

Because inflammation is thought to be involved in sarcoidosis, your doctor may prescribe medicines to reduce inflammation or treat an overactive immune system that may be causing too much inflammation in the body. Some of the medicines include:

- Corticosteroids
- Disease-modifying antirheumatic drugs (DMARDs)
- Monoclonal antibodies (mAbs)
- Antibiotics
- Antimalarials
- Colchicine
- Corticotropin
- Pentoxifylline

Chapter 35

Pancreatitis

What Is Pancreatitis?

Pancreatitis is inflammation of the pancreas. The pancreas is a large gland behind the stomach, close to the first part of the small intestine, called the duodenum. The pancreas has two main functions—to make insulin and to make digestive juices, or enzymes, to help you digest food. These enzymes digest food in the intestine. Pancreatitis occurs when the enzymes damage the pancreas, which causes inflammation. Pancreatitis can be acute or chronic. Either form is serious and can lead to complications.

Acute Pancreatitis

Acute pancreatitis occurs suddenly and is a short-term condition. Most people with acute pancreatitis get better, and it goes away in several days with treatment. Some people can have a more severe form of acute pancreatitis, which requires a lengthy hospital stay.

Chronic Pancreatitis

Chronic pancreatitis is a long-lasting condition. The pancreas does not heal or improve. Instead, it gets worse over time, which can lead to lasting damage to your pancreas.

This chapter includes text excerpted from "Pancreatitis," National Institute of Diabetes and Digestive and Kidney Diseases (NIDDK), November 2017.

How Common Is Pancreatitis?

Acute pancreatitis is becoming more common, for reasons that are not clear. Each year, about 275,000 hospital stays for acute pancreatitis occur in the United States. Although pancreatitis is rare in children, the number of children with acute pancreatitis has grown. Chronic pancreatitis is less common, with about 86,000 hospital stays per year.

Who Is More Likely to Get Pancreatitis?

Certain groups of people are more likely to get acute or chronic pancreatitis than others:

- Men are more likely to get pancreatitis than women.
- African Americans have a higher risk of getting pancreatitis.
- People with a family history of pancreatitis have a higher risk.
- People with a personal or family history of gallstones also have a higher risk.

People with Certain Health Conditions

You are more likely to get pancreatitis if you have one of the following health conditions:

- Diabetes
- Gallstones
- High triglycerides
- Genetic disorders of the pancreas
- Certain autoimmune conditions
- Cystic fibrosis (CF)

People with Other Health Concerns

You are also more likely to get pancreatitis if you:

- have obesity
- are a heavy alcohol user
- are a smoker

What Are the Complications of Pancreatitis?

Both acute and chronic pancreatitis can lead to complications that include:

- Narrowing or blockage in a bile or pancreatic duct
- Leakage from the pancreatic duct
- Pancreatic pseudocysts
- Damage to your pancreas
- Heart, lung, or kidney failure
- Death

Acute Pancreatitis

Repeat episodes of acute pancreatitis may lead to chronic pancreatitis. Other complications of acute pancreatitis include:

- Dehydration
- Bleeding
- Infection

Chronic Pancreatitis

Complications of chronic pancreatitis include:

- Chronic pain in your abdomen
- Maldigestion, when you can't digest food properly
- Malnutrition and malabsorption
- Problems with how well your pancreas works
- Scars in your pancreas
- Diabetes
- Pancreatic cancer, which is more likely in people with both diabetes and pancreatitis
- Osteopenia, osteoporosis, and bone fractures

What Are the Symptoms of Pancreatitis?

The main symptom of acute and chronic pancreatitis is pain in your upper abdomen that may spread to your back. People with acute or chronic pancreatitis may feel the pain in different ways.

Acute Pancreatitis

Acute pancreatitis usually starts with pain that:

- begins slowly or suddenly in your upper abdomen
- sometimes spreads to your back
- can be mild or severe
- may last for several days

Other symptoms may include:

- Fever
- Nausea and vomiting
- Fast heartbeat
- Swollen or tender abdomen

People with acute pancreatitis usually look and feel seriously ill and need to see a doctor right away.

Chronic Pancreatitis

Most people with chronic pancreatitis feel pain in the upper abdomen, although some people have no pain at all.
The pain may:

- Spread to your back
- Become constant and severe
- Become worse after eating
- Go away as your condition gets worse

People with chronic pancreatitis may not have symptoms until they have complications.
Other symptoms may include:

- Diarrhea
- Nausea
- Greasy, foul-smelling stools
- Vomiting
- Weight loss

Seek Care Right Away for Pancreatitis

Seek care right away for the following symptoms of severe pancreatitis:

- Pain or tenderness in the abdomen that is severe or becomes worse
- Nausea and vomiting
- Fever or chills
- Fast heartbeat
- Shortness of breath
- Yellowish color of the skin or whites of the eyes, called jaundice

These symptoms may be a sign of:

- Serious infection
- Inflammation
- Blockage of the pancreas, gallbladder, or a bile and pancreatic duct

Left untreated, these problems can be fatal.

What Causes Pancreatitis

The most common causes of both acute and chronic pancreatitis are:

- Gallstones
- Heavy alcohol use
- Genetic disorders of your pancreas
- Some medicines

Other causes include:

- Infections, such as viruses or parasites
- Injury to your abdomen
- Pancreatic cancer
- Having a procedure called endoscopic retrograde cholangiopancreatography (ERCP) to treat another condition
- Pancreas divisum

Acute Pancreatitis

The most common cause of acute pancreatitis is having gallstones. Gallstones cause inflammation of your pancreas as stones pass through and get stuck in a bile or pancreatic duct. This condition is called gallstone pancreatitis.

Chronic Pancreatitis

The most common causes of chronic pancreatitis are:

- Heavy alcohol use
- Genetic disorders of your pancreas

Other causes include:

- Blockage in your pancreatic duct
- High levels of blood fats, called lipids
- High level of calcium in your blood

In many cases, doctors can't find the cause of pancreatitis. This is called idiopathic pancreatitis.

How Do Doctors Diagnose Pancreatitis?

To diagnose pancreatitis and find its causes, doctors use:

- Your medical history
- A physical exam
- Lab and imaging tests

A healthcare professional will ask:

- About your symptoms
- If you have a history of health conditions or concerns that make you more likely to get pancreatitis—including medicines you are taking
- If you have a personal or family medical history of pancreatitis or gallstones

During a physical exam, the healthcare professional will:

- Examine your body
- Check your abdomen for pain, swelling, or tenderness

What Tests Do Healthcare Professionals Use to Diagnose Pancreatitis?

Healthcare professionals may use lab or imaging tests to diagnose pancreatitis and find its causes. Diagnosing chronic pancreatitis can be hard in the early stages. Your doctor will also test for other conditions that have similar symptoms, such as peptic ulcers or pancreatic cancer.

Lab Tests

Lab tests to help diagnose pancreatitis include the following:

Blood tests. A healthcare professional may take a blood sample from you and send the sample to a lab to test for:

- High amylase and lipase levels—digestive enzymes made in your pancreas

- High blood glucose, also called blood sugar

- High levels of blood fats, called lipids

- Signs of infection or inflammation of the bile ducts, pancreas, gallbladder, or liver

- Pancreatic cancer

Stool tests. Your doctor may test a stool sample to find out if a person has fat malabsorption.

Imaging Tests

Healthcare professionals also use imaging tests to diagnose pancreatitis. A technician performs most tests in an outpatient center, a hospital, or a doctor's office. You don't need anesthesia, a medicine to keep you calm, for most of these tests.

Ultrasound. Ultrasound uses a device called a transducer, which bounces safe, painless sound waves off your organs to create a picture of their structure. Ultrasound can find gallstones.

Computed tomography (CT) scan. CT scans create pictures of your pancreas, gallbladder, and bile ducts. CT scans can show pancreatitis or pancreatic cancer.

Magnetic resonance cholangiopancreatography (MRCP). MRCP uses a magnetic resonance imaging (MRI) machine, which creates pictures of your organs and soft tissues without X-rays. Your doctor or a specialist may use MRCP to look at your pancreas, gallbladder, and bile ducts for causes of pancreatitis.

Endoscopic ultrasound (EUS). Your doctor inserts an endoscope—a thin, flexible tube—down your throat, through your stomach, and into your small intestine. The doctor turns on an ultrasound attachment to create pictures of your pancreas and bile ducts. Your doctor may send you to a gastroenterologist to perform this test.

Pancreatic function test (PFT). Your doctor may use this test to measure how your pancreas responds to secretin, a hormone made by the small intestine. This test is done only at some centers in the United States.

How Do Healthcare Professionals Treat Pancreatitis?

Treatment for acute or chronic pancreatitis may include:

- A hospital stay to treat dehydration with intravenous (IV) fluids and if you can swallow them, fluids by mouth

- Pain medicine, and antibiotics by mouth or through an IV if you have an infection in your pancreas

- A low-fat diet, or nutrition by feeding tube or IV if you can't eat

Your doctor may send you to a gastroenterologist or surgeon for one of the following treatments, depending on the type of pancreatitis that you have.

Acute Pancreatitis

Mild acute pancreatitis usually goes away in a few days with rest and treatment. If your pancreatitis is more severe, your treatment may also include:

Surgery. Your doctor may recommend surgery to remove the gallbladder, called cholecystectomy, if gallstones cause your pancreatitis. Having surgery within a few days after you are admitted to the hospital lowers the chance of complications. If you have severe pancreatitis, your doctor may advise delaying surgery to first treat complications.

Procedures. Your doctor or specialist will drain fluid in your abdomen if you have an abscess or infected pseudocyst, or a large pseudocyst causing pain or bleeding. Your doctor may remove damaged tissue from your pancreas.

Endoscopic retrograde cholangiopancreatography (ERCP).
Doctors use ERCP to treat both acute and chronic pancreatitis. ERCP combines upper gastrointestinal endoscopy and X-rays to treat narrowing or blockage of a bile or pancreatic duct. Your gastroenterologist may use ERCP to remove gallstones blocking the bile or pancreatic ducts.

Chronic Pancreatitis

Treatment for chronic pancreatitis may help relieve pain, improve how well the pancreas works, and manage complications. Your doctor may prescribe or provide the following:

Medicines and vitamins. Your doctor may give you enzyme pills to help with digestion, or vitamins A, D, E, and K if you have malabsorption. He or she may also give you vitamin B_{12} shots if you need them.

Treatment for diabetes. Chronic pancreatitis may cause diabetes. If you get diabetes, your doctor and healthcare team will work with you to create an eating plan and a routine of medicine, blood glucose monitoring, and regular checkups.

Surgery. Your doctor may recommend surgery to relieve pressure or blockage in your pancreatic duct, or to remove a damaged or infected part of your pancreas. Surgery is done in a hospital, where you may have to stay a few days.

In patients who do not get better with other treatments, surgeons may perform surgery to remove your whole pancreas, followed by islet autotransplantation. Islets are groups of cells in your pancreas that make hormones, including insulin. After removing your pancreas, doctors will take islets from your pancreas and transplant them into your liver. The islets will begin to make hormones and release them into your bloodstream.

Procedures. Your doctor may suggest a nerve block, which is a shot of numbing medicine through your skin and directly into nerves that carry the pain message from your pancreas. If you have stones blocking your pancreatic duct, your doctor may use a procedure to break up and remove the stones.

How Can I Help Manage My Pancreatitis?
Stop Drinking Alcohol

Healthcare professionals strongly advise people with pancreatitis to stop drinking alcohol, even if your pancreatitis is mild or in the early stages. Continuing to drink alcohol when you have acute pancreatitis can lead to:

- More episodes of acute pancreatitis

- Chronic pancreatitis

When people with chronic pancreatitis caused by alcohol use continue to drink alcohol, the condition is more likely to lead to severe complications and even death.

Talk with your healthcare professional if you need help to stop drinking alcohol.

Stop Smoking

Healthcare professionals strongly advise people with pancreatitis to stop smoking, even if your pancreatitis is mild or in the early stages. Smoking with acute pancreatitis, especially if it's caused by alcohol use, greatly raises the chances that your pancreatitis will become chronic. Smoking with pancreatitis also may raise your risk of pancreatic cancer. Talk with your healthcare professional if you need help to stop smoking.

How Can I Help Prevent Pancreatitis?

You can't prevent pancreatitis, but you can take steps to help you stay healthy.

Maintain a Healthy Weight or Lose Weight Safely

Maintaining a healthy lifestyle and a healthy weight—or losing weight if needed—can help to:

- Make your pancreas work better

- Lower your chance of getting gallstones, a leading cause of pancreatitis

- Prevent obesity—a risk factor for pancreatitis

- Prevent diabetes—a risk factor for pancreatitis

Avoid Alcohol Use

Alcohol use can cause acute and chronic pancreatitis. Talk with your healthcare professional if you need help to stop drinking alcohol.

Avoid Smoking

Smoking is a common risk factor for pancreatitis—and the chances of getting pancreatitis are even higher in people who smoke and drink alcohol. Talk with your healthcare professional if you need help to stop smoking.

Can What I Eat Help or Prevent Pancreatitis?

During pancreatitis treatment, your doctor may tell you not to eat or drink for a while. Instead, your doctor may use a feeding tube to give you nutrition. Once you may start eating again, he or she will prescribe a healthy, low-fat eating plan that includes small, frequent meals. If you have pancreatitis, drink plenty of fluids and limit caffeine. Healthcare professionals strongly advise people with pancreatitis not to drink any alcohol, even if your pancreatitis is mild.

Having an eating plan high in fat and calories can lead to high levels of fat in your blood, which raises your risk of pancreatitis. You can lower your chances of getting pancreatitis by sticking with a low-fat, healthy eating plan.

Part Six

Cancers of the Gastrointestinal Tract

Chapter 36

Gastrointestinal Carcinoid Tumors

A gastrointestinal (GI) carcinoid tumor is cancer that forms in the lining of the gastrointestinal tract. The gastrointestinal tract is part of the body's digestive system. It helps to digest food, takes nutrients (vitamins, minerals, carbohydrates, fats, proteins, and water) from food to be used by the body and helps pass waste material out of the body. The GI tract is made up of these and other organs:

- Stomach

- Small intestine (duodenum, jejunum, and ileum)

- Colon

- Rectum

Gastrointestinal carcinoid tumors form from a certain type of neuroendocrine cell (a type of cell that is like a nerve cell and a hormone-making cell). These cells are scattered throughout the chest and abdomen but most are found in the GI tract. Neuroendocrine cells make hormones that help control digestive juices and the muscles used in moving food through the stomach and intestines. A GI carcinoid tumor may also make hormones and release them into the body.

This chapter includes text excerpted from "Gastrointestinal Carcinoid Tumors Treatment (PDQ®)—Patient Version," National Cancer Institute (NCI), February 16, 2018.

GI carcinoid tumors are rare and most grow very slowly. Most of them occur in the small intestine, rectum, and appendix. Sometimes more than one tumor will form.

Health history can affect the risk of gastrointestinal carcinoid tumors. Anything that increases a person's chance of developing a disease is called a risk factor. Having a risk factor does not mean that you will get cancer; not having risk factors doesn't mean that you will not get cancer. Talk to your doctor if you think you may be at risk.

Risk factors for GI carcinoid tumors include the following:

- Having a family history of multiple endocrine neoplasia type 1 (MEN1) syndrome or neurofibromatosis type 1 (NF1) syndrome

- Having certain conditions that affect the stomach's ability to make stomach acid, such as atrophic gastritis, pernicious anemia, or Zollinger-Ellison syndrome (ZES)

Signs and Symptoms of Gastrointestinal Carcinoid Tumors

Signs and symptoms may be caused by the growth of the tumor and/ or the hormones the tumor makes. Some tumors, especially tumors of the stomach or appendix, may not cause signs or symptoms. Carcinoid tumors are often found during tests or treatments for other conditions.

Carcinoid tumors in the small intestine (duodenum, jejunum, and ileum), colon, and rectum sometimes cause signs or symptoms as they grow or because of the hormones they make. Other conditions may cause the same signs or symptoms. Check with your doctor if you have any of the following:

Duodenum

Signs and symptoms of GI carcinoid tumors in the duodenum (first part of the small intestine, that connects to the stomach) may include the following:

- Abdominal pain

- Constipation

- Diarrhea

- Change in stool color

- Nausea

- Vomiting

- Jaundice (yellowing of the skin and whites of the eyes)
- Heartburn

Jejunum and Ileum

Signs and symptoms of GI carcinoid tumors in the jejunum (middle part of the small intestine) and ileum (last part of the small intestine, that connects to the colon) may include the following:

- Abdominal pain
- Weight loss for no known reason
- Feeling very tired
- Feeling bloated
- Diarrhea
- Nausea
- Vomiting

Colon

Signs and symptoms of GI carcinoid tumors in the colon may include the following:

- Abdominal pain
- Weight loss for no known reason

Rectum

Signs and symptoms of GI carcinoid tumors in the rectum may include the following:

- Blood in the stool
- Pain in the rectum
- Constipation

Carcinoid syndrome may occur if the tumor spreads to the liver or other parts of the body. The hormones made by gastrointestinal carcinoid tumors are usually destroyed by liver enzymes in the blood. If the tumor has spread to the liver and the liver enzymes cannot destroy the extra hormones made by the tumor, high amounts of these hormones may remain in the body and cause carcinoid syndrome. This can also happen if tumor cells enter the blood. Signs and symptoms of carcinoid syndrome include the following:

- Redness or a feeling of warmth in the face and neck.
- Abdominal pain
- Feeling bloated
- Diarrhea
- Wheezing or other trouble breathing
- Fast heartbeat

These signs and symptoms may be caused by gastrointestinal carcinoid tumors or by other conditions. Talk to your doctor if you have any of these signs or symptoms.

Diagnosis of Gastrointestinal Carcinoid Tumors

Imaging studies and tests that examine the blood and urine are used to detect (find) and diagnose gastrointestinal carcinoid tumors. The following tests and procedures may be used:

- **Physical exam and history:** An exam of the body to check general signs of health, including checking for signs of disease, such as lumps or anything else that seems unusual. A history of the patient's health habits and past illnesses and treatments will also be taken.

- **Blood chemistry studies:** A procedure in which a blood sample is checked to measure the amounts of certain substances, such as hormones, released into the blood by organs and tissues in the body. An unusual (higher or lower than normal) amount of a substance can be a sign of disease. The blood sample is checked to see if it contains a hormone produced by carcinoid tumors. This test is used to help diagnose carcinoid syndrome.

- **Tumor marker test:** A procedure in which a sample of blood, urine, or tissue is checked to measure the amounts of certain substances, such as chromogranin A, made by organs, tissues, or tumor cells in the body. Chromogranin A is a tumor marker. It has been linked to neuroendocrine tumors when found in increased levels in the body.

- **Twenty-four-hour urine test:** A test in which urine is collected for 24 hours to measure the amounts of certain substances, such as 5-hydroxyindoleacetic acid (5-HIAA) or serotonin (hormone). An unusual (higher or lower than normal) amount of a substance can be a sign of disease in the organ or tissue that makes it. This test is used to help diagnose carcinoid syndrome.

- **Metaiodobenzylguanidine (MIBG) scan:** A procedure used to find neuroendocrine tumors, such as carcinoid tumors. A very small amount of radioactive material called MIBG (metaiodobenzylguanidine) is injected into a vein and travels through the bloodstream. Carcinoid tumors take up the radioactive material and are detected by a device that measures radiation.

- **Computed tomography (CT) scan (CAT scan):** A procedure that makes a series of detailed pictures of areas inside the body, taken from different angles. The pictures are made by a computer linked to an X-ray machine. A dye may be injected into a vein or swallowed to help the organs or tissues show up more clearly. This procedure is also called computed tomography, computerized tomography, or computerized axial tomography.

- **Magnetic resonance imaging (MRI):** A procedure that uses a magnet, radio waves, and a computer to make a series of detailed pictures of areas inside the body. This procedure is also called nuclear magnetic resonance imaging.

- **Positron emission tomography (PET) scan:** A procedure to find malignant tumor cells in the body. A small amount of radioactive glucose (sugar) is injected into a vein. The PET scanner rotates around the body and makes a picture of where glucose is being used in the body. Malignant tumor cells show up brighter in the picture because they are more active and take up more glucose than normal cells.

- **Endoscopic ultrasound (EUS):** A procedure in which an endoscope is inserted into the body, usually through the mouth or rectum. An endoscope is a thin, tube-like instrument with a light and a lens for viewing. A probe at the end of the endoscope is used to bounce high-energy sound waves (ultrasound) off internal tissues or organs, such as the stomach, small intestine, colon, or rectum, and make echoes. The echoes form a picture of body tissues called a sonogram. This procedure is also called endosonography.

- **Upper endoscopy:** A procedure to look at organs and tissues inside the body to check for abnormal areas. An endoscope is inserted through the mouth and passed through the esophagus into the stomach. Sometimes the endoscope also is passed from the stomach into the small intestine. An endoscope is a thin, tube-like instrument with a light and a lens for viewing. It may also have a tool to remove tissue or lymph node samples, which are checked under a microscope for signs of disease.

- **Colonoscopy:** A procedure to look inside the rectum and colon for polyps, abnormal areas, or cancer. A colonoscope is inserted through the rectum into the colon. A colonoscope is a thin, tube-like instrument with a light and a lens for viewing. It may also have a tool to remove polyps or tissue samples, which are checked under a microscope for signs of cancer.

- **Capsule endoscopy:** A procedure used to see all of the small intestine. The patient swallows a capsule that contains a tiny camera. As the capsule moves through the gastrointestinal tract, the camera takes pictures and sends them to a receiver worn on the outside of the body.

- **Biopsy:** The removal of cells or tissues so they can be viewed under a microscope to check for signs of cancer. Tissue samples may be taken during endoscopy and colonoscopy.

Certain factors affect prognosis (chance of recovery) and treatment options. The prognosis (chance of recovery) and treatment options depend on the following:

- Where the tumor is in the gastrointestinal tract

- The size of the tumor

- Whether the cancer has spread from the stomach and intestines to other parts of the body, such as the liver or lymph nodes

- Whether the patient has carcinoid syndrome or has carcinoid heart syndrome

- Whether the cancer can be completely removed by surgery

- Whether the cancer is newly diagnosed or has recurred

Stages of Gastrointestinal Carcinoid Tumors

After a gastrointestinal carcinoid tumor has been diagnosed, tests are done to find out if cancer cells have spread within the stomach and intestines or to other parts of the body. Staging is the process used to find out how far the cancer has spread. The information gathered from the staging process determines the stage of the disease. The results of tests and procedures used to diagnose gastrointestinal (GI) carcinoid tumors may also be used for staging.

A bone scan may be done to check if there are rapidly dividing cells, such as cancer cells, in the bone. A very small amount of radioactive material is injected into a vein and travels through the bloodstream. The radioactive material collects in the bones with cancer and is detected by a scanner.

The metastatic tumor is the same type of tumor as the primary tumor. For example, if a gastrointestinal (GI) carcinoid tumor spreads to the liver, the tumor cells in the liver are actually GI carcinoid tumor cells. The disease is metastatic GI carcinoid tumor, not liver cancer.

The plan for cancer treatment depends on where the carcinoid tumor is found and whether it can be removed by surgery. For many cancers it is important to know the stage of the cancer in order to plan treatment. However, the treatment of gastrointestinal carcinoid tumors is not based on the stage of the cancer. Treatment depends mainly on whether the tumor can be removed by surgery and if the tumor has spread.

Treatment is based on whether the tumor:

- can be completely removed by surgery

- has spread to other parts of the body

- has come back after treatment. The tumor may come back in the stomach or intestines or in other parts of the body.

- has not gotten better with treatment

Treatment for Gastrointestinal Carcinoid Tumors

There are different types of treatment for patients with gastrointestinal carcinoid tumors. Different types of treatment are available for patients with gastrointestinal carcinoid tumor. Some treatments are standard (the currently used treatment), and some are being tested in clinical trials. A treatment clinical trial is a research study meant to help improve current treatments or obtain information on new treatments for patients with cancer. When clinical trials show that a new treatment is better than the standard treatment, the new treatment may become the standard treatment. Patients may want to think about taking part in a clinical trial. Some clinical trials are open only to patients who have not started treatment.

Four types of standard treatment are used:

Surgery

Treatment of GI carcinoid tumors usually includes surgery. One of the following surgical procedures may be used:

- **Endoscopic resection:** Surgery to remove a small tumor that is on the inside lining of the GI tract. An endoscope is inserted through the mouth and passed through the esophagus to the stomach and sometimes, the duodenum. An endoscope is a thin, tube-like instrument with a light, a lens for viewing, and a tool for removing tumor tissue.

- **Local excision:** Surgery to remove the tumor and a small amount of normal tissue around it.

- **Resection:** Surgery to remove part or all of the organ that contains cancer. Nearby lymph nodes may also be removed.

- **Cryosurgery:** A treatment that uses an instrument to freeze and destroy carcinoid tumor tissue. This type of treatment is also called cryotherapy. The doctor may use ultrasound to guide the instrument.

- **Radiofrequency ablation:** The use of a special probe with tiny electrodes that release high-energy radio waves (similar to microwaves) that kill cancer cells. The probe may be inserted through the skin or through an incision (cut) in the abdomen.

- **Liver transplant:** Surgery to remove the whole liver and replace it with a healthy donated liver.

- **Hepatic artery embolization (HAE):** A procedure to embolize (block) the hepatic artery, which is the main blood vessel that brings blood into the liver. Blocking the flow of blood to the liver helps kill cancer cells growing there.

Radiation Therapy

Radiation therapy is a cancer treatment that uses high-energy X-rays or other types of radiation to kill cancer cells or keep them from growing. There are two types of radiation therapy:

- External radiation therapy uses a machine outside the body to send radiation toward the cancer.

- Internal radiation therapy uses a radioactive substance sealed in needles, seeds, wires, or catheters that are placed directly into or near the cancer.

Radiopharmaceutical therapy is a type of internal radiation therapy. Radiation is given to the tumor using a drug that has a radioactive substance, such as iodine 131 (I-131), attached to it. The radioactive substance kills the tumor cells. External and internal radiation therapy are used to treat gastrointestinal carcinoid tumors that have spread to other parts of the body.

Chemotherapy

Chemotherapy is a cancer treatment that uses drugs to stop the growth of cancer cells, either by killing the cells or by stopping the cells from dividing. When chemotherapy is taken by mouth or injected into a vein or muscle, the drugs enter the bloodstream and can reach cancer cells throughout the body (systemic chemotherapy). When chemotherapy is placed directly into the cerebrospinal fluid, an organ, or a body cavity such as the abdomen, the drugs mainly affect cancer cells in those areas (regional chemotherapy). Chemoembolization of the hepatic artery is a type of regional chemotherapy that may be used to treat a gastrointestinal carcinoid tumor that has spread to the liver. The anticancer drug is injected into the hepatic artery through a catheter (thin tube). The drug is mixed with a substance that embolizes (blocks) the artery, and cuts off blood flow to the tumor. Most of the anticancer drug is trapped near the tumor and only a small amount of the drug reaches other parts of the body. The blockage may be temporary or permanent, depending on the substance used to block the artery. The tumor is prevented from getting the oxygen and nutrients it needs to grow. The liver continues to receive blood from the hepatic portal vein, which carries blood from the stomach and intestine.

The way the chemotherapy is given depends on the type and stage of the cancer being treated.

Hormone Therapy

Hormone therapy with a somatostatin analogue is a treatment that stops extra hormones from being made. GI carcinoid tumors are treated with octreotide or lanreotide which are injected under the skin or into the muscle. Octreotide and lanreotide may also have a small effect on stopping tumor growth.

521

Treatment for carcinoid syndrome may also be needed. Treatment of carcinoid syndrome may include the following:

- Hormone therapy with a somatostatin analogue stops extra hormones from being made. Carcinoid syndrome is treated with octreotide or lanreotide to lessen flushing and diarrhea. Octreotide and lanreotide may also help slow tumor growth.

- Interferon therapy stimulates the body's immune system to work better and lessens flushing and diarrhea. Interferon may also help slow tumor growth.

- Taking medicine for diarrhea

- Taking medicine for skin rashes

- Taking medicine to breathe easier

- Taking medicine before having anesthesia for a medical procedure

Other ways to help treat carcinoid syndrome include avoiding things that cause flushing or difficulty breathing such as alcohol, nuts, certain cheeses and foods with capsaicin, such as chili peppers. Avoiding stressful situations and certain types of physical activity can also help treat carcinoid syndrome. For some patients with carcinoid heart syndrome, a heart valve replacement may be done.

Treatment Options for Gastrointestinal Carcinoid Tumors

Carcinoid Tumors in the Stomach

Treatment of gastrointestinal (GI) carcinoid tumors in the stomach may include the following:

- Endoscopic surgery (resection) for small tumors

- Surgery (resection) to remove part or all of the stomach. Nearby lymph nodes for larger tumors, tumors that grow deep into the stomach wall, or tumors that are growing and spreading quickly may also be removed.

For patients with GI carcinoid tumors in the stomach and multiple endocrine neoplasia type 1 (MEN1) syndrome, treatment may also include:

- Surgery (resection) to remove tumors in the duodenum (first part of the small intestine, that connects to the stomach)

- Hormone therapy

Carcinoid Tumors in the Small Intestine

It is not clear what the best treatment is for GI carcinoid tumors in the duodenum (first part of the small intestine, that connects to the stomach). Treatment may include the following:

- Endoscopic surgery (resection) for small tumors

- Surgery (local excision) to remove slightly larger tumors

- Surgery (resection) to remove the tumor and nearby lymph nodes

Treatment of GI carcinoid tumors in the jejunum (middle part of the small intestine) and ileum (last part of the small intestine, that connects to the colon) may include the following:

- Surgery (resection) to remove the tumor and the membrane that connects the intestines to the back of the abdominal wall. Nearby lymph nodes are also removed.

- A second surgery to remove the membrane that connects the intestines to the back of the abdominal wall, if any tumor remains or the tumor continues to grow

- Hormone therapy

Carcinoid Tumors in the Appendix

Treatment of GI carcinoid tumors in the appendix may include the following:

- Surgery (resection) to remove the appendix

- Surgery (resection) to remove the right side of the colon including the appendix. Nearby lymph nodes are also removed.

Carcinoid Tumors in the Colon

Treatment of GI carcinoid tumors in the colon may include the following:

- Surgery (resection) to remove part of the colon and nearby lymph nodes, in order to remove as much of the cancer as possible

Carcinoid Tumors in the Rectum

Treatment of GI carcinoid tumors in the rectum may include the following:

- Endoscopic surgery (resection) for tumors that are smaller than one centimeter

- Surgery (resection) for tumors that are larger than two centimeters or that have spread to the muscle layer of the rectal wall. This may be either:

  - surgery to remove part of the rectum

  - surgery to remove the anus, the rectum, and part of the colon through an incision made in the abdomen

It is not clear what the best treatment is for tumors that are one to two centimeters. Treatment may include the following:

- Endoscopic surgery (resection)

- Surgery (resection) to remove part of the rectum

- Surgery (resection) to remove the anus, the rectum, and part of the colon through an incision made in the abdomen

Metastatic Gastrointestinal Carcinoid Tumors

Distant Metastases

Treatment of distant metastases of GI carcinoid tumors is usually palliative therapy to relieve symptoms and improve quality of life (QOL). Treatment may include the following:

- Surgery (resection) to remove as much of the tumor as possible

- Hormone therapy

- Radiopharmaceutical therapy

- External radiation therapy for cancer that has spread to the bone, brain, or spinal cord

- A clinical trial of a new treatment

Liver Metastases

Treatment of cancer that has spread to the liver may include the following:

- Surgery (local excision) to remove the tumor from the liver
- Hepatic artery embolization
- Cryosurgery
- Radiofrequency ablation
- Liver transplant

Recurrent Gastrointestinal Carcinoid Tumors

Treatment of recurrent GI carcinoid tumors may include the following:

- Surgery (local excision) to remove part or all of the tumor
- A clinical trial of a new treatment

Chapter 37

Esophageal Cancer

Esophageal cancer is a disease in which malignant (cancer) cells form in the tissues of the esophagus. The esophagus is the hollow, muscular tube that moves food and liquid from the throat to the stomach. The wall of the esophagus is made up of several layers of tissue, including mucous membrane, muscle, and connective tissue. Esophageal cancer starts on the inside lining of the esophagus and spreads outward through the other layers as it grows.

The two most common forms of esophageal cancer are named for the type of cells that become malignant (cancerous):

- **Squamous cell carcinoma:** Cancer that forms in squamous cells, the thin, flat cells lining the esophagus. This cancer is most often found in the upper and middle part of the esophagus, but can occur anywhere along the esophagus. This is also called epidermoid carcinoma.

- **Adenocarcinoma:** Cancer that begins in glandular (secretory) cells. Glandular cells in the lining of the esophagus produce and release fluids such as mucus. Adenocarcinomas usually form in the lower part of the esophagus, near the stomach.

Smoking, heavy alcohol use, and Barrett esophagus can increase the risk of esophageal cancer. Anything that increases your risk of getting a disease is called a risk factor. Having a risk factor does not mean that you will get cancer; not having risk factors doesn't mean

This chapter includes text excerpted from "Esophageal Cancer Treatment (PDQ®)—Patient Version," National Cancer Institute (NCI), September 7, 2018.

that you will not get cancer. Talk with your doctor if you think you may be at risk. Risk factors include the following:

- Tobacco use

- Heavy alcohol use

- Barrett esophagus (A condition in which the cells lining the lower part of the esophagus have changed or been replaced with abnormal cells that could lead to cancer of the esophagus.)

- Older age

Signs and Symptoms of Esophageal Cancer

Signs and symptoms of esophageal cancer are weight loss and painful or difficult swallowing. These and other signs and symptoms may be caused by esophageal cancer or by other conditions. Check with your doctor if you have any of the following:

- Painful or difficult swallowing

- Weight loss

- Pain behind the breastbone

- Hoarseness and cough

- Indigestion and heartburn

- A lump under the skin

Diagnosis of Esophageal Cancer

Tests that examine the esophagus are used to detect (find) and diagnose esophageal cancer. The following tests and procedures may be used:

- **Physical exam and history:** An exam of the body to check general signs of health, including checking for signs of disease, such as lumps or anything else that seems unusual. A history of the patient's health habits and past illnesses and treatments will also be taken.

- **Chest X-ray:** An X-ray of the organs and bones inside the chest. An X-ray is a type of energy beam that can go through the body and onto film, making a picture of areas inside the body.

- **Barium swallow:** A series of X-rays of the esophagus and stomach. The patient drinks a liquid that contains barium (a silver-white metallic compound). The liquid coats the esophagus and stomach, and X-rays are taken. This procedure is also called an upper GI series.

- **Esophagoscopy:** A procedure to look inside the esophagus to check for abnormal areas. An esophagoscope is inserted through the mouth or nose and down the throat into the esophagus. An esophagoscope is a thin, tube-like instrument with a light and a lens for viewing. It may also have a tool to remove tissue samples, which are checked under a microscope for signs of cancer. When the esophagus and stomach are looked at, it is called an upper endoscopy.

- **Biopsy:** The removal of cells or tissues so they can be viewed under a microscope by a pathologist to check for signs of cancer. The biopsy is usually done during an esophagoscopy. Sometimes a biopsy shows changes in the esophagus that are not cancer but may lead to cancer.

Certain factors affect prognosis (chance of recovery) and treatment options. The prognosis (chance of recovery) and treatment options depend on the following:

- The stage of the cancer (whether it affects part of the esophagus, involves the whole esophagus, or has spread to other places in the body)

- Whether the tumor can be completely removed by surgery

- The patient's general health

When esophageal cancer is found very early, there is a better chance of recovery. Esophageal cancer is often in an advanced stage when it is diagnosed. At later stages, esophageal cancer can be treated but rarely can be cured. Taking part in one of the clinical trials being done to improve treatment should be considered.

Stages of Esophageal Cancer

After esophageal cancer has been diagnosed, tests are done to find out if cancer cells have spread within the esophagus or to other parts of the body. The process used to find out if cancer cells have spread within the esophagus or to other parts of the body is called staging. The information gathered from the staging process determines the stage of the disease. It is important to know the stage in order to plan treatment. The following tests and procedures may be used in the staging process:

- Endoscopic ultrasound (EUS)

- Computed tomography (CT) scan (CAT scan)

- Positron emission tomography (PET) scan

- Magnetic resonance imaging (MRI)

- Thoracoscopy

- Laparoscopy

- Ultrasound exam

The metastatic tumor is the same type of cancer as the primary tumor. For example, if esophageal cancer spreads to the lung, the cancer cells in the lung are actually esophageal cancer cells. The disease is metastatic esophageal cancer, not lung cancer.

The grade of the tumor is also used to describe the cancer and plan treatment. The grade of the tumor describes how abnormal the cancer cells look under a microscope and how quickly the tumor is likely to grow and spread. Grades one to three are used to describe esophageal cancer:

- In grade 1, the cancer cells look more like normal cells under a microscope and grow and spread more slowly than grade 2 and 3 cancer cells.

- In grade 2, the cancer cells look more abnormal under a microscope and grow and spread more quickly than grade 1 cancer cells.

- In grade 3, the cancer cells look more abnormal under a microscope and grow and spread more quickly than grade 1 and 2 cancer cells.

The following stages are used for squamous cell carcinoma of the esophagus:

Stage 0

In stage 0, abnormal cells are found in the mucosa or submucosa layer of the esophagus wall. These abnormal cells may become cancer and spread into nearby normal tissue. Stage 0 is also called high-grade dysplasia.

Stage I

Stage I is divided into stage IA and stage IB, depending on where the cancer is found.

- Stage IA: Cancer has formed in the mucosa or submucosa layer of the esophagus wall. The cancer cells are grade 1. Grade 1 cancer cells look more like normal cells under a microscope and grow and spread more slowly than grade 2 and 3 cancer cells.

- Stage IB: Cancer has formed:
  - in the mucosa or submucosa layer of the esophagus wall. The cancer cells are grade 2 and 3
  - in the mucosa or submucosa layer and spread into the muscle layer or the connective tissue layer of the esophagus wall. The cancer cells are grade 1. The tumor is in the lower esophagus or it is not known where the tumor is.

Grade 1 cancer cells look more like normal cells under a microscope and grow and spread more slowly than grade 2 and 3 cancer cells.

Stage II

Stage II is divided into stage IIA and stage IIB, depending on where the cancer has spread.

- Stage IIA: Cancer has spread:
  - into the muscle layer or the connective tissue layer of the esophagus wall. The cancer cells are grade 1. The tumor is in either the upper or middle esophagus; or
  - into the muscle layer or the connective tissue layer of the esophagus wall. The cancer cells are grade 2 and 3. The tumor is in the lower esophagus or it is not known where the tumor is.

Grade 1 cancer cells look more like normal cells under a microscope and grow and spread more slowly than grade 2 and 3 cancer cells.

- Stage IIB: Cancer:
- has spread into the muscle layer or the connective tissue layer of the esophagus wall. The cancer cells are grade 2 and 3. Grade 2 and 3 cancer cells look more abnormal under a microscope and grow and spread more quickly than grade 1 cancer cells. The tumor is in either the upper or middle esophagus; or

- is in the mucosa or submucosa layer and may have spread into the muscle layer of the esophagus wall. Cancer is found in one or two lymph nodes near the tumor.

Stage III

Stage III is divided into stage IIIA, stage IIIB, and stage IIIC, depending on where the cancer has spread.

- Stage IIIA: Cancer:
  - is in the mucosa or submucosa layer and may have spread into the muscle layer of the esophagus wall. Cancer is found in three to six lymph nodes near the tumor; or
  - has spread into the connective tissue layer of the esophagus wall. Cancer is found in one or two lymph nodes near the tumor; or
  - has spread into the diaphragm, pleura (tissue that covers the lungs and lines the inner wall of the chest cavity), or sac around the heart. The cancer can be removed by surgery.
- Stage IIIB: Cancer has spread into the connective tissue layer of the esophagus wall. Cancer is found in three to six lymph nodes near the tumor.
- Stage IIIC: Cancer has spread:
  - into the diaphragm, pleura (tissue that covers the lungs and lines the inner wall of the chest cavity), or sac around the heart. The cancer can be removed by surgery. Cancer is found in one to six lymph nodes near the tumor; or
  - into other nearby organs such as the aorta, trachea, or spine, and the cancer cannot be removed by surgery; or
  - to seven or more lymph nodes near the tumor.

Stage IV

In Stage IV, cancer has spread to other parts of the body.

Recurrent Esophageal Cancer

Recurrent esophageal cancer is cancer that has recurred (come back) after it has been treated. The cancer may come back in the esophagus or in other parts of the body.

Treatment Option Overview for Esophageal Cancer

Different types of treatment are available for patients with esophageal cancer. Some treatments are standard (the currently used treatment), and some are being tested in clinical trials. A treatment clinical trial is a research study meant to help improve current treatments or obtain information on new treatments for patients with cancer. When clinical trials show that a new treatment is better than the standard treatment, the new treatment may become the standard treatment. Patients may want to think about taking part in a clinical trial. Some clinical trials are open only to patients who have not started treatment.

Patients have special nutritional needs during treatment for esophageal cancer. Many people with esophageal cancer find it hard to eat because they have trouble swallowing. The esophagus may be narrowed by the tumor or as a side effect of treatment. Some patients may receive nutrients directly into a vein. Others may need a feeding tube (a flexible plastic tube that is passed through the nose or mouth into the stomach) until they are able to eat on their own.

Six types of standard treatment are used:

Surgery

Surgery is the most common treatment for cancer of the esophagus. Part of the esophagus may be removed in an operation called an esophagectomy.

The doctor will connect the remaining healthy part of the esophagus to the stomach so the patient can still swallow. A plastic tube or part of the intestine may be used to make the connection. Lymph nodes near the esophagus may also be removed and viewed under a microscope to see if they contain cancer. If the esophagus is partly blocked by the tumor, an expandable metal stent (tube) may be placed inside the esophagus to help keep it open.

Small, early-stage cancer and high-grade dysplasia of the esophagus may be removed by endoscopic resection. An endoscope (a thin, tube-like instrument with a light and a lens for viewing) is inserted through a small incision (cut) in the skin or through an opening in the body, such as the mouth. A tool attached to the endoscope is used to remove tissue.

Radiation Therapy

Radiation therapy is a cancer treatment that uses high-energy X-rays or other types of radiation to kill cancer cells or keep them from growing. There are two types of radiation therapy:

- External radiation therapy uses a machine outside the body to send radiation toward the cancer

- Internal radiation therapy uses a radioactive substance sealed in needles, seeds, wires, or catheters that are placed directly into or near the cancer

The way the radiation therapy is given depends on the type and stage of the cancer being treated. External and internal radiation therapy are used to treat esophageal cancer. A plastic tube may be inserted into the esophagus to keep it open during radiation therapy. This is called intraluminal intubation and dilation.

Chemotherapy

Chemotherapy is a cancer treatment that uses drugs to stop the growth of cancer cells, either by killing the cells or by stopping them from dividing. When chemotherapy is taken by mouth or injected into a vein or muscle, the drugs enter the bloodstream and can reach cancer cells throughout the body (systemic chemotherapy). When chemotherapy is placed directly into the cerebrospinal fluid, an organ, or a body cavity such as the abdomen, the drugs mainly affect cancer cells in those areas (regional chemotherapy). The way the chemotherapy is given depends on the type and stage of the cancer being treated.

Chemoradiation Therapy

Chemoradiation therapy combines chemotherapy and radiation therapy to increase the effects of both.

Laser Therapy

Laser therapy is a cancer treatment that uses a laser beam (a narrow beam of intense light) to kill cancer cells.

Electrocoagulation

Electrocoagulation is the use of an electric current to kill cancer cells.

Treatment Options by Stage for Esophageal Cancer

Stage 0

Treatment of stage 0 may include the following:

- Surgery
- Endoscopic resection

Stage I

Treatment of stage I esophageal squamous cell carcinoma or adenocarcinoma may include the following:

- Chemoradiation therapy followed by surgery
- Surgery alone

Stage II

Treatment of stage II esophageal squamous cell carcinoma or adenocarcinoma may include the following:

- Chemoradiation therapy followed by surgery
- Surgery alone
- Chemotherapy followed by surgery
- Chemoradiation therapy alone

Stage III

Treatment of stage III esophageal squamous cell carcinoma or adenocarcinoma may include the following:

- Chemoradiation therapy followed by surgery
- Chemotherapy followed by surgery
- Chemoradiation therapy alone

Stage IV

Treatment of stage IV esophageal squamous cell carcinoma or adenocarcinoma may include the following:

- Chemoradiation therapy followed by surgery

- Chemotherapy

- Laser surgery or electrocoagulation as palliative therapy to relieve symptoms and improve quality of life (QOL)

- An esophageal stent as palliative therapy to relieve symptoms and improve quality of life

- External or internal radiation therapy as palliative therapy to relieve symptoms and improve quality of life

- Clinical trials of chemotherapy

- A clinical trial of targeted therapy combined with chemotherapy

Chapter 38

Gastric Cancer

Gastric cancer is a disease in which malignant (cancer) cells form in the lining of the stomach. The stomach is a J-shaped organ in the upper abdomen. It is part of the digestive system, which processes nutrients (vitamins, minerals, carbohydrates, fats, proteins, and water) in foods that are eaten and helps pass waste material out of the body. Food moves from the throat to the stomach through a hollow, muscular tube called the esophagus. After leaving the stomach, partly-digested food passes into the small intestine and then into the large intestine.

The wall of the stomach is made up of five layers of tissue. From the innermost layer to the outermost layer, the layers of the stomach wall are: mucosa, submucosa, muscle, subserosa (connective tissue), and serosa. Gastric cancer begins in the mucosa and spreads through the outer layers as it grows.

Stromal tumors of the stomach begin in supporting connective tissue and are treated differently from gastric cancer.

Age, diet, and stomach disease can affect the risk of developing gastric cancer. Anything that increases your risk of getting a disease is called a risk factor. Having a risk factor does not mean that you will get cancer; not having risk factors doesn't mean that you will not get cancer. Talk with your doctor if you think you may be at risk. Risk factors for gastric cancer include the following:

- Having any of the following medical conditions:

  - *Helicobacter pylori* (*H. pylori*) infection of the stomach

---

This chapter includes text excerpted from "Gastric Cancer Treatment (PDQ®)— Patient Version," National Cancer Institute (NCI), August 16, 2018.

- Chronic gastritis (inflammation of the stomach)

- Pernicious anemia

- Intestinal metaplasia (a condition in which the normal stomach lining is replaced with the cells that line the intestines)

- Familial adenomatous polyposis (FAP) or gastric polyps

- Eating a diet high in salted, smoked foods and low in fruits and vegetables

- Eating foods that have not been prepared or stored properly

- Being older or male

- Smoking cigarettes

- Having a mother, father, sister, or brother who has had stomach cancer

Signs and Symptoms of Gastric Cancer

Symptoms of gastric cancer include indigestion and stomach discomfort or pain. These and other signs and symptoms may be caused by gastric cancer or by other conditions.

In the early stages of gastric cancer, the following symptoms may occur:

- Indigestion and stomach discomfort

- A bloated feeling after eating

- Mild nausea

- Loss of appetite

- Heartburn

In more advanced stages of gastric cancer, the following signs and symptoms may occur:

- Blood in the stool

- Vomiting

- Weight loss for no known reason

- Stomach pain

- Jaundice (yellowing of eyes and skin)

- Ascites (buildup of fluid in the abdomen)

- Trouble swallowing

Check with your doctor if you have any of these problems.

Diagnosis of Gastric Cancer

Tests that examine the stomach and esophagus are used to detect (find) and diagnose gastric cancer. The following tests and procedures may be used:

- **Physical exam and history:** An exam of the body to check general signs of health, including checking for signs of disease, such as lumps or anything else that seems unusual. A history of the patient's health habits and past illnesses and treatments will also be taken.

- **Blood chemistry studies:** A procedure in which a blood sample is checked to measure the amounts of certain substances released into the blood by organs and tissues in the body. An unusual (higher or lower than normal) amount of a substance can be a sign of disease.

- **Complete blood count (CBC):** A procedure in which a sample of blood is drawn and checked for the following:

  - The number of red blood cells (RBCs), white blood cells (WBCs), and platelets

  - The amount of hemoglobin (the protein that carries oxygen) in the RBCs

  - The portion of the sample made up of RBCs

- **Upper endoscopy:** A procedure to look inside the esophagus, stomach, and duodenum (first part of the small intestine) to check for abnormal areas. An endoscope (a thin, lighted tube) is passed through the mouth and down the throat into the esophagus.

- **Barium swallow:** A series of X-rays of the esophagus and stomach. The patient drinks a liquid that contains barium (a silver-white metallic compound). The liquid coats the esophagus and stomach, and X-rays are taken. This procedure is also called an upper GI series.

- **Computed tomography (CT) scan (CAT scan):** A procedure that makes a series of detailed pictures of areas inside the body, taken from different angles. The pictures are made by a computer linked to an X-ray machine. A dye may be injected into a vein or swallowed to help the organs or tissues show up more clearly. This procedure is also called computerized tomography or computerized axial tomography.

- **Biopsy:** The removal of cells or tissues so they can be viewed under a microscope to check for signs of cancer. A biopsy of the stomach is usually done during the endoscopy.

The sample of tissue may be checked to measure how many *HER2* genes there are and how much HER2 protein is being made. If there are more *HER2* genes or higher levels of HER2 protein than normal, the cancer is called HER2 positive. HER2-positive gastric cancer may be treated with a monoclonal antibody (mAb) that targets the HER2 protein.

The sample of tissue may also be checked for *Helicobacter pylori* (*H. pylori*) infection.

Certain factors affect prognosis (chance of recovery) and treatment options. The prognosis (chance of recovery) and treatment options depend on the following:

- The stage of the cancer (whether it is in the stomach only or has spread to lymph nodes or other places in the body)

- The patient's general health

When gastric cancer is found very early, there is a better chance of recovery. Gastric cancer is often in an advanced stage when it is diagnosed. At later stages, gastric cancer can be treated but rarely can be cured. Taking part in one of the clinical trials being done to improve treatment should be considered.

Stages of Gastric Cancer

After gastric cancer has been diagnosed, tests are done to find out if cancer cells have spread within the stomach or to other parts of the body. The process used to find out if cancer has spread within the stomach or to other parts of the body is called staging. The information gathered from the staging process determines the stage of the disease. It is important to know the stage in order to plan treatment.

The following tests and procedures may be used in the staging process:

- Endoscopic ultrasound (EUS)

- Computed tomography (CT) scan (CAT scan)

- Positron emission tomography (PET) scan

- Magnetic resonance imaging (MRI) with gadolinium

- Laparoscopy

The metastatic tumor is the same type of cancer as the primary tumor. For example, if gastric cancer spreads to the liver, the cancer cells in the liver are actually gastric cancer cells. The disease is metastatic gastric cancer, not liver cancer.

The following stages are used for gastric cancer:

Stage 0

In stage 0, abnormal cells are found in the mucosa (innermost layer) of the stomach wall. These abnormal cells may become cancer and spread into nearby normal tissue. Stage 0 is also called carcinoma in situ.

Stage I

Stage I is divided into stages IA and IB.

- Stage IA: Cancer has formed in the mucosa (innermost layer) of the stomach wall and may have spread to the submucosa (layer of tissue next to the mucosa).

- Stage IB: Cancer

  - has formed in the mucosa (innermost layer) of the stomach wall and may have spread to the submucosa (layer of tissue next to the mucosa). Cancer has spread to one or two nearby lymph nodes; or

  - has formed in the mucosa of the stomach wall and has spread to the muscle layer.

Stage II

Stage II gastric cancer is divided into stages IIA and IIB.

- Stage IIA: Cancer

  - may have spread to the submucosa (layer of tissue next to the mucosa) of the stomach wall. Cancer has spread to three to six nearby lymph nodes; or

- has spread to the muscle layer of the stomach wall. Cancer has spread to one or two nearby lymph nodes; or

- has spread to the subserosa (layer of connective tissue next to the muscle layer) of the stomach wall.

- Stage IIB: Cancer

  - may have spread to the submucosa (layer of tissue next to the mucosa) of the stomach wall. Cancer has spread to 7–15 nearby lymph nodes; or

  - has spread to the muscle layer of the stomach wall. Cancer has spread to three to six nearby lymph nodes; or

  - has spread to the subserosa (layer of connective tissue next to the muscle layer) of the stomach wall. Cancer has spread to one or two nearby lymph nodes; or

  - has spread to the serosa (outermost layer) of the stomach wall.

Stage III

Stage III gastric cancer is divided into stages IIIA, IIIB, and IIIC.

- Stage IIIA: Cancer has spread

  - to the muscle layer of the stomach wall. Cancer has spread to 7–15 nearby lymph nodes; or

  - to the subserosa (layer of connective tissue next to the muscle layer) of the stomach wall. Cancer has spread to three to six nearby lymph nodes; or

  - to the serosa (outermost layer) of the stomach wall. Cancer has spread to one to six nearby lymph nodes; or

  - to nearby organs, such as the spleen, colon, liver, diaphragm, pancreas, abdomen wall, adrenal gland, kidney, or small intestine, or to the back of the abdomen.

- Stage IIIB: Cancer

  - may have spread to the submucosa (layer of tissue next to the mucosa) or to the muscle layer of the stomach wall. Cancer has spread to 16 or more nearby lymph nodes; or

  - has spread to the subserosa (layer of connective tissue next to the muscle layer) or to the serosa (outermost layer) of the stomach wall. Cancer has spread to 7–15 nearby lymph nodes; or

- has spread from the stomach to nearby organs, such as the spleen, colon, liver, diaphragm, pancreas, abdomen wall, adrenal gland, kidney, or small intestine, or to the back of the abdomen. Cancer has spread to one to six nearby lymph nodes.
- Stage IIIC: Cancer has spread
  - to the subserosa (layer of connective tissue next to the muscle layer) or to the serosa (outermost layer) of the stomach wall. Cancer has spread to 16 or more nearby lymph nodes; or
  - from the stomach into nearby organs, such as the spleen, colon, liver, diaphragm, pancreas, abdomen wall, adrenal gland, kidney, or small intestine, or to the back of the abdomen. Cancer has spread to seven or more nearby lymph nodes.

Stage IV

In stage IV, cancer has spread to other parts of the body, such as the lungs, liver, distant lymph nodes, and the tissue that lines the abdomen wall.

Recurrent Gastric Cancer

Recurrent gastric cancer is cancer that has recurred (come back) after it has been treated. The cancer may come back in the stomach or in other parts of the body such as the liver or lymph nodes.

Treatment Option Overview for Gastric Cancer

Different types of treatments are available for patients with gastric cancer. Some treatments are standard (the currently used treatment), and some are being tested in clinical trials. A treatment clinical trial is a research study meant to help improve current treatments or obtain information on new treatments for patients with cancer. When clinical trials show that a new treatment is better than the standard treatment, the new treatment may become the standard treatment. Patients may want to think about taking part in a clinical trial. Some clinical trials are open only to patients who have not started treatment.

Five types of standard treatment are used:

Surgery

Surgery is a common treatment of all stages of gastric cancer. The following types of surgery may be used:

- **Subtotal gastrectomy:** Removal of the part of the stomach that contains cancer, nearby lymph nodes, and parts of other tissues and organs near the tumor. The spleen may be removed. The spleen is an organ in the upper abdomen that filters the blood and removes old blood cells.

- **Total gastrectomy:** Removal of the entire stomach, nearby lymph nodes, and parts of the esophagus, small intestine, and other tissues near the tumor. The spleen may be removed. The esophagus is connected to the small intestine so the patient can continue to eat and swallow.

If the tumor is blocking the stomach but the cancer cannot be completely removed by standard surgery, the following procedures may be used:

- **Endoluminal stent placement:** A procedure to insert a stent (a thin, expandable tube) in order to keep a passage (such as arteries or the esophagus) open. For tumors blocking the passage into or out of the stomach, surgery may be done to place a stent from the esophagus to the stomach or from the stomach to the small intestine to allow the patient to eat normally.

- **Endoluminal laser therapy:** A procedure in which an endoscope (a thin, lighted tube) with a laser attached is inserted into the body. A laser is an intense beam of light that can be used as a knife.

- **Gastrojejunostomy:** Surgery to remove the part of the stomach with cancer that is blocking the opening into the small intestine. The stomach is connected to the jejunum (a part of the small intestine) to allow food and medicine to pass from the stomach into the small intestine.

Chemotherapy

Chemotherapy is a cancer treatment that uses drugs to stop the growth of cancer cells, either by killing the cells or by stopping them from dividing. When chemotherapy is taken by mouth or injected into a vein or muscle, the drugs enter the bloodstream and can reach cancer cells throughout the body (systemic chemotherapy). When chemotherapy is placed directly into the cerebrospinal fluid, an organ, or a body cavity such as the abdomen, the drugs mainly affect cancer cells in those areas (regional chemotherapy). The way the chemotherapy is given depends on the type and stage of the cancer being treated.

Radiation Therapy

Radiation therapy is a cancer treatment that uses high-energy X-rays or other types of radiation to kill cancer cells or keep them from growing. There are two types of radiation therapy:

- External radiation therapy uses a machine outside the body to send radiation toward the cancer.

- Internal radiation therapy uses a radioactive substance sealed in needles, seeds, wires, or catheters that are placed directly into or near the cancer.

The way the radiation therapy is given depends on the type and stage of the cancer being treated. External radiation therapy is used to treat gastric cancer.

Chemoradiation

Chemoradiation therapy combines chemotherapy and radiation therapy to increase the effects of both. Chemoradiation given after surgery, to lower the risk that the cancer will come back, is called adjuvant therapy. Chemoradiation given before surgery, to shrink the tumor (neoadjuvant therapy), is being studied.

Targeted Therapy

Targeted therapy is a type of treatment that uses drugs or other substances to identify and attack specific cancer cells without harming normal cells. Monoclonal antibody (mAb) therapy is a type of targeted therapy used in the treatment of gastric cancer.

Monoclonal antibody therapy uses antibodies made in the laboratory from a single type of immune system cell. These antibodies can identify substances on cancer cells or normal substances that may help cancer cells grow. The antibodies attach to the substances and kill the cancer cells, block their growth, or keep them from spreading. Monoclonal antibodies (mAbs) are given by infusion. They may be used alone or to carry drugs, toxins, or radioactive material directly to cancer cells. For stage IV gastric cancer and gastric cancer that has recurred, monoclonal antibodies, such as trastuzumab or ramucirumab, may be given. Trastuzumab blocks the effect of the growth factor protein HER2, which sends growth signals to gastric cancer cells. Ramucirumab blocks the effect of the protein vascular endothelial growth factor (VEGF) and may prevent the growth of new blood vessels that tumors need to grow.

Treatment Options by Stage for Gastric Cancer

Stage 0

Treatment of stage 0 is usually surgery (total or subtotal gastrectomy).

Stage I

Treatment of stage I gastric cancer may include the following:

- Surgery (total or subtotal gastrectomy)

- Surgery (total or subtotal gastrectomy) followed by chemoradiation therapy

- A clinical trial of chemoradiation therapy given before surgery

Stage II

Treatment of stage II gastric cancer may include the following:

- Surgery (total or subtotal gastrectomy)

- Surgery (total or subtotal gastrectomy) followed by chemoradiation therapy or chemotherapy

- Chemotherapy given before and after surgery

- A clinical trial of surgery followed by chemoradiation therapy testing new anticancer drugs

- A clinical trial of chemoradiation therapy given before surgery

Stage III

Treatment of stage III gastric cancer may include the following:

- Surgery (total gastrectomy)

- Surgery followed by chemoradiation therapy or chemotherapy

- Chemotherapy given before and after surgery

- A clinical trial of surgery followed by chemoradiation therapy testing new anticancer drugs

- A clinical trial of chemoradiation therapy given before surgery

Stage IV and Recurrent Gastric Cancer

Treatment of stage IV or recurrent gastric cancer may include the following:

- Chemotherapy as palliative therapy to relieve symptoms and improve the quality of life (QOL)

- Targeted therapy with a monoclonal antibody with or without chemotherapy

- Endoluminal laser therapy or endoluminal stent placement to relieve a blockage in the stomach, or gastrojejunostomy to bypass the blockage

- Radiation therapy as palliative therapy to stop bleeding, relieve pain, or shrink a tumor that is blocking the stomach

- Surgery as palliative therapy to stop bleeding or shrink a tumor that is blocking the stomach

- A clinical trial of new combinations of chemotherapy as palliative therapy to relieve symptoms and improve the quality of life

Chapter 39

Small Intestine Cancer

Small intestine cancer is a rare disease in which malignant (cancer) cells form in the tissues of the small intestine. The small intestine is part of the body's digestive system, which also includes the esophagus, stomach, and large intestine. The digestive system removes and processes nutrients (vitamins, minerals, carbohydrates, fats, proteins, and water) from foods and helps pass waste material out of the body. The small intestine is a long tube that connects the stomach to the large intestine. It folds many times to fit inside the abdomen.

There are five types of small intestine cancer. The types of cancer found in the small intestine are adenocarcinoma, sarcoma, carcinoid tumors, gastrointestinal stromal tumor, and lymphoma.

Adenocarcinoma starts in glandular cells in the lining of the small intestine and is the most common type of small intestine cancer. Most of these tumors occur in the part of the small intestine near the stomach. They may grow and block the intestine.

Leiomyosarcoma starts in the smooth muscle cells of the small intestine. Most of these tumors occur in the part of the small intestine near the large intestine.

Diet and health history can affect the risk of developing small intestine cancer. Anything that increases your risk of getting a disease is called a risk factor. Having a risk factor does not mean that you will get cancer; not having risk factors doesn't mean that you will not get

This chapter includes text excerpted from "Small Intestine Cancer Treatment (PDQ®)—Patient Version," National Cancer Institute (NCI), May 11, 2018.

cancer. Talk with your doctor if you think you may be at risk. Risk factors for small intestine cancer include the following:

- Eating a high-fat diet
- Having Crohn disease
- Having celiac disease
- Having familial adenomatous polyposis (FAP)

Signs and Symptoms of Small Intestine Cancer

Signs and symptoms of small intestine cancer include unexplained weight loss and abdominal pain. These and other signs and symptoms may be caused by small intestine cancer or by other conditions. Check with your doctor if you have any of the following:

- Pain or cramps in the middle of the abdomen
- Weight loss with no known reason
- A lump in the abdomen
- Blood in the stool

Tests that examine the small intestine are used to detect (find), diagnose, and stage small intestine cancer. Procedures that make pictures of the small intestine and the area around it help diagnose small intestine cancer and show how far the cancer has spread. The process used to find out if cancer cells have spread within and around the small intestine is called staging.

In order to plan treatment, it is important to know the type of small intestine cancer and whether the tumor can be removed by surgery. Tests and procedures to detect, diagnose, and stage small intestine cancer are usually done at the same time. The following tests and procedures may be used:

- **Physical exam and history:** An exam of the body to check general signs of health, including checking for signs of disease, such as lumps or anything else that seems unusual. A history of the patient's health habits and past illnesses and treatments will also be taken.

- **Blood chemistry studies:** A procedure in which a blood sample is checked to measure the amounts of certain substances released into the blood by organs and tissues in the body. An unusual (higher or lower than normal) amount of a substance can be a sign of disease.

- **Liver function tests:** A procedure in which a blood sample is checked to measure the amounts of certain substances released into the blood by the liver. A higher than normal amount of a substance can be a sign of liver disease that may be caused by small intestine cancer.

- **Endoscopy:** A procedure to look at organs and tissues inside the body to check for abnormal areas. There are different types of endoscopy:

  - **Upper endoscopy:** A procedure to look at the inside of the esophagus, stomach, and duodenum (first part of the small intestine, near the stomach). An endoscope is inserted through the mouth and into the esophagus, stomach, and duodenum. An endoscope is a thin, tube-like instrument with a light and a lens for viewing. It may also have a tool to remove tissue samples, which are checked under a microscope for signs of cancer.

  - **Capsule endoscopy:** A procedure to look at the inside of the small intestine. A capsule that is about the size of a large pill and contains a light and a tiny wireless camera is swallowed by the patient. The capsule travels through the digestive tract, including the small intestine, and sends many pictures of the inside of the digestive tract to a recorder that is worn around the waist or over the shoulder. The pictures are sent from the recorder to a computer and viewed by the doctor who checks for signs of cancer. The capsule passes out of the body during a bowel movement.

  - **Double balloon endoscopy (DBE):** A procedure to look at the inside of the small intestine. A special instrument made up of two tubes (one inside the other) is inserted through the mouth or rectum and into the small intestine. The inside tube (an endoscope with a light and lens for viewing) is moved through part of the small intestine and a balloon at the end of it is inflated to keep the endoscope in place. Next, the outer tube is moved through the small intestine to reach the end of the endoscope, and a balloon at the end of the outer tube is inflated to keep it in place. Then, the balloon at the end of the endoscope is deflated and the endoscope is moved through the next part of the small intestine. These steps are repeated many times as the tubes move through the small intestine. The doctor is able to see the inside of the small intestine through the endoscope and use a tool to remove samples of abnormal tissue. The tissue samples are checked under a microscope for signs of cancer. This procedure may be done if the results of a capsule endoscopy are abnormal. This procedure is also called double balloon enteroscopy.

- **Laparotomy:** A surgical procedure in which an incision (cut) is made in the wall of the abdomen to check the inside of the abdomen for signs of disease. The size of the incision depends on the reason the laparotomy is being done. Sometimes organs or lymph nodes are removed or tissue samples are taken and checked under a microscope for signs of disease.

- **Biopsy:** The removal of cells or tissues so they can be viewed under a microscope to check for signs of cancer. This may be done during an endoscopy or laparotomy. The sample is checked by a pathologist to see if it contains cancer cells.

- **Upper gastrointestinal (GI) series with small bowel follow-through:** A series of X-rays of the esophagus, stomach, and small bowel. The patient drinks a liquid that contains barium (a silver-white metallic compound). The liquid coats the esophagus, stomach, and small bowel. X-rays are taken at different times as the barium travels through the upper GI tract and small bowel.

- **Computed tomography (CT) scan (CAT scan):** A procedure that makes a series of detailed pictures of areas inside the body, taken from different angles. The pictures are made by a computer linked to an X-ray machine. A dye may be injected into a vein or swallowed to help the organs or tissues show up more clearly. This procedure is also called computerized tomography or computerized axial tomography.

- **Magnetic resonance imaging (MRI):** A procedure that uses a magnet, radio waves, and a computer to make a series of detailed pictures of areas inside the body. This procedure is also called nuclear magnetic resonance imaging (NMRI).

Certain factors affect prognosis (chance of recovery) and treatment options. The prognosis (chance of recovery) and treatment options depend on the following:

- The type of small intestine cancer

- Whether the cancer is in the inner lining of the small intestine only or has spread into or beyond the wall of the small intestine

- Whether the cancer has spread to other places in the body, such as the lymph nodes, liver, or peritoneum (tissue that lines the wall of the abdomen and covers most of the organs in the abdomen)
- Whether the cancer can be completely removed by surgery
- Whether the cancer is newly diagnosed or has recurred

Stages of Small Intestine Cancer

Tests and procedures to stage small intestine cancer are usually done at the same time as diagnosis. Staging is used to find out how far the cancer has spread, but treatment decisions are not based on stage.

There are three ways that cancer spreads in the body. Cancer can spread through tissue, the lymph system, and the blood:

- **Tissue.** The cancer spreads from where it began by growing into nearby areas.
- **Lymph system.** The cancer spreads from where it began by getting into the lymph system. The cancer travels through the lymph vessels to other parts of the body.
- **Blood.** The cancer spreads from where it began by getting into the blood. The cancer travels through the blood vessels to other parts of the body.

Cancer may spread from where it began to other parts of the body. When cancer spreads to another part of the body, it is called metastasis. Cancer cells break away from where they began (the primary tumor) and travel through the lymph system or blood.

- **Lymph system.** The cancer gets into the lymph system, travels through the lymph vessels, and forms a tumor (metastatic tumor) in another part of the body.
- **Blood.** The cancer gets into the blood, travels through the blood vessels, and forms a tumor (metastatic tumor) in another part of the body.

The metastatic tumor is the same type of cancer as the primary tumor. For example, if small intestine cancer spreads to the liver, the cancer cells in the liver are actually small intestine cancer cells. The disease is metastatic small intestine cancer, not liver cancer. Small intestine cancer is grouped according to whether or not the tumor can be completely removed by surgery. Treatment depends on whether the tumor can be removed by surgery and if the cancer is being treated as a primary tumor or is metastatic cancer.

Recurrent Small Intestine Cancer

Recurrent small intestine cancer is cancer that has recurred (come back) after it has been treated. The cancer may come back in the small intestine or in other parts of the body.

Treatment Option Overview for Small Intestine Cancer

Different types of treatments are available for patients with small intestine cancer. Some treatments are standard (the currently used treatment), and some are being tested in clinical trials. A treatment clinical trial is a research study meant to help improve current treatments or obtain information on new treatments for patients with cancer. When clinical trials show that a new treatment is better than the standard treatment, the new treatment may become the standard treatment. Patients may want to think about taking part in a clinical trial. Some clinical trials are open only to patients who have not started treatment.

Three types of standard treatments used are:

Surgery

Surgery is the most common treatment of small intestine cancer. One of the following types of surgery may be done:

- **Resection:** Surgery to remove part or all of an organ that contains cancer. The resection may include the small intestine and nearby organs (if the cancer has spread). The doctor may remove the section of the small intestine that contains cancer and perform an anastomosis (joining the cut ends of the intestine together). The doctor will usually remove lymph nodes near the small intestine and examine them under a microscope to see whether they contain cancer.

- **Bypass:** Surgery to allow food in the small intestine to go around (bypass) a tumor that is blocking the intestine but cannot be removed.

After the doctor removes all the cancer that can be seen at the time of the surgery, some patients may be given radiation therapy after

554

surgery to kill any cancer cells that are left. Treatment given after the surgery, to lower the risk that the cancer will come back, is called adjuvant therapy.

Radiation Therapy

Radiation therapy is a cancer treatment that uses high-energy X-rays or other types of radiation to kill cancer cells or keep them from growing. There are two types of radiation therapy:

- External radiation therapy uses a machine outside the body to send radiation toward the cancer.

- Internal radiation therapy uses a radioactive substance sealed in needles, seeds, wires, or catheters that are placed directly into or near the cancer.

The way the radiation therapy is given depends on the type of the cancer being treated. External radiation therapy is used to treat small intestine cancer.

Chemotherapy

Chemotherapy is a cancer treatment that uses drugs to stop the growth of cancer cells, either by killing the cells or by stopping them from dividing. When chemotherapy is taken by mouth or injected into a vein or muscle, the drugs enter the bloodstream and can reach cancer cells throughout the body (systemic chemotherapy). When chemotherapy is placed directly into the cerebrospinal fluid, an organ, or a body cavity such as the abdomen, the drugs mainly affect cancer cells in those areas (regional chemotherapy). The way the chemotherapy is given depends on the type and stage of the cancer being treated.

Treatment Options for Small Intestine Cancer

Small Intestine Adenocarcinoma

When possible, treatment of small intestine adenocarcinoma will be surgery to remove the tumor and some of the normal tissue around it.

Treatment of small intestine adenocarcinoma that cannot be removed by surgery may include the following:

- Surgery to bypass the tumor

- Radiation therapy as palliative therapy to relieve symptoms and improve the patient's quality of life (QOL)

- A clinical trial of radiation therapy with radiosensitizers, with or without chemotherapy

- A clinical trial of new anticancer drugs

- A clinical trial of biologic therapy

Small Intestine Leiomyosarcoma

When possible, treatment of small intestine leiomyosarcoma will be surgery to remove the tumor and some of the normal tissue around it.

Treatment of small intestine leiomyosarcoma that cannot be removed by surgery may include the following:

- Surgery (to bypass the tumor) and radiation therapy

- Surgery, radiation therapy, or chemotherapy as palliative therapy to relieve symptoms and improve the patient's quality of life

- A clinical trial of new anticancer drugs

- A clinical trial of biologic therapy

Recurrent Small Intestine Cancer

Treatment of recurrent small intestine cancer that has spread to other parts of the body is usually a clinical trial of new anticancer drugs or biologic therapy.

Treatment of locally recurrent small intestine cancer may include the following:

- Surgery

- Radiation therapy or chemotherapy as palliative therapy to relieve symptoms and improve the patient's quality of life

- A clinical trial of radiation therapy with radiosensitizers, with or without chemotherapy

Chapter 40

Colon Cancer

Colon cancer is a disease in which malignant (cancer) cells form in the tissues of the colon. The colon is part of the body's digestive system. The digestive system removes and processes nutrients (vitamins, minerals, carbohydrates, fats, proteins, and water) from foods and helps pass waste material out of the body. The digestive system is made up of the esophagus, stomach, and the small and large intestines. The colon (large bowel) is the first part of the large intestine and is about five feet long. Together, the rectum and anal canal make up the last part of the large intestine and are about six to eight inches long. The anal canal ends at the anus (the opening of the large intestine to the outside of the body).

Health history affects the risk of developing colon cancer. Anything that increases your chance of getting a disease is called a risk factor. Having a risk factor does not mean that you will get cancer; not having risk factors doesn't mean that you will not get cancer. Talk to your doctor if you think you may be at risk for colorectal cancer.

Risk factors for colorectal cancer include the following:

- Having a family history of colon or rectal cancer in a first-degree relative (parent, sibling, or child)

- Having a personal history of cancer of the colon, rectum, or ovary

- Having a personal history of high-risk adenomas (colorectal polyps that are one centimeter or larger in size or that have cells that look abnormal under a microscope)

This chapter includes text excerpted from "Colon Cancer Treatment (PDQ®)—Patient Version," National Cancer Institute (NCI), August 17, 2018.

- Having inherited changes in certain genes that increase the risk of familial adenomatous polyposis (FAP) or Lynch syndrome (Hereditary nonpolyposis colorectal cancer (HNPCC))

- Having a personal history of chronic ulcerative colitis or Crohn disease for eight years or more

- Having three or more alcoholic drinks per day.

- Smoking cigarettes

- Being black

- Being obese

Older age is a main risk factor for most cancers. The chance of getting cancer increases as you get older.

Signs and Symptoms of Colon Cancer

Signs of colon cancer include blood in the stool or a change in bowel habits. These and other signs and symptoms may be caused by colon cancer or by other conditions. Check with your doctor if you have any of the following:

- A change in bowel habits

- Blood (either bright red or very dark) in the stool

- Diarrhea, constipation, or feeling that the bowel does not empty all the way

- Stools that are narrower than usual

- Frequent gas pains, bloating, fullness, or cramps

- Weight loss for no known reason

- Feeling very tired

- Vomiting

Diagnosis of Colon Cancer

Tests that examine the colon and rectum are used to detect (find) and diagnose colon cancer. The following tests and procedures may be used:

- **Physical exam and history:** An exam of the body to check general signs of health, including checking for signs of disease, such as lumps or anything else that seems unusual. A history of the patient's health habits and past illnesses and treatments will also be taken.

- **Digital rectal exam (DRE):** An exam of the rectum. The doctor or nurse inserts a lubricated, gloved finger into the rectum to feel for lumps or anything else that seems unusual.

- **Fecal occult blood test (FOBT):** A test to check stool (solid waste) for blood that can only be seen with a microscope. A small sample of stool is placed on a special card or in a special container and returned to the doctor or laboratory for testing. Blood in the stool may be a sign of polyps, cancer, or other conditions.

There are two types of FOBTs:

- **Guaiac FOBT:** The sample of stool on the special card is tested with a chemical. If there is blood in the stool, the special card changes color.

- **Immunochemical FOBT:** A liquid is added to the stool sample. This mixture is injected into a machine that contains antibodies that can detect blood in the stool. If there is blood in the stool, a line appears in a window in the machine. This test is also called fecal immunochemical test or FIT.

- **Barium enema:** A series of X-rays of the lower gastrointestinal tract. A liquid that contains barium (a silver-white metallic compound) is put into the rectum. The barium coats the lower gastrointestinal tract and X-rays are taken. This procedure is also called a lower GI series.

- **Sigmoidoscopy:** A procedure to look inside the rectum and sigmoid (lower) colon for polyps (small areas of bulging tissue), other abnormal areas, or cancer. A sigmoidoscope is inserted through the rectum into the sigmoid colon. A sigmoidoscope is a thin, tube-like instrument with a light and a lens for viewing. It may also have a tool to remove polyps or tissue samples, which are checked under a microscope for signs of cancer.

- **Colonoscopy:** A procedure to look inside the rectum and colon for polyps, abnormal areas, or cancer. A colonoscope is inserted through the rectum into the colon. A colonoscope is a thin, tube-like instrument with a light and a lens for viewing. It may also have a tool to remove polyps or tissue samples, which are checked under a microscope for signs of cancer.

- **Virtual colonoscopy (VC):** A procedure that uses a series of X-rays called computed tomography (CT) to make a series of pictures of the colon. A computer puts the pictures together to create detailed images that may show polyps and anything else that seems unusual on the inside surface of the colon. This test is also called colonography or CT colonography.

- **Biopsy:** The removal of cells or tissues so they can be viewed under a microscope by a pathologist to check for signs of cancer.

Certain factors affect prognosis (chance of recovery) and treatment options. The prognosis (chance of recovery) and treatment options depend on the following:

- The stage of the cancer (whether the cancer is in the inner lining of the colon only or has spread through the colon wall, or has spread to lymph nodes or other places in the body)

- Whether the cancer has blocked or made a hole in the colon

- Whether there are any cancer cells left after surgery

- Whether the cancer has recurred

- The patient's general health

The prognosis also depends on the blood levels of carcinoembryonic antigen (CEA) before treatment begins. CEA is a substance in the blood that may be increased when cancer is present.

Stages of Colon Cancer

After colon cancer has been diagnosed, tests are done to find out if cancer cells have spread within the colon or to other parts of the body. The process used to find out if cancer has spread within the colon or to other parts of the body is called staging. The information gathered from the staging process determines the stage of the disease. It is important to know the stage in order to plan treatment.

The following tests and procedures may be used in the staging process:

- Computed tomography (CT) scan (CAT scan)

- Magnetic resonance imaging (MRI)

- Positron emission tomography (PET) scan

- Chest X-ray

- Surgery

- Lymph node biopsy

- Complete blood count (CBC)

- Carcinoembryonic antigen (CEA) assay

The metastatic tumor is the same type of cancer as the primary tumor. For example, if colon cancer spreads to the lung, the cancer cells in the lung are actually colon cancer cells. The disease is metastatic colon cancer, not lung cancer.

The following stages are used for colon cancer:

Stage 0

In stage 0, abnormal cells are found in the mucosa (innermost layer) of the colon wall. These abnormal cells may become cancer and spread into nearby normal tissue. Stage 0 is also called carcinoma in situ.

Stage I

In stage I colon cancer, cancer has formed in the mucosa (innermost layer) of the colon wall and has spread to the submucosa (layer of tissue next to the mucosa) or to the muscle layer of the colon wall.

Stage II

Stage II colon cancer is divided into stages IIA, IIB, and IIC.

- Stage IIA: Cancer has spread through the muscle layer of the colon wall to the serosa (outermost layer) of the colon wall.

- Stage IIB: Cancer has spread through the serosa (outermost layer) of the colon wall to the tissue that lines the organs in the abdomen (visceral peritoneum).

- Stage IIC: Cancer has spread through the serosa (outermost layer) of the colon wall to nearby organs.

Stage III

Stage III colon cancer is divided into stages IIIA, IIIB, and IIIC. In stage IIIA, cancer has spread:

- through the mucosa (innermost layer) of the colon wall to the submucosa (layer of tissue next to the mucosa) or to the muscle

561

layer of the colon wall. Cancer has spread to one to three nearby lymph nodes or cancer cells have formed in tissue near the lymph nodes

- through the mucosa (innermost layer) of the colon wall to the submucosa (layer of tissue next to the mucosa). Cancer has spread to four to six nearby lymph nodes.

In stage IIIB, cancer has spread:

- through the muscle layer of the colon wall to the serosa (outermost layer) of the colon wall or has spread through the serosa to the tissue that lines the organs in the abdomen (visceral peritoneum). Cancer has spread to one to three nearby lymph nodes or cancer cells have formed in tissue near the lymph nodes; or

- to the muscle layer or to the serosa (outermost layer) of the colon wall. Cancer has spread to four to six nearby lymph nodes

- through the mucosa (innermost layer) of the colon wall to the submucosa (layer of tissue next to the mucosa) or to the muscle layer of the colon wall. Cancer has spread to seven or more nearby lymph nodes.

In stage IIIC, cancer has spread:

- through the serosa (outermost layer) of the colon wall to the tissue that lines the organs in the abdomen (visceral peritoneum). Cancer has spread to four to six nearby lymph nodes.

- through the muscle layer of the colon wall to the serosa (outermost layer) of the colon wall or has spread through the serosa to the tissue that lines the organs in the abdomen (visceral peritoneum). Cancer has spread to seven or more nearby lymph nodes.

- through the serosa (outermost layer) of the colon wall to nearby organs. Cancer has spread to one or more nearby lymph nodes or cancer cells have formed in tissue near the lymph nodes.

Stage IV

Stage IV colon cancer is divided into stages IVA, IVB, and IVC.

- Stage IVA: Cancer has spread to one area or organ that is not near the colon, such as the liver, lung, ovary, or a distant lymph node.

- Stage IVB: Cancer has spread to more than one area or organ that is not near the colon, such as the liver, lung, ovary, or a distant lymph node.

- Stage IVC: Cancer has spread to the tissue that lines the wall of the abdomen and may have spread to other areas or organs.

Recurrent Colon Cancer

Recurrent colon cancer is cancer that has recurred (come back) after it has been treated. The cancer may come back in the colon or in other parts of the body, such as the liver, lungs, or both.

Treatment Option Overview for Colon Cancer

Different types of treatment are available for patients with colon cancer. Some treatments are standard (the currently used treatment), and some are being tested in clinical trials. A treatment clinical trial is a research study meant to help improve current treatments or obtain information on new treatments for patients with cancer. When clinical trials show that a new treatment is better than the standard treatment, the new treatment may become the standard treatment. Patients may want to think about taking part in a clinical trial. Some clinical trials are open only to patients who have not started treatment.

Six types of standard treatment are used:

Surgery

Surgery (removing the cancer in an operation) is the most common treatment for all stages of colon cancer. A doctor may remove the cancer using one of the following types of surgery:

- **Local excision:** If the cancer is found at a very early stage, the doctor may remove it without cutting through the abdominal wall. Instead, the doctor may put a tube with a cutting tool through the rectum into the colon and cut the cancer out. This is called a local excision. If the cancer is found in a polyp (a small bulging area of tissue), the operation is called a polypectomy.

- **Resection of the colon with anastomosis:** If the cancer is larger, the doctor will perform a partial colectomy (removing the cancer and a small amount of healthy tissue around it). The doctor may then perform an anastomosis (sewing the healthy parts of the colon together). The doctor will also usually remove lymph nodes near the colon and examine them under a microscope to see whether they contain cancer.

- **Resection of the colon with colostomy:** If the doctor is not able to sew the two ends of the colon back together, a stoma (an opening) is made on the outside of the body for waste to pass through. This procedure is called a colostomy. A bag is placed around the stoma to collect the waste. Sometimes the colostomy is needed only until the lower colon has healed, and then it can be reversed. If the doctor needs to remove the entire lower colon, however, the colostomy may be permanent.

After the doctor removes all the cancer that can be seen at the time of the surgery, some patients may be given chemotherapy or radiation therapy after surgery to kill any cancer cells that are left. Treatment given after the surgery, to lower the risk that the cancer will come back, is called adjuvant therapy.

Radiofrequency Ablation

Radiofrequency ablation is the use of a special probe with tiny electrodes that kill cancer cells. Sometimes the probe is inserted directly through the skin and only local anesthesia is needed. In other cases, the probe is inserted through an incision in the abdomen. This is done in the hospital with general anesthesia.

Cryosurgery

Cryosurgery is a treatment that uses an instrument to freeze and destroy abnormal tissue. This type of treatment is also called cryotherapy.

Chemotherapy

Chemotherapy is a cancer treatment that uses drugs to stop the growth of cancer cells, either by killing the cells or by stopping them from dividing. When chemotherapy is taken by mouth or injected into a vein or muscle, the drugs enter the bloodstream and can reach cancer cells throughout the body (systemic chemotherapy). When chemotherapy is placed directly into the cerebrospinal fluid, an organ, or a body cavity such as the abdomen, the drugs mainly affect cancer cells in those areas (regional chemotherapy).

Chemoembolization of the hepatic artery may be used to treat cancer that has spread to the liver. This involves blocking the hepatic artery (the main artery that supplies blood to the liver) and inject-ing anticancer drugs between the blockage and the liver. The liver's arteries then deliver the drugs throughout the liver. Only a small amount of the drug reaches other parts of the body. The blockage may be temporary or permanent, depending on what is used to block the artery. The liver continues to receive some blood from the hepatic portal vein, which carries blood from the stomach and intestine. The way the chemotherapy is given depends on the type and stage of the cancer being treated.

Radiation Therapy

Radiation therapy is a cancer treatment that uses high-energy X-rays or other types of radiation to kill cancer cells or keep them from growing. There are two types of radiation therapy:

- External radiation therapy uses a machine outside the body to send radiation toward the cancer.

- Internal radiation therapy uses a radioactive substance sealed in needles, seeds, wires, or catheters that are placed directly into or near the cancer.

The way the radiation therapy is given depends on the type and stage of the cancer being treated. External radiation therapy is used as palliative therapy to relieve symptoms and improve quality of life.

Targeted Therapy

Targeted therapy is a type of treatment that uses drugs or other substances to identify and attack specific cancer cells without harming normal cells.

Types of targeted therapies used in the treatment of colon cancer include the following:

- **Monoclonal antibodies (mAbs):** Monoclonal antibodies are made in the laboratory from a single type of immune system cell. These antibodies can identify substances on cancer cells or normal substances that may help cancer cells grow. The antibodies attach to the substances and kill the cancer cells, block their growth, or keep them from spreading. Monoclonal antibodies are given by infusion. They may be used alone or to carry drugs, toxins, or radioactive material directly to cancer cells.

There are different types of monoclonal antibody (mAb) therapy:

- **Vascular endothelial growth factor (VEGF) inhibitor therapy:** Cancer cells make a substance called VEGF, which causes new blood vessels to form (angiogenesis) and helps the cancer grow. VEGF inhibitors block VEGF and stop new blood vessels from forming. This may kill cancer cells because they need new blood vessels to grow. Bevacizumab and ramucirumab are VEGF inhibitors and angiogenesis inhibitors.

- **Epidermal growth factor receptor (EGFR) inhibitor therapy:** EGFRs are proteins found on the surface of certain cells, including cancer cells. Epidermal growth factor attaches to the EGFR on the surface of the cell and causes the cells to grow and divide. EGFR inhibitors block the receptor and stop the epidermal growth factor from attaching to the cancer cell. This stops the cancer cell from growing and dividing. Cetuximab and panitumumab are EGFR inhibitors.

- **Immune checkpoint inhibitor therapy:** PD-1 is a protein on the surface of T cells that helps keep the body's immune responses in check. When PD-1 attaches to another protein called PDL-1 on a cancer cell, it stops the T cell from killing the cancer cell. PD-1 inhibitors attach to PDL-1 and allow the T cells to kill cancer cells. Pembrolizumab is a type of immune checkpoint inhibitor.

- **Angiogenesis inhibitors:** Angiogenesis inhibitors stop the growth of new blood vessels that tumors need to grow.

  - Ziv-aflibercept is a vascular endothelial growth factor trap that blocks an enzyme needed for the growth of new blood vessels in tumors.

  - Regorafenib is used to treat colorectal cancer that has spread to other parts of the body and has not gotten better with other treatment. It blocks the action of certain proteins, including vascular endothelial growth factor. This may help keep cancer cells from growing and may kill them. It may also prevent the growth of new blood vessels that tumors need to grow.

Treatment Options for Colon Cancer

Stage 0

Treatment of stage 0 (carcinoma in situ) may include the following types of surgery:

- Local excision or simple polypectomy
- Resection and anastomosis. This is done when the tumor is too large to remove by local excision

Stage I

Treatment of stage I colon cancer usually includes the following:

- Resection and anastomosis

Stage II

Treatment of stage II colon cancer may include the following:

- Resection and anastomosis

Stage III

Treatment of stage III colon cancer may include the following:

- Resection and anastomosis which may be followed by chemotherapy
- Clinical trials of new chemotherapy regimens after surgery

Stage IV and Recurrent Colon Cancer

Treatment of stage IV and recurrent colon cancer may include the following:

- Local excision for tumors that have recurred
- Resection with or without anastomosis
- Surgery to remove parts of other organs, such as the liver, lungs, and ovaries, where the cancer may have recurred or spread. Treatment of cancer that has spread to the liver may also include the following:

- Chemotherapy given before surgery to shrink the tumor, after surgery, or both before and after

- Radiofrequency ablation or cryosurgery, for patients who cannot have surgery

- Chemoembolization of the hepatic artery

- Radiation therapy or chemotherapy may be offered to some patients as palliative therapy to relieve symptoms and improve quality of life

- Chemotherapy and/or targeted therapy with a monoclonal antibody (mAb) or an angiogenesis inhibitor

- Clinical trials of chemotherapy and/or targeted therapy

Chapter 41

Rectal Cancer

Rectal cancer is a disease in which malignant (cancer) cells form in the tissues of the rectum. The rectum is part of the body's digestive system. The digestive system takes in nutrients (vitamins, minerals, carbohydrates, fats, proteins, and water) from foods and helps pass waste material out of the body. The digestive system is made up of the esophagus, stomach, and the small and large intestines. The colon (large bowel) is the first part of the large intestine and is about five feet long. Together, the rectum and anal canal make up the last part of the large intestine and are six to eight inches long. The anal canal ends at the anus (the opening of the large intestine to the outside of the body).

Health history affects the risk of developing rectal cancer. Anything that increases your chance of getting a disease is called a risk factor. Having a risk factor does not mean that you will get cancer; not having risk factors doesn't mean that you will not get cancer. Talk to your doctor if you think you may be at risk for colorectal cancer.

Risk factors for colorectal cancer include the following:

- Having a family history of colon or rectal cancer in a first-degree relative (parent, sibling, or child)

- Having a personal history of cancer of the colon, rectum, or ovary

- Having a personal history of high-risk adenomas (colorectal polyps that are one centimeter or larger in size or that have cells that look abnormal under a microscope)

This chapter includes text excerpted from "Rectal Cancer Treatment (PDQ®)—Patient Version," National Cancer Institute (NCI), August 17, 2018.

- Having inherited changes in certain genes that increase the risk of familial adenomatous polyposis (FAP) or Lynch syndrome (LS) (Hereditary nonpolyposis colorectal cancer (HNPCC))

- Having a personal history of chronic ulcerative colitis (UC) or Crohn disease for eight years or more

- Having three or more alcoholic drinks per day

- Smoking cigarettes

- Being black

- Being obese

Older age is a main risk factor for most cancers. The chance of getting cancer increases as you get older.

Signs and Symptoms of Rectal Cancer

Signs of rectal cancer include a change in bowel habits or blood in the stool. These and other signs and symptoms may be caused by rectal cancer or by other conditions. Check with your doctor if you have any of the following:

- Blood (either bright red or very dark) in the stool
- A change in bowel habits
  - Diarrhea
  - Constipation
  - Feeling that the bowel does not empty completely
  - Stools that are narrower or have a different shape than usual
- General abdominal discomfort (frequent gas pains, bloating, fullness, or cramps)
- Change in appetite
- Weight loss for no known reason
- Feeling very tired

Diagnosis of Rectal Cancer

Tests that examine the rectum and colon are used to detect (find) and diagnose rectal cancer. Tests used to diagnose rectal cancer include the following:

- **Physical exam and history:** An exam of the body to check general signs of health, including checking for signs of disease, such as lumps or anything else that seems unusual. A history of the patient's health habits and past illnesses and treatments will also be taken.

- **Digital rectal exam (DRE):** An exam of the rectum. The doctor or nurse inserts a lubricated, gloved finger into the lower part of the rectum to feel for lumps or anything else that seems unusual. In women, the vagina may also be examined.

- **Colonoscopy:** A procedure to look inside the rectum and colon for polyps (small pieces of bulging tissue), abnormal areas, or cancer. A colonoscope is a thin, tube-like instrument with a light and a lens for viewing. It may also have a tool to remove polyps or tissue samples, which are checked under a microscope for signs of cancer.

- **Biopsy:** The removal of cells or tissues so they can be viewed under a microscope to check for signs of cancer. Tumor tissue that is removed during the biopsy may be checked to see if the patient is likely to have the gene mutation that causes HNPCC. This may help to plan treatment. The following tests may be used:

  - **Reverse transcription–polymerase chain reaction (RT–PCR) test:** A laboratory test in which cells in a sample of tissue are studied using chemicals to look for certain changes in the structure or function of genes.

  - **Immunohistochemistry:** A test that uses antibodies to check for certain antigens in a sample of tissue. The antibody is usually linked to a radioactive substance or a dye that causes the tissue to light up under a microscope. This type of test may be used to tell the difference between different types of cancer.

- **Carcinoembryonic antigen (CEA) assay:** A test that measures the level of CEA in the blood. CEA is released into the bloodstream from both cancer cells and normal cells. When found in higher than normal amounts, it can be a sign of rectal cancer or other conditions.

Certain factors affect prognosis (chance of recovery) and treatment options. The prognosis (chance of recovery) and treatment options depend on the following:

- The stage of the cancer (whether it affects the inner lining of the rectum only, involves the whole rectum, or has spread to lymph nodes, nearby organs, or other places in the body)

- Whether the tumor has spread into or through the bowel wall

- Where the cancer is found in the rectum

- Whether the bowel is blocked or has a hole in it

- Whether all of the tumor can be removed by surgery

- The patient's general health

- Whether the cancer has just been diagnosed or has recurred (come back)

Stages of Rectal Cancer

After rectal cancer has been diagnosed, tests are done to find out if cancer cells have spread within the rectum or to other parts of the body. The process used to find out whether cancer has spread within the rectum or to other parts of the body is called staging. The information gathered from the staging process determines the stage of the disease. It is important to know the stage in order to plan treatment.

The following tests and procedures may be used in the staging process:

- Chest X-ray

- Colonoscopy

- Computed tomography (CT) scan (CAT scan)

- Magnetic resonance imaging (MRI)

- Positron emission tomography (PET) scan

- Endorectal ultrasound

The metastatic tumor is the same type of cancer as the primary tumor. For example, if rectal cancer spreads to the lung, the cancer cells in the lung are actually rectal cancer cells. The disease is metastatic rectal cancer, not lung cancer.

The following stages are used for rectal cancer:

Stage 0

In stage 0 rectal cancer, abnormal cells are found in the mucosa (innermost layer) of the rectum wall. These abnormal cells may become cancer and spread into nearby normal tissue. Stage 0 is also called carcinoma in situ.

Stage I

In stage I rectal cancer, cancer has formed in the mucosa (innermost layer) of the rectum wall and has spread to the submucosa (layer of tissue next to the mucosa) or to the muscle layer of the rectum wall.

Stage II

Stage II rectal cancer is divided into stages IIA, IIB, and IIC.

- Stage IIA: Cancer has spread through the muscle layer of the rectum wall to the serosa (outermost layer) of the rectum wall.

- Stage IIB: Cancer has spread through the serosa (outermost layer) of the rectum wall to the tissue that lines the organs in the abdomen (visceral peritoneum).

- Stage IIC: Cancer has spread through the serosa (outermost layer) of the rectum wall to nearby organs.

Stage III

Stage III rectal cancer is divided into stages IIIA, IIIB, and IIIC. In stage IIIA, cancer has spread:

- through the mucosa (innermost layer) of the rectum wall to the submucosa (layer of tissue next to the mucosa) or to the muscle layer of the rectum wall. Cancer has spread to one to three nearby lymph nodes or cancer cells have formed in tissue near the lymph nodes

- through the mucosa (innermost layer) of the rectum wall to the submucosa (layer of tissue next to the mucosa). Cancer has spread to four to six nearby lymph nodes.

In stage IIIB, cancer has spread:

- through the muscle layer of the rectum wall to the serosa (outermost layer) of the rectum wall or has spread through the serosa to the tissue that lines the organs in the abdomen (visceral peritoneum). Cancer has spread to one to three nearby lymph nodes or cancer cells have formed in tissue near the lymph nodes; or

- to the muscle layer or to the serosa (outermost layer) of the rectum wall. Cancer has spread to four to six nearby lymph nodes; or

- through the mucosa (innermost layer) of the rectum wall to the submucosa (layer of tissue next to the mucosa) or to the muscle layer of the rectum wall. Cancer has spread to seven or more nearby lymph nodes.

In stage IIIC, cancer has spread:

- through the serosa (outermost layer) of the rectum wall to the tissue that lines the organs in the abdomen (visceral peritoneum). Cancer has spread to four to six nearby lymph nodes.

- through the muscle layer of the rectum wall to the serosa (outermost layer) of the rectum wall or has spread through the serosa to the tissue that lines the organs in the abdomen (visceral peritoneum). Cancer has spread to seven or more nearby lymph nodes.

- through the serosa (outermost layer) of the rectum wall to nearby organs. Cancer has spread to one or more nearby lymph nodes or cancer cells have formed in tissue near the lymph nodes.

Stage IV

Stage IV rectal cancer is divided into stages IVA, IVB, and IVC.

- Stage IVA: Cancer has spread to one area or organ that is not near the rectum, such as the liver, lung, ovary, or a distant lymph node.

- Stage IVB: Cancer has spread to more than one area or organ that is not near the rectum, such as the liver, lung, ovary, or a distant lymph node.

- Stage IVC: Cancer has spread to the tissue that lines the wall of the abdomen and may have spread to other areas or organs.

Recurrent Rectal Cancer

Recurrent rectal cancer is cancer that has recurred (come back) after it has been treated. The cancer may come back in the rectum or in other parts of the body, such as the colon, pelvis, liver, or lungs.

Treatment Option Overview for Rectal Cancer

Different types of treatment are available for patients with rectal cancer. Some treatments are standard (the currently used treatment), and some are being tested in clinical trials. A treatment clinical trial is a research study meant to help improve current treatments or obtain information on new treatments for patients with cancer. When clinical trials show that a new treatment is better than the standard treatment, the new treatment may become the standard treatment. Patients may want to think about taking part in a clinical trial. Some clinical trials are open only to patients who have not started.

Five types of standard treatment are used:

Surgery

Surgery is the most common treatment for all stages of rectal cancer. The cancer is removed using one of the following types of surgery:

- **Polypectomy:** If the cancer is found in a polyp (a small piece of bulging tissue), the polyp is often removed during a colonoscopy.

- **Local excision:** If the cancer is found on the inside surface of the rectum and has not spread into the wall of the rectum, the cancer and a small amount of surrounding healthy tissue is removed.

- **Resection:** If the cancer has spread into the wall of the rectum, the section of the rectum with cancer and nearby healthy tissue is removed. Sometimes the tissue between the rectum and the abdominal wall is also removed. The lymph nodes near the rectum are removed and checked under a microscope for signs of cancer.

- **Radiofrequency ablation:** The use of a special probe with tiny electrodes that kill cancer cells. Sometimes the probe is inserted directly through the skin and only local anesthesia is needed. In other cases, the probe is inserted through an incision in the abdomen. This is done in the hospital with general anesthesia.

- **Cryosurgery:** A treatment that uses an instrument to freeze and destroy abnormal tissue. This type of treatment is also called cryotherapy.

- **Pelvic exenteration:** If the cancer has spread to other organs near the rectum, the lower colon, rectum, and bladder are removed. In women, the cervix, vagina, ovaries, and nearby lymph nodes may be removed. In men, the prostate may be removed. Artificial openings (stoma) are made for urine and stool to flow from the body to a collection bag.

After the cancer is removed, the surgeon will either:

- do an anastomosis (sew the healthy parts of the rectum together, sew the remaining rectum to the colon, or sew the colon to the anus); or

- make a stoma (an opening) from the rectum to the outside of the body for waste to pass through. This procedure is done if the cancer is too close to the anus and is called a colostomy. A bag is placed around the stoma to collect the waste. Sometimes the colostomy is needed only until the rectum has healed, and then it can be reversed. If the entire rectum is removed, however, the colostomy may be permanent.

Radiation therapy and/or chemotherapy may be given before surgery to shrink the tumor, make it easier to remove the cancer, and help with bowel control after surgery. Treatment given before surgery is called neoadjuvant therapy. After all the cancer that can be seen at the time of the surgery is removed, some patients may be given radiation therapy and/or chemotherapy after surgery to kill any cancer cells that are left. Treatment given after the surgery, to lower the risk that the cancer will come back, is called adjuvant therapy.

Radiation Therapy

Radiation therapy is a cancer treatment that uses high-energy X-rays or other types of radiation to kill cancer cells or keep them from growing. There are two types of radiation therapy:

- External radiation therapy uses a machine outside the body to send radiation toward the cancer.

- Internal radiation therapy uses a radioactive substance sealed in needles, seeds, wires, or catheters that are placed directly into or near the cancer.

The way the radiation therapy is given depends on the type and stage of the cancer being treated. External radiation therapy is used to treat rectal cancer.

Short-course preoperative radiation therapy is used in some types of rectal cancer. This treatment uses fewer and lower doses of radiation than standard treatment, followed by surgery several days after the last dose.

Chemotherapy

Chemotherapy is a cancer treatment that uses drugs to stop the growth of cancer cells, either by killing the cells or by stopping the cells from dividing. When chemotherapy is taken by mouth or injected into a vein or muscle, the drugs enter the bloodstream and can reach cancer cells throughout the body (systemic chemotherapy). When chemotherapy is placed directly in the cerebrospinal fluid, an organ, or a body cavity such as the abdomen, the drugs mainly affect cancer cells in those areas (regional chemotherapy).

Chemoembolization of the hepatic artery is a type of regional chemotherapy that may be used to treat cancer that has spread to the liver. This is done by blocking the hepatic artery (the main artery that supplies blood to the liver) and injecting anticancer drugs between the blockage and the liver. The liver's arteries then carry the drugs into the liver. Only a small amount of the drug reaches other parts of the body. The blockage may be temporary or permanent, depending on what is used to block the artery. The liver continues to receive some blood from the hepatic portal vein, which carries blood from the stomach and intestine.

The way the chemotherapy is given depends on the type and stage of the cancer being treated.

Active Surveillance

Active surveillance is closely following a patient's condition without giving any treatment unless there are changes in test results. It is used to find early signs that the condition is getting worse. In active surveillance, patients are given certain exams and tests to check if the cancer is growing. When the cancer begins to grow, treatment is given to cure the cancer. Tests include the following:

- Digital rectal exam
- MRI
- Endoscopy
- Sigmoidoscopy
- CT scan
- Carcinoembryonic antigen (CEA) assay

Targeted Therapy

Targeted therapy is a type of treatment that uses drugs or other substances to identify and attack specific cancer cells without harming normal cells.

Types of targeted therapies used in the treatment of rectal cancer include the following:

- **Monoclonal antibodies (mAbs):** Monoclonal antibody (mAb) therapy is a type of targeted therapy being used for the treatment of rectal cancer. Monoclonal antibody therapy uses antibodies made in the laboratory from a single type of immune system cell. These antibodies can identify substances on cancer cells or normal substances that may help cancer cells grow. The antibodies attach to the substances and kill the cancer cells, block their growth, or keep them from spreading. Monoclonal antibodies are given by infusion. They may be used alone or to carry drugs, toxins, or radioactive material directly to cancer cells.

There are different types of monoclonal antibody therapy:

- **Vascular endothelial growth factor (VEGF) inhibitor therapy:** Cancer cells make a substance called VEGF, which causes new blood vessels to form (angiogenesis) and helps the cancer grow. VEGF inhibitors block VEGF and stop new blood vessels from forming. This may kill cancer cells because they need new blood vessels to grow. Bevacizumab and ramucirumab are VEGF inhibitors and angiogenesis inhibitors.

- **Epidermal growth factor receptor (EGFR) inhibitor therapy:** EGFRs are proteins found on the surface of certain cells, including cancer cells. Epidermal growth factor attaches to the EGFR on the surface of the cell and causes the cells to grow and divide. EGFR inhibitors block the receptor and stop the epidermal growth factor from attaching to the cancer cell. This stops the cancer cell from growing and dividing. Cetuximab and panitumumab are EGFR inhibitors.

- **Immune checkpoint inhibitor therapy:** PD-1 is a protein on the surface of T cells that helps keep the body's immune responses in check. When PD-1 attaches to another protein called PDL-1 on a cancer cell, it stops the T cell from killing the cancer cell. PD-1 inhibitors attach to PDL-1 and allow the T cells to kill cancer cells. Pembrolizumab is a type of immune checkpoint inhibitor.

- **Angiogenesis inhibitors:** Angiogenesis inhibitors stop the growth of new blood vessels that tumors need to grow.

  - Ziv-aflibercept is a vascular endothelial growth factor trap that blocks an enzyme needed for the growth of new blood vessels in tumors.

  - Regorafenib is used to treat colorectal cancer that has spread to other parts of the body and has not gotten better with other treatment. It blocks the action of certain proteins, including vascular endothelial growth factor. This may help keep cancer cells from growing and may kill them. It may also prevent the growth of new blood vessels that tumors need to grow.

Treatment Options by Stage for Rectal Cancer

Stage 0

Treatment of stage 0 may include the following:

- Simple polypectomy
- Local excision
- Resection (when the tumor is too large to remove by local excision)

Stage I

Treatment of stage I rectal cancer may include the following:

- Local excision
- Resection
- Resection with radiation therapy and chemotherapy after surgery

Stages II and III

Treatment of stage II and stage III rectal cancer may include the following:

- Surgery
- Chemotherapy combined with radiation therapy, followed by surgery
- Short-course radiation therapy followed by surgery and chemotherapy

- Resection followed by chemotherapy combined with radiation therapy

- Chemotherapy combined with radiation therapy, followed by active surveillance. Surgery may be done if the cancer recurs (comes back)

- A clinical trial of a new treatment

Stage IV and Recurrent Rectal Cancer

Treatment of stage IV and recurrent rectal cancer may include the following:

- Surgery with or without chemotherapy or radiation therapy

- Systemic chemotherapy with or without targeted therapy (a monoclonal antibody or angiogenesis inhibitor)

- Chemotherapy to control the growth of the tumor

- Radiation therapy, chemotherapy, or a combination of both, as palliative therapy to relieve symptoms and improve the quality of life (QOL)

- Placement of a stent to help keep the rectum open if it is partly blocked by the tumor, as palliative therapy to relieve symptoms and improve the quality of life

- A clinical trial of a new anticancer drug

Treatment of rectal cancer that has spread to other organs depends on where the cancer has spread.

- Treatment for areas of cancer that have spread to the liver includes the following:

  - Surgery to remove the tumor. Chemotherapy may be given before surgery, to shrink the tumor

  - Cryosurgery or radiofrequency ablation

  - Chemoembolization and/or systemic chemotherapy

  - A clinical trial of chemoembolization combined with radiation therapy to the tumors in the liver

Chapter 42

Gallbladder Cancer

Gallbladder cancer is a rare disease in which malignant (cancer) cells are found in the tissues of the gallbladder. The gallbladder is a pear-shaped organ that lies just under the liver in the upper abdomen. The gallbladder stores bile, a fluid made by the liver to digest fat. When food is being broken down in the stomach and intestines, bile is released from the gallbladder through a tube called the common bile duct, which connects the gallbladder and liver to the first part of the small intestine.

The wall of the gallbladder has four main layers of tissue:

1. Mucosal (inner) layer

2. Muscle layer

3. Connective tissue layer

4. Serosal (outer) layer

Primary gallbladder cancer starts in the inner layer and spreads through the outer layers as it grows. Being female can increase the risk of developing gallbladder cancer. Anything that increases your chance of getting a disease is called a risk factor. Having a risk factor does not mean that you will get cancer; not having risk factors doesn't mean

This chapter contains text excerpted from the following sources: Text in this chapter begins with excerpts from "Gallbladder Cancer Symptoms, Tests, Prognosis, and Stages (PDQ®)—Patient Version," National Cancer Institute (NCI), March 22, 2018; Text beginning with the heading "Treatment Options Overview" is excerpted from "Gallbladder Cancer Treatment (PDQ®)—Patient Version," National Cancer Institute (NCI), March 22, 2018.

that you will not get cancer. Talk with your doctor if you think you may be at risk. Risk factors for gallbladder cancer include the following:

- Being female
- Being Native American

Signs and Symptoms of Gallbladder Cancer

Signs and symptoms of gallbladder cancer include jaundice, fever, and pain. These and other signs and symptoms may be caused by gallbladder cancer or by other conditions. Check with your doctor if you have any of the following:

- Jaundice (yellowing of the skin and whites of the eyes)
- Pain above the stomach
- Fever
- Nausea and vomiting
- Bloating
- Lumps in the abdomen

Gallbladder cancer is difficult to detect and diagnose for the following reasons:

- There are no signs or symptoms in the early stages of gallbladder cancer.
- The symptoms of gallbladder cancer, when present, are like the symptoms of many other illnesses.
- The gallbladder is hidden behind the liver.

Gallbladder cancer is sometimes found when the gallbladder is removed for other reasons. Patients with gallstones rarely develop gallbladder cancer.

Diagnosis of Gallbladder Cancer

Tests that examine the gallbladder and nearby organs are used to detect (find), diagnose, and stage gallbladder cancer. Procedures that make pictures of the gallbladder and the area around it help diagnose gallbladder cancer and show how far the cancer has spread. The process used to find out if cancer cells have spread within and around the gallbladder is called staging. In order to plan treatment, it is important to know if the gallbladder cancer can be removed by surgery. Tests and procedures to detect, diagnose, and stage gallbladder cancer are usually done at the same time. The following tests and procedures may be used:

- **Physical exam and history:** An exam of the body to check general signs of health, including checking for signs of disease, such as lumps or anything else that seems unusual. A history of the patient's health habits and past illnesses and treatments will also be taken.

- **Liver function tests:** A procedure in which a blood sample is checked to measure the amounts of certain substances released into the blood by the liver. A higher than normal amount of a substance can be a sign of liver disease that may be caused by gallbladder cancer.

- **Blood chemistry studies:** A procedure in which a blood sample is checked to measure the amounts of certain substances released into the blood by organs and tissues in the body. An unusual (higher or lower than normal) amount of a substance can be a sign of disease.

- **Computerized tomography (CT) scan (CAT scan):** A procedure that makes a series of detailed pictures of areas inside the body, such as the chest, abdomen, and pelvis, taken from different angles. The pictures are made by a computer linked to an X-ray machine. A dye may be injected into a vein or swallowed to help the organs or tissues show up more clearly. This procedure is also called computed tomography, computerized tomography, or computerized axial tomography.

- **Ultrasound exam:** A procedure in which high-energy sound waves (ultrasound) are bounced off internal tissues or organs and make echoes. The echoes form a picture of body tissues called a sonogram. An abdominal ultrasound is done to diagnose gallbladder cancer.

- **Percutaneous transhepatic cholangiography (PTC):** A procedure used to X-ray the liver and bile ducts. A thin needle is inserted through the skin below the ribs and into the liver. Dye is injected into the liver or bile ducts and an X-ray is taken. If a blockage is found, a thin, flexible tube called a stent is sometimes left in the liver to drain bile into the small intestine or a collection bag outside the body.

- **Endoscopic retrograde cholangiopancreatography (ERCP):** A procedure used to X-ray the ducts (tubes) that carry bile from the liver to the gallbladder and from the gallbladder to the small intestine. Sometimes gallbladder cancer causes these ducts to narrow and block or slow the flow of bile, causing jaundice. An endoscope (a thin, lighted tube) is passed through the mouth, esophagus, and stomach into the first part of the small intestine. A catheter (a smaller tube) is then inserted through the endoscope into the bile ducts. A dye is injected through the catheter into the ducts and an X-ray is taken. If the ducts are blocked by a tumor, a fine tube may be inserted into the duct to unblock it. This tube (or stent) may be left in place to keep the duct open. Tissue samples may also be taken.

- **Magnetic resonance imaging (MRI) with gadolinium:** A procedure that uses a magnet, radio waves, and a computer to make a series of detailed pictures of areas inside the body. A substance called gadolinium is injected into a vein. The gadolinium collects around the cancer cells so they show up brighter in the picture. This procedure is also called nuclear magnetic resonance imaging (NMRI).

- **Endoscopic ultrasound (EUS):** A procedure in which an endoscope is inserted into the body, usually through the mouth or rectum. An endoscope is a thin, tube-like instrument with a light and a lens for viewing. A probe at the end of the endoscope is used to bounce high-energy sound waves (ultrasound) off internal tissues or organs and make echoes. The echoes form a picture of body tissues called a sonogram. This procedure is also called endosonography.

- **Laparoscopy:** A surgical procedure to look at the organs inside the abdomen to check for signs of disease. Small incisions (cuts) are made in the wall of the abdomen and a laparoscope (a thin, lighted tube) is inserted into one of the incisions. Other instruments may be inserted through the same or other incisions to perform procedures such as removing organs or taking tissue samples for biopsy. The laparoscopy helps to find out if the cancer is within the gallbladder only or has spread to nearby tissues and if it can be removed by surgery.

- **Biopsy:** The removal of cells or tissues so they can be viewed under a microscope by a pathologist to check for signs of cancer. The biopsy may be done after surgery to remove the tumor. If the tumor clearly cannot be removed by surgery, the biopsy may be done using a fine needle to remove cells from the tumor.

Certain factors affect the prognosis (chance of recovery) and treatment options. The prognosis (chance of recovery) and treatment options depend on the following:

- The stage of the cancer (whether the cancer has spread from the gallbladder to other places in the body)
- Whether the cancer can be completely removed by surgery
- The type of gallbladder cancer (how the cancer cell looks under a microscope)
- Whether the cancer has just been diagnosed or has recurred (come back)

Treatment may also depend on the age and general health of the patient and whether the cancer is causing signs or symptoms. Gallbladder cancer can be cured only if it is found before it has spread, when it can be removed by surgery. If the cancer has spread, palliative treatment can improve the patient's quality of life by controlling the symptoms and complications of this disease. Taking part in one of the clinical trials being done to improve treatment should be considered.

Stages of Gallbladder Cancer

Tests and procedures to stage gallbladder cancer are usually done at the same time as diagnosis.

The metastatic tumor is the same type of cancer as the primary tumor. For example, if gallbladder cancer spreads to the liver, the cancer cells in the liver are actually gallbladder cancer cells. The disease is metastatic gallbladder cancer, not liver cancer. The following stages are used for gallbladder cancer:

Stage 0

In stage 0, abnormal cells are found in the mucosa (innermost layer) of the gallbladder wall. These abnormal cells may become cancer and spread into nearby normal tissue. Stage 0 is also called carcinoma in situ.

Stage I

In stage I, cancer has formed in the mucosa (innermost layer) of the gallbladder wall and may have spread to the muscle layer of the gallbladder wall.

Stage II

Stage II is divided into stages IIA and IIB, depending on where the cancer has spread in the gallbladder.

- In stage IIA, cancer has spread through the muscle layer to the connective tissue layer of the gallbladder wall on the side of the gallbladder that is not near the liver.

- In stage IIB, cancer has spread through the muscle layer to the connective tissue layer of the gallbladder wall on the same side as the liver. Cancer has not spread to the liver.

Stage III

Stage III is divided into stages IIIA and IIIB, depending on where the cancer has spread.

- In stage IIIA, cancer has spread through the connective tissue layer of the gallbladder wall and one or more of the following is true:

  - Cancer has spread to the serosa (layer of tissue that covers the gallbladder)

  - Cancer has spread to the liver

  - Cancer has spread to one nearby organ or structure (such as the stomach, small intestine, colon, pancreas, or the bile ducts outside the liver)

- In stage IIIB, cancer has formed in the mucosa (innermost layer) of the gallbladder wall and may have spread to the muscle, connective tissue, or serosa (layer of tissue that covers the gallbladder) and may have also spread to the liver or to one nearby organ or structure (such as the stomach, small intestine, colon, pancreas, or the bile ducts outside the liver). Cancer has spread to one to three nearby lymph nodes.

Stage IV

Stage IV is divided into stages IVA and IVB.

- In stage IVA, cancer has spread to the portal vein or hepatic artery or to two or more organs or structures other than the liver. Cancer may have spread to one to three nearby lymph nodes.

- In stage IVB, cancer may have spread to nearby organs or structures. Cancer has spread:
  - to four or more nearby lymph nodes
  - to other parts of the body, such as the peritoneum and liver

For gallbladder cancer, stages are also grouped according to how the cancer may be treated. There are two treatment groups:

Localized

Cancer is found in the wall of the gallbladder and can be completely removed by surgery.

Unresectable, Recurrent, or Metastatic

Unresectable cancer cannot be removed completely by surgery. Most patients with gallbladder cancer have unresectable cancer. Recurrent cancer is cancer that has recurred (come back) after it has been treated. Gallbladder cancer may come back in the gallbladder or in other parts of the body. Metastasis is the spread of cancer from the primary site (place where it started) to other places in the body. Metastatic gallbladder cancer may spread to surrounding tissues, organs, throughout the abdominal cavity, or to distant parts of the body.

Treatment Options Overview for Gallbladder Cancer

There are different types of treatment for patients with gallbladder cancer. Different types of treatments are available for patients with gallbladder cancer. Some treatments are standard (the currently used treatment), and some are being tested in clinical trials. A treatment clinical trial is a research study meant to help improve current treatments or obtain information on new treatments for patients with cancer. When clinical trials show that a new treatment is better than the standard treatment, the new treatment may become the standard treatment. Patients may want to think about taking part in a clinical trial. Some clinical trials are open only to patients who have not started treatment.

Three types of standard treatment are used:

Surgery

Gallbladder cancer may be treated with a cholecystectomy, surgery to remove the gallbladder and some of the tissues around it.

Nearby lymph nodes may be removed. A laparoscope is sometimes used to guide gallbladder surgery. The laparoscope is attached to a video camera and inserted through an incision (port) in the abdomen. Surgical instruments are inserted through other ports to perform the surgery. Because there is a risk that gallbladder cancer cells may spread to these ports, tissue surrounding the port sites may also be removed.

If the cancer has spread and cannot be removed, the following types of palliative surgery may relieve symptoms:

- **Biliary bypass:** If the tumor is blocking the bile duct and bile is building up in the gallbladder, a biliary bypass may be done. During this operation, the doctor will cut the gallbladder or bile duct in the area before the blockage and sew it to the small intestine to create a new pathway around the blocked area.

- **Endoscopic stent placement:** If the tumor is blocking the bile duct, surgery may be done to put in a stent (a thin tube) to drain bile that has built up in the area. The doctor may place the stent through a catheter that drains the bile into a bag on the outside of the body or the stent may go around the blocked area and drain the bile into the small intestine.

- **Percutaneous transhepatic biliary drainage (PTBD):** A procedure done to drain bile when there is a blockage and endoscopic stent placement is not possible. An X-ray of the liver and bile ducts is done to locate the blockage. Images made by ultrasound are used to guide placement of a stent, which is left in the liver to drain bile into the small intestine or a collection bag outside the body. This procedure may be done to relieve jaundice before surgery.

Radiation Therapy

Radiation therapy is a cancer treatment that uses high-energy X-rays or other types of radiation to kill cancer cells or keep them from growing. There are two types of radiation therapy:

- External radiation therapy uses a machine outside the body to send radiation toward the cancer.

- Internal radiation therapy uses a radioactive substance sealed in needles, seeds, wires, or catheters that are placed directly into or near the cancer.

The way the radiation therapy is given depends on the type and stage of the cancer being treated. External radiation therapy is used to treat gallbladder cancer.

Chemotherapy

Chemotherapy is a cancer treatment that uses drugs to stop the growth of cancer cells, either by killing the cells or by stopping the cells from dividing. When chemotherapy is taken by mouth or injected into a vein or muscle, the drugs enter the bloodstream and can reach cancer cells throughout the body (systemic chemotherapy). When chemotherapy is placed directly into the cerebrospinal fluid, an organ, or a body cavity such as the abdomen, the drugs mainly affect cancer cells in those areas (regional chemotherapy). The way the chemotherapy is given depends on the type and stage of the cancer being treated.

New types of treatment are being tested in clinical trials.

Radiation Sensitizers

Clinical trials are studying ways to improve the effect of radiation therapy on tumor cells, including the following:

- **Hyperthermia therapy:** A treatment in which body tissue is exposed to high temperatures to damage and kill cancer cells or to make cancer cells more sensitive to the effects of radiation therapy and certain anticancer drugs.

- **Radiosensitizers:** Drugs that make tumor cells more sensitive to radiation therapy. Giving radiation therapy together with radiosensitizers may kill more tumor cells.

Treatment for gallbladder cancer may cause side effects.

Treatment Options for Gallbladder Cancer

Localized Gallbladder Cancer

Treatment of localized gallbladder cancer may include the following:

- Surgery to remove the gallbladder and some of the tissue around it. Part of the liver and nearby lymph nodes may also be removed. Radiation therapy with or without chemotherapy may follow surgery.

- Radiation therapy with or without chemotherapy

- A clinical trial of radiation therapy with radiosensitizers

Unresectable, Recurrent, or Metastatic Gallbladder Cancer

Treatment of unresectable, recurrent, or metastatic gallbladder cancer is usually within a clinical trial. Treatment may include the following:

- Percutaneous transhepatic biliary drainage or the placement of stents to relieve symptoms caused by blocked bile ducts. This may be followed by radiation therapy as palliative treatment.

- Surgery as palliative treatment to relieve symptoms caused by blocked bile ducts

- Chemotherapy

- A clinical trial of new ways to give palliative radiation therapy, such as giving it together with hyperthermia therapy, radiosensitizers, or chemotherapy

- A clinical trial of new drugs and drug combinations

Chapter 43

Pancreatic Cancer

Pancreatic cancer is a disease in which malignant (cancer) cells form in the tissues of the pancreas. The pancreas is a gland about six inches long that is shaped like a thin pear lying on its side. The wider end of the pancreas is called the head, the middle section is called the body, and the narrow end is called the tail. The pancreas lies between the stomach and the spine.

The pancreas has two main jobs in the body:

- To make juices that help digest (break down) food

- To make hormones, such as insulin and glucagon, that help control blood sugar levels. Both of these hormones help the body use and store the energy it gets from food.

The digestive juices are made by exocrine pancreas cells and the hormones are made by endocrine pancreas cells. About 95 percent of pancreatic cancers begin in exocrine cells.

Smoking and health history can affect the risk of pancreatic cancer. Anything that increases your risk of getting a disease is called a risk factor. Having a risk factor does not mean that you will get cancer; not having risk factors doesn't mean that you will not get cancer. Talk with your doctor if you think you may be at risk.

Risk factors for pancreatic cancer include the following:

- Smoking

- Being very overweight

This chapter includes text excerpted from "Pancreatic Cancer Treatment (PDQ®)—Patient Version," National Cancer Institute (NCI), May 23, 2018.

- Having a personal history of diabetes or chronic pancreatitis
- Having a family history of pancreatic cancer or pancreatitis
- Having certain hereditary conditions, such as:
  - Multiple endocrine neoplasia type 1 (MEN1) syndrome.
  - Hereditary nonpolyposis colon cancer (HNPCC; Lynch syndrome)
  - von Hippel-Lindau syndrome (VHL)
  - Peutz-Jeghers syndrome (PJS)
  - Hereditary breast and ovarian cancer syndrome
  - Familial atypical multiple mole melanoma (FAMMM) syndrome

Signs and Symptoms of Pancreatic Cancer

Signs and symptoms of pancreatic cancer include jaundice, pain, and weight loss. Pancreatic cancer may not cause early signs or symptoms. Signs and symptoms may be caused by pancreatic cancer or by other conditions. Check with your doctor if you have any of the following:

- Jaundice (yellowing of the skin and whites of the eyes)
- Light-colored stools
- Dark urine
- Pain in the upper or middle abdomen and back
- Weight loss for no known reason
- Loss of appetite
- Feeling very tired

Pancreatic cancer is difficult to detect and diagnose for the following reasons:

- There aren't any noticeable signs or symptoms in the early stages of pancreatic cancer.
- The signs and symptoms of pancreatic cancer, when present, are like the signs and symptoms of many other illnesses.
- The pancreas is hidden behind other organs such as the stomach, small intestine, liver, gallbladder, spleen, and bile ducts.

Diagnosis of Pancreatic Cancer

Tests that examine the pancreas are used to detect (find), diagnose, and stage pancreatic cancer. Pancreatic cancer is usually diagnosed with tests and procedures that make pictures of the pancreas and the area around it. The process used to find out if cancer cells have spread within and around the pancreas is called staging. Tests and procedures to detect, diagnose, and stage pancreatic cancer are usually done at the same time. In order to plan treatment, it is important to know the stage of the disease and whether or not the pancreatic cancer can be removed by surgery.

The following tests and procedures may be used:

- **Physical exam and history:** An exam of the body to check general signs of health, including checking for signs of disease, such as lumps or anything else that seems unusual. A history of the patient's health habits and past illnesses and treatments will also be taken.

- **Blood chemistry studies:** A procedure in which a blood sample is checked to measure the amounts of certain substances, such as bilirubin, released into the blood by organs and tissues in the body. An unusual (higher or lower than normal) amount of a substance can be a sign of disease.

- **Tumor marker test:** A procedure in which a sample of blood, urine, or tissue is checked to measure the amounts of certain substances, such as cancer antigen 19-9 (CA 19-9), and carcinoembryonic antigen (CEA), made by organs, tissues, or tumor cells in the body. Certain substances are linked to specific types of cancer when found in increased levels in the body. These are called tumor markers.

- **Magnetic resonance imaging (MRI):** A procedure that uses a magnet, radio waves, and a computer to make a series of detailed pictures of areas inside the body. This procedure is also called nuclear magnetic resonance imaging (NMRI).

- **Computed tomography (CT) scan (CAT scan):** A procedure that makes a series of detailed pictures of areas inside the body, taken from different angles. The pictures are made by a computer linked to an X-ray machine. A dye may be injected into a vein or swallowed to help the organs or tissues show up more clearly. This procedure is also called computed tomography, computerized tomography, or computerized axial tomography. A spiral or helical CT scan makes a series of very detailed pictures of areas inside the body using an X-ray machine that scans the body in a spiral path.

- **Positron emission tomography (PET) scan:** A procedure to find malignant tumor cells in the body. A small amount of radioactive glucose (sugar) is injected into a vein. The PET scanner rotates around the body and makes a picture of where glucose is being used in the body. Malignant tumor cells show up brighter in the picture because they are more active and take up more glucose than normal cells do. A PET scan and CT scan may be done at the same time. This is called a PET-CT.

- **Abdominal ultrasound:** An ultrasound exam used to make pictures of the inside of the abdomen. The ultrasound transducer is pressed against the skin of the abdomen and directs high-energy sound waves (ultrasound) into the abdomen. The sound waves bounce off the internal tissues and organs and make echoes. The transducer receives the echoes and sends them to a computer, which uses the echoes to make pictures called sonograms. The picture can be printed to be looked at later.

- **Endoscopic ultrasound (EUS):** A procedure in which an endoscope is inserted into the body, usually through the mouth or rectum. An endoscope is a thin, tube-like instrument with a light and a lens for viewing. A probe at the end of the endoscope is used to bounce high-energy sound waves (ultrasound) off internal tissues or organs and make echoes. The echoes form a picture of body tissues called a sonogram. This procedure is also called endosonography.

- **Endoscopic retrograde cholangiopancreatography (ERCP):** A procedure used to X-ray the ducts (tubes) that carry bile from the liver to the gallbladder and from the gallbladder to the small intestine. Sometimes pancreatic cancer causes these ducts to narrow and block or slow the flow of bile, causing jaundice. An endoscope (a thin, lighted tube) is passed through the mouth, esophagus, and stomach into the first part of the small intestine. A catheter (a smaller tube) is then inserted through the endoscope into the pancreatic ducts. A dye is injected through the catheter into the ducts and an X-ray is taken. If the ducts are blocked by a tumor, a fine tube may be inserted into the duct to unblock it. This tube (or stent) may be left in place to keep the duct open. Tissue samples may also be taken.

- **Percutaneous transhepatic cholangiography (PTC):** A procedure used to X-ray the liver and bile ducts. A thin needle is inserted through the skin below the ribs and into the liver. Dye is injected into the liver or bile ducts and an X-ray is taken. If a blockage is found, a thin, flexible tube called a stent is sometimes left in the liver to drain bile into the small intestine or a collection bag outside the body. This test is done only if ERCP cannot be done.

- **Laparoscopy:** A surgical procedure to look at the organs inside the abdomen to check for signs of disease. Small incisions (cuts) are made in the wall of the abdomen and a laparoscope (a thin, lighted tube) is inserted into one of the incisions. The laparoscope may have an ultrasound probe at the end in order to bounce high-energy sound waves off internal organs, such as the pancreas. This is called laparoscopic ultrasound. Other instruments may be inserted through the same or other incisions to perform procedures such as taking tissue samples from the pancreas or a sample of fluid from the abdomen to check for cancer.

- **Biopsy:** The removal of cells or tissues so they can be viewed under a microscope by a pathologist to check for signs of cancer. There are several ways to do a biopsy for pancreatic cancer. A fine needle or a core needle may be inserted into the pancreas during an X-ray or ultrasound to remove cells. Tissue may also be removed during a laparoscopy or surgery to remove the tumor.

Certain factors affect prognosis (chance of recovery) and treatment options. The prognosis (chance of recovery) and treatment options depend on the following:

- Whether or not the tumor can be removed by surgery

- The stage of the cancer (the size of the tumor and whether the cancer has spread outside the pancreas to nearby tissues or lymph nodes or to other places in the body)

- The patient's general health

- Whether the cancer has just been diagnosed or has recurred (come back)

Pancreatic cancer can be controlled only if it is found before it has spread, when it can be completely removed by surgery. If the cancer

595

has spread, palliative treatment can improve the patient's quality of life by controlling the symptoms and complications of this disease.

Stages of Pancreatic Cancer

Tests and procedures to stage pancreatic cancer are usually done at the same time as diagnosis. The process used to find out if cancer has spread within the pancreas or to other parts of the body is called staging. The information gathered from the staging process determines the stage of the disease. It is important to know the stage of the disease in order to plan treatment. The results of some of the tests used to diagnose pancreatic cancer are often also used to stage the disease.

The metastatic tumor is the same type of cancer as the primary tumor. For example, if pancreatic cancer spreads to the liver, the cancer cells in the liver are actually pancreatic cancer cells. The disease is metastatic pancreatic cancer, not liver cancer.

The following stages are used for pancreatic cancer:

Stage 0

In stage 0, abnormal cells are found in the lining of the pancreas. These abnormal cells may become cancer and spread into nearby normal tissue. Stage 0 is also called carcinoma in situ.

Stage I

In stage I, cancer has formed and is found in the pancreas only. Stage I is divided into stages IA and IB, depending on the size of the tumor.

- Stage IA: The tumor is two centimeters or smaller.

- Stage IB: The tumor is larger than two centimeters but not larger than four centimeters.

Stage II

Stage II is divided into stages IIA and IIB, depending on the size of the tumor and where the cancer has spread.

- Stage IIA: The tumor is larger than four centimeters.

- Stage IIB: The tumor is any size and cancer has spread to one to three nearby lymph nodes.

Stage III

In stage III, the tumor is any size and cancer has spread to:

- four or more nearby lymph nodes; or
- the major blood vessels near the pancreas.

Stage IV

In stage IV, the tumor is any size and cancer has spread to other parts of the body, such as the liver, lung, or peritoneal cavity (the body cavity that contains most of the organs in the abdomen).

Recurrent Pancreatic Cancer

Recurrent pancreatic cancer is cancer that has recurred (come back) after it has been treated. The cancer may come back in the pancreas or in other parts of the body.

Treatment Option Overview for Pancreatic Cancer

There are different types of treatment for patients with pancreatic cancer.

Different types of treatment are available for patients with pancreatic cancer. Some treatments are standard (the currently used treatment), and some are being tested in clinical trials. A treatment clinical trial is a research study meant to help improve current treatments or obtain information on new treatments for patients with cancer. When clinical trials show that a new treatment is better than the standard treatment, the new treatment may become the standard treatment. Patients may want to think about taking part in a clinical trial. Some clinical trials are open only to patients who have not started treatment.

Five types of standard treatment are used:

Surgery

One of the following types of surgery may be used to take out the tumor:

- **Whipple procedure:** A surgical procedure in which the head of the pancreas, the gallbladder, part of the stomach, part of the small intestine, and the bile duct are removed. Enough of the pancreas is left to produce digestive juices and insulin.

597

- **Total pancreatectomy:** This operation removes the whole pancreas, part of the stomach, part of the small intestine, the common bile duct, the gallbladder, the spleen, and nearby lymph nodes.

- **Distal pancreatectomy:** Surgery to remove the body and the tail of the pancreas. The spleen may also be removed if cancer has spread to the spleen.

If the cancer has spread and cannot be removed, the following types of palliative surgery may be done to relieve symptoms and improve quality of life:

- **Biliary bypass:** If cancer is blocking the bile duct and bile is building up in the gallbladder, a biliary bypass may be done. During this operation, the doctor will cut the gallbladder or bile duct in the area before the blockage and sew it to the small intestine to create a new pathway around the blocked area.

- **Endoscopic stent placement:** If the tumor is blocking the bile duct, surgery may be done to put in a stent (a thin tube) to drain bile that has built up in the area. The doctor may place the stent through a catheter that drains the bile into a bag on the outside of the body or the stent may go around the blocked area and drain the bile into the small intestine.

- **Gastric bypass:** If the tumor is blocking the flow of food from the stomach, the stomach may be sewn directly to the small intestine so the patient can continue to eat normally.

Radiation Therapy

Radiation therapy is a cancer treatment that uses high-energy X-rays or other types of radiation to kill cancer cells or keep them from growing. There are two types of radiation therapy:

- External radiation therapy uses a machine outside the body to send radiation toward the cancer.

- Internal radiation therapy uses a radioactive substance sealed in needles, seeds, wires, or catheters that are placed directly into or near the cancer.

The way the radiation therapy is given depends on the type and stage of the cancer being treated. External radiation therapy is used to treat pancreatic cancer.

Chemotherapy

Chemotherapy is a cancer treatment that uses drugs to stop the growth of cancer cells, either by killing the cells or by stopping them from dividing. When chemotherapy is taken by mouth or injected into a vein or muscle, the drugs enter the bloodstream and can reach cancer cells throughout the body (systemic chemotherapy). When chemotherapy is placed directly into the cerebrospinal fluid, an organ, or a body cavity such as the abdomen, the drugs mainly affect cancer cells in those areas (regional chemotherapy). Combination chemotherapy is treatment using more than one anticancer drug. The way the chemotherapy is given depends on the type and stage of the cancer being treated.

Chemoradiation Therapy

Chemoradiation therapy combines chemotherapy and radiation therapy to increase the effects of both.

Targeted Therapy

Targeted therapy is a type of treatment that uses drugs or other substances to identify and attack specific cancer cells without harming normal cells. Tyrosine kinase inhibitors (TKIs) are targeted therapy drugs that block signals needed for tumors to grow. Erlotinib is a type of TKI used to treat pancreatic cancer. There are treatments for pain caused by pancreatic cancer. Pain can occur when the tumor presses on nerves or other organs near the pancreas. When pain medicine is not enough, there are treatments that act on nerves in the abdomen to relieve the pain. The doctor may inject medicine into the area around affected nerves or may cut the nerves to block the feeling of pain. Radiation therapy with or without chemotherapy can also help relieve pain by shrinking the tumor. Patients with pancreatic cancer have special nutritional needs. Surgery to remove the pancreas may affect its ability to make pancreatic enzymes that help to digest food. As a result, patients may have problems digesting food and absorbing nutrients into the body. To prevent malnutrition, the doctor may prescribe medicines that replace these enzymes.

Treatment Options by Stage for Pancreatic Cancer

Stages I and II

Treatment of stage I and stage II pancreatic cancer may include the following:

- Surgery

- Surgery followed by chemotherapy

- Surgery followed by chemoradiation

- A clinical trial of combination chemotherapy

- A clinical trial of chemotherapy and targeted therapy, with or without chemoradiation

- A clinical trial of chemotherapy and/or radiation therapy before surgery

Stage III

Treatment of stage III pancreatic cancer may include the following:

- Palliative surgery or stent placement to bypass blocked areas in ducts or the small intestine

- Chemotherapy followed by chemoradiation

- Chemoradiation followed by chemotherapy

- Chemotherapy with or without targeted therapy

- A clinical trial of new anticancer therapies together with chemotherapy or chemoradiation

- A clinical trial of radiation therapy given during surgery or internal radiation therapy

Stage IV

Treatment of stage IV pancreatic cancer may include the following:

- Palliative treatments to relieve pain, such as nerve blocks, and other supportive care

- Palliative surgery or stent placement to bypass blocked areas in ducts or the small intestine

- Chemotherapy with or without targeted therapy

- Clinical trials of new anticancer agents with or without chemotherapy

Treatment Options for Recurrent Pancreatic Cancer

Treatment of recurrent pancreatic cancer may include the following:

- Palliative surgery or stent placement to bypass blocked areas in ducts or the small intestine
- Palliative radiation therapy to shrink the tumor
- Other palliative medical care to reduce symptoms, such as nerve blocks to relieve pain
- Chemotherapy
- Clinical trials of chemotherapy, new anticancer therapies, or biologic therapy

Chapter 44

Pancreatic Neuroendocrine Tumors

Pancreatic neuroendocrine tumors form in hormone-making cells (islet cells) of the pancreas. The pancreas is a gland about six inches long that is shaped like a thin pear lying on its side. The wider end of the pancreas is called the head, the middle section is called the body, and the narrow end is called the tail. The pancreas lies behind the stomach and in front of the spine.

There are two kinds of cells in the pancreas:

1. Endocrine pancreas cells make several kinds of hormones (chemicals that control the actions of certain cells or organs in the body), such as insulin to control blood sugar. They cluster together in many small groups (islets) throughout the pancreas. Endocrine pancreas cells are also called islet cells or islets of Langerhans. Tumors that form in islet cells are called islet cell tumors, pancreatic endocrine tumors, or pancreatic neuroendocrine tumors (pancreatic NETs).

2. Exocrine pancreas cells make enzymes that are released into the small intestine to help the body digest food. Most of the pancreas is made of ducts with small sacs at the end of the ducts, which are lined with exocrine cells.

Pancreatic neuroendocrine tumors (NETs) may be benign (not cancer) or malignant (cancer). When pancreatic NETs are malignant, they are called pancreatic endocrine cancer or islet cell carcinoma.

This chapter includes text excerpted from "Pancreatic Neuroendocrine Tumors (Islet Cell Tumors) Treatment (PDQ®)—Patient Version," National Cancer Institute (NCI), March 22, 2018.

Pancreatic NETs are much less common than pancreatic exocrine tumors and have a better prognosis. Pancreatic NETs may or may not cause signs or symptoms.

Pancreatic NETs may be functional or nonfunctional:

- Functional tumors make extra amounts of hormones, such as gastrin, insulin, and glucagon, that cause signs and symptoms.

- Nonfunctional tumors do not make extra amounts of hormones. Signs and symptoms are caused by the tumor as it spreads and grows. Most nonfunctional tumors are malignant (cancer).

Most pancreatic NETs are functional tumors. There are different kinds of functional pancreatic NETs. Pancreatic NETs make different kinds of hormones such as gastrin, insulin, and glucagon. Functional pancreatic NETs include the following:

- **Gastrinoma:** A tumor that forms in cells that make gastrin. Gastrin is a hormone that causes the stomach to release an acid that helps digest food. Both gastrin and stomach acid are increased by gastrinomas. When increased stomach acid, stomach ulcers, and diarrhea are caused by a tumor that makes gastrin, it is called Zollinger-Ellison syndrome. A gastrinoma usually forms in the head of the pancreas and sometimes forms in the small intestine. Most gastrinomas are malignant (cancer).

- **Insulinoma:** A tumor that forms in cells that make insulin. Insulin is a hormone that controls the amount of glucose (sugar) in the blood. It moves glucose into the cells, where it can be used by the body for energy. Insulinomas are usually slow-growing tumors that rarely spread. An insulinoma forms in the head, body, or tail of the pancreas. Insulinomas are usually benign (not cancer).

- **Glucagonoma:** A tumor that forms in cells that make glucagon. Glucagon is a hormone that increases the amount of glucose in the blood. It causes the liver to break down glycogen. Too much glucagon causes hyperglycemia (high blood sugar). A glucagonoma usually forms in the tail of the pancreas. Most glucagonomas are malignant (cancer).

- **Other types of tumors:** There are other rare types of functional pancreatic NETs that make hormones, including hormones that control the balance of sugar, salt, and water in the body. These tumors include:

- VIPomas, which make vasoactive intestinal peptide. VIPoma may also be called Verner-Morrison syndrome.

- Somatostatinomas, which make somatostatin

These other types of tumors are grouped together because they are treated in much the same way.

Having certain syndromes can increase the risk of pancreatic NETs. Anything that increases your risk of getting a disease is called a risk factor. Having a risk factor does not mean that you will get cancer; not having risk factors doesn't mean that you will not get cancer. Talk with your doctor if you think you may be at risk. Multiple endocrine neoplasia type 1 (MEN1) syndrome is a risk factor for pancreatic NETs.

Signs and Symptoms of Pancreatic Neuroendocrine Tumors

Signs or symptoms can be caused by the growth of the tumor and/ or by hormones the tumor makes or by other conditions. Some tumors may not cause signs or symptoms. Check with your doctor if you have any of these problems.

Signs and Symptoms of a Nonfunctional Pancreatic NET

A nonfunctional pancreatic NET may grow for a long time without causing signs or symptoms. It may grow large or spread to other parts of the body before it causes signs or symptoms, such as:

- Diarrhea

- Indigestion

- A lump in the abdomen

- Pain in the abdomen or back

- Yellowing of the skin and whites of the eyes

Signs and Symptoms of a Functional Pancreatic NET

The signs and symptoms of a functional pancreatic NET depend on the type of hormone being made.

Too much gastrin may cause:

- Stomach ulcers that keep coming back

- Pain in the abdomen, which may spread to the back. The pain may come and go and it may go away after taking an antacid

- The flow of stomach contents back into the esophagus (gastroesophageal reflux)

- Diarrhea

Too much insulin may cause:

- Low blood sugar. This can cause blurred vision, headache, and feeling lightheaded, tired, weak, shaky, nervous, irritable, sweaty, confused, or hungry.

- Fast heartbeat

Too much glucagon may cause:

- Skin rash on the face, stomach, or legs

- High blood sugar. This can cause headaches, frequent urination, dry skin and mouth, or feeling hungry, thirsty, tired, or weak

- Blood clots. Blood clots in the lung can cause shortness of breath, cough, or pain in the chest. Blood clots in the arm or leg can cause pain, swelling, warmth, or redness of the arm or leg

- Diarrhea

- Weight loss for no known reason

- Sore tongue or sores at the corners of the mouth

Too much vasoactive intestinal peptide (VIP) may cause:

- Very large amounts of watery diarrhea

- Dehydration. This can cause feeling thirsty, making less urine, dry skin and mouth, headaches, dizziness, or feeling tired

- Low potassium level in the blood. This can cause muscle weakness, aching, or cramps, numbness and tingling, frequent urination, fast heartbeat, and feeling confused or thirsty.

- Cramps or pain in the abdomen

- Weight loss for no known reason

Too much somatostatin may cause:

- High blood sugar. This can cause headaches, frequent urination, dry skin and mouth, or feeling hungry, thirsty, tired, or weak

- Diarrhea

- Steatorrhea (very foul-smelling stool that floats)

- Gallstones

- Yellowing of the skin and whites of the eyes

- Weight loss for no known reason

Diagnosis of Pancreatic Neuroendocrine Tumors

Lab tests and imaging tests are used to detect (find) and diagnose pancreatic NETs. The following tests and procedures may be used:

- **Physical exam and history:** An exam of the body to check general signs of health, including checking for signs of disease, such as lumps or anything else that seems unusual. A history of the patient's health habits and past illnesses and treatments will also be taken.

- **Blood chemistry studies:** A procedure in which a blood sample is checked to measure the amounts of certain substances, such as glucose (sugar), released into the blood by organs and tissues in the body. An unusual (higher or lower than normal) amount of a substance can be a sign of disease.

- **Chromogranin A (CgA) test:** A test in which a blood sample is checked to measure the amount of CgA in the blood. A higher than normal amount of CgA and normal amounts of hormones such as gastrin, insulin, and glucagon can be a sign of a nonfunctional pancreatic NET.

- **Abdominal computerized tomography (CT) scan (CAT scan):** A procedure that makes a series of detailed pictures of the abdomen, taken from different angles. The pictures are made by a computer linked to an X-ray machine. A dye may be injected into a vein or swallowed to help the organs or tissues show up more clearly. This procedure is also called computed tomography, computerized tomography, or computerized axial tomography.

- **Magnetic resonance imaging (MRI):** A procedure that uses a magnet, radio waves, and a computer to make a series of detailed pictures of areas inside the body. This procedure is also called nuclear magnetic resonance imaging (NMRI).

- **Somatostatin receptor scintigraphy (SRS):** A type of radionuclide scan that may be used to find small pancreatic

NETs. A small amount of radioactive octreotide (a hormone that attaches to tumors) is injected into a vein and travels through the blood. The radioactive octreotide attaches to the tumor and a special camera that detects radioactivity is used to show where the tumors are in the body. This procedure is also called octreotide scan and SRS.

- **Endoscopic ultrasound (EUS):** A procedure in which an endoscope is inserted into the body, usually through the mouth or rectum. An endoscope is a thin, tube-like instrument with a light and a lens for viewing. A probe at the end of the endoscope is used to bounce high-energy sound waves (ultrasound) off internal tissues or organs and make echoes. The echoes form a picture of body tissues called a sonogram. This procedure is also called endosonography.

- **Endoscopic retrograde cholangiopancreatography (ERCP):** A procedure used to X-ray the ducts (tubes) that carry bile from the liver to the gallbladder and from the gallbladder to the small intestine. Sometimes pancreatic cancer causes these ducts to narrow and block or slow the flow of bile, causing jaundice. An endoscope is passed through the mouth, esophagus, and stomach into the first part of the small intestine. An endoscope is a thin, tube-like instrument with a light and a lens for viewing. A catheter (a smaller tube) is then inserted through the endoscope into the pancreatic ducts. A dye is injected through the catheter into the ducts and an X-ray is taken. If the ducts are blocked by a tumor, a fine tube may be inserted into the duct to unblock it. This tube (or stent) may be left in place to keep the duct open. Tissue samples may also be taken and checked under a microscope for signs of cancer.

- **Angiogram:** A procedure to look at blood vessels and the flow of blood. A contrast dye is injected into the blood vessel. As the contrast dye moves through the blood vessel, X-rays are taken to see if there are any blockages.

- **Laparotomy:** A surgical procedure in which an incision (cut) is made in the wall of the abdomen to check the inside of the abdomen for signs of disease. The size of the incision depends on the reason the laparotomy is being done. Sometimes organs are removed or tissue samples are taken and checked under a microscope for signs of disease.

- **Intraoperative ultrasound:** A procedure that uses high-energy sound waves (ultrasound) to create images of internal organs or tissues during surgery. A transducer placed directly on the organ or tissue is used to make the sound waves, which create echoes. The transducer receives the echoes and sends them to a computer, which uses the echoes to make pictures called sonograms.

- **Biopsy:** The removal of cells or tissues so they can be viewed under a microscope by a pathologist to check for signs of cancer. There are several ways to do a biopsy for pancreatic NETs. Cells may be removed using a fine or wide needle inserted into the pancreas during an X-ray or ultrasound. Tissue may also be removed during a laparoscopy (a surgical incision made in the wall of the abdomen).

- **Bone scan:** A procedure to check if there are rapidly dividing cells, such as cancer cells, in the bone. A very small amount of radioactive material is injected into a vein and travels through the bloodstream. The radioactive material collects in bones with cancer and is detected by a scanner.

Other kinds of lab tests are used to check for the specific type of pancreatic NETs. The following tests and procedures may be used:

Gastrinoma

- **Fasting serum gastrin test:** A test in which a blood sample is checked to measure the amount of gastrin in the blood. This test is done after the patient has had nothing to eat or drink for at least eight hours. Conditions other than gastrinoma can cause an increase in the amount of gastrin in the blood.

- **Basal acid output test:** A test to measure the amount of acid made by the stomach. The test is done after the patient has had nothing to eat or drink for at least eight hours. A tube is inserted through the nose or throat, into the stomach. The stomach contents are removed and four samples of gastric acid are removed through the tube. These samples are used to find out the amount of gastric acid made during the test and the pH level of the gastric secretions.

- **Secretin stimulation test:** If the basal acid output test result is not normal, a secretin stimulation test may be done. The tube is moved into the small intestine and samples are taken from the small intestine after a drug called secretin is injected. Secretin causes the small intestine to make acid. When there is a gastrinoma, the secretin causes an increase in how much gastric acid is made and the level of gastrin in the blood.

- **Somatostatin receptor scintigraphy:** A type of radionuclide scan that may be used to find small pancreatic NETs. A small amount of radioactive octreotide (a hormone that attaches to tumors) is injected into a vein and travels through the blood. The radioactive octreotide attaches to the tumor and a special camera that detects radioactivity is used to show where the tumors are in the body. This procedure is also called octreotide scan and SRS.

Insulinoma

- **Fasting serum glucose and insulin test:** A test in which a blood sample is checked to measure the amounts of glucose (sugar) and insulin in the blood. The test is done after the patient has had nothing to eat or drink for at least 24 hours.

Glucagonoma

- **Fasting serum glucagon test:** A test in which a blood sample is checked to measure the amount of glucagon in the blood. The test is done after the patient has had nothing to eat or drink for at least eight hours.

Other Tumor Types

- VIPoma

  - **Serum VIP (Vasoactive intestinal peptide) test:** A test in which a blood sample is checked to measure the amount of VIP.

  - **Blood chemistry studies:** A procedure in which a blood sample is checked to measure the amounts of certain substances released into the blood by organs and tissues in the body. An unusual (higher or lower than normal) amount of a substance can be a sign of disease. In VIPoma, there is a lower than normal amount of potassium.

  - **Stool analysis:** A stool sample is checked for a higher than normal sodium (salt) and potassium levels.

- Somatostatinoma

  - **Fasting serum somatostatin test:** A test in which a blood sample is checked to measure the amount of somatostatin in the blood. The test is done after the patient has had nothing to eat or drink for at least eight hours.

  - **Somatostatin receptor scintigraphy:** A type of radionuclide scan that may be used to find small pancreatic NETs. A small amount of radioactive octreotide (a hormone that attaches to tumors) is injected into a vein and travels through the blood. The radioactive octreotide attaches to the tumor and a special camera that detects radioactivity is used to show where the tumors are in the body. This procedure is also called octreotide scan and SRS.

Certain factors affect prognosis (chance of recovery) and treatment options. Pancreatic NETs can often be cured. The prognosis (chance of recovery) and treatment options depend on the following:

- The type of cancer cell
- Where the tumor is found in the pancreas
- Whether the tumor has spread to more than one place in the pancreas or to other parts of the body
- Whether the patient has MEN1 syndrome
- The patient's age and general health
- Whether the cancer has just been diagnosed or has recurred (come back)

Stages of Pancreatic Neuroendocrine Tumors

The plan for cancer treatment depends on where the NET is found in the pancreas and whether it has spread. The process used to find out if cancer has spread within the pancreas or to other parts of the body is called staging. The results of the tests and procedures used to diagnose pancreatic neuroendocrine tumors (NETs) are also used to find out whether the cancer has spread.

Although there is a standard staging system for pancreatic NETs, it is not used to plan treatment. Treatment of pancreatic NETs is based on the following:

- Whether the cancer is found in one place in the pancreas

- Whether the cancer is found in several places in the pancreas

- Whether the cancer has spread to lymph nodes near the pancreas or to other parts of the body such as the liver, lung, peritoneum, or bone

The metastatic tumor is the same type of tumor as the primary tumor. For example, if a pancreatic neuroendocrine tumor spreads to the liver, the tumor cells in the liver are actually neuroendocrine tumor cells. The disease is metastatic pancreatic neuroendocrine tumor, not liver cancer.

Treatment Option Overview for Pancreatic Neuroendocrine Tumors

Different types of treatments are available for patients with pancreatic neuroendocrine tumors (NETs). Some treatments are standard (the currently used treatment), and some are being tested in clinical trials. A treatment clinical trial is a research study meant to help improve current treatments or obtain information on new treatments for patients with cancer. When clinical trials show that a new treatment is better than the standard treatment, the new treatment may become the standard treatment. Patients may want to think about taking part in a clinical trial. Some clinical trials are open only to patients who have not started treatment.

Six types of standard treatment are used:

Surgery

An operation may be done to remove the tumor. One of the following types of surgery may be used:

- **Enucleation:** Surgery to remove the tumor only. This may be done when cancer occurs in one place in the pancreas.

- **Pancreatoduodenectomy:** A surgical procedure in which the head of the pancreas, the gallbladder, nearby lymph nodes and part of the stomach, small intestine, and bile duct are removed. Enough of the pancreas is left to make digestive juices and insulin. The organs removed during this procedure depend on the patient's condition. This is also called the Whipple procedure.

- **Distal pancreatectomy:** Surgery to remove the body and tail of the pancreas. The spleen may also be removed if cancer has spread to the spleen.

- **Total gastrectomy:** Surgery to remove the whole stomach.

- **Parietal cell vagotomy:** Surgery to cut the nerve that causes stomach cells to make acid.

- **Liver resection:** Surgery to remove part or all of the liver.

- **Radiofrequency ablation:** The use of a special probe with tiny electrodes that kill cancer cells. Sometimes the probe is inserted directly through the skin and only local anesthesia is needed. In other cases, the probe is inserted through an incision in the abdomen. This is done in the hospital with general anesthesia.

- **Cryosurgical ablation:** A procedure in which tissue is frozen to destroy abnormal cells. This is usually done with a special instrument that contains liquid nitrogen or liquid carbon dioxide. The instrument may be used during surgery or laparoscopy or inserted through the skin. This procedure is also called cryoablation.

Chemotherapy

Chemotherapy is a cancer treatment that uses drugs to stop the growth of cancer cells, either by killing the cells or by stopping them from dividing. When chemotherapy is taken by mouth or injected into a vein or muscle, the drugs enter the bloodstream and can reach cancer cells throughout the body (systemic chemotherapy). When chemotherapy is placed directly into the cerebrospinal fluid, an organ, or a body cavity such as the abdomen, the drugs mainly affect cancer cells in those areas (regional chemotherapy). Combination chemotherapy is the use of more than one anticancer drug. The way the chemotherapy is given depends on the type of the cancer being treated.

Hormone Therapy

Hormone therapy is a cancer treatment that removes hormones or blocks their action and stops cancer cells from growing. Hormones are substances made by glands in the body and circulated in the bloodstream. Some hormones can cause certain cancers to grow. If tests show that the cancer cells have places where hormones can attach (receptors), drugs, surgery, or radiation therapy is used to reduce the production of hormones or block them from working.

613

Hepatic Arterial Occlusion or Chemoembolization

Hepatic arterial occlusion uses drugs, small particles, or other agents to block or reduce the flow of blood to the liver through the hepatic artery (the major blood vessel that carries blood to the liver). This is done to kill cancer cells growing in the liver. The tumor is prevented from getting the oxygen and nutrients it needs to grow. The liver continues to receive blood from the hepatic portal vein, which carries blood from the stomach and intestine.

Chemotherapy delivered during hepatic arterial occlusion is called chemoembolization. The anticancer drug is injected into the hepatic artery through a catheter (thin tube). The drug is mixed with the substance that blocks the artery and cuts off blood flow to the tumor. Most of the anticancer drug is trapped near the tumor and only a small amount of the drug reaches other parts of the body. The blockage may be temporary or permanent, depending on the substance used to block the artery.

Targeted Therapy

Targeted therapy is a type of treatment that uses drugs or other substances to identify and attack specific cancer cells without harming normal cells. Certain types of targeted therapies are being studied in the treatment of pancreatic NETs.

Supportive Care

Supportive care is given to lessen the problems caused by the disease or its treatment. Supportive care for pancreatic NETs may include treatment for the following:

- Stomach ulcers may be treated with drug therapy such as:
  - Proton pump inhibitor drugs such as omeprazole, lansoprazole, or pantoprazole
  - Histamine blocking drugs such as cimetidine, ranitidine, or famotidine
  - Somatostatin-type drugs such as octreotide
- Diarrhea may be treated with:
  - Intravenous (IV) fluids with electrolytes such as potassium or chloride
  - Somatostatin-type drugs such as octreotide

- Low blood sugar may be treated by having small, frequent meals or with drug therapy to maintain a normal blood sugar level.

- High blood sugar may be treated with drugs taken by mouth or insulin by injection.

Treatment Options for Pancreatic Neuroendocrine Tumors

Gastrinoma

Treatment of gastrinoma may include supportive care and the following:

- For symptoms caused by too much stomach acid, treatment may be a drug that decreases the amount of acid made by the stomach

- For a single tumor in the head of the pancreas:

  - Surgery to remove the tumor

  - Surgery to cut the nerve that causes stomach cells to make acid and treatment with a drug that decreases stomach acid

  - Surgery to remove the whole stomach (rare)

- For a single tumor in the body or tail of the pancreas, treatment is usually surgery to remove the body or tail of the pancreas.

- For several tumors in the pancreas, treatment is usually surgery to remove the body or tail of the pancreas. If tumor remains after surgery, treatment may include either:

- Surgery to cut the nerve that causes stomach cells to make acid and treatment with a drug that decreases stomach acid

- Surgery to remove the whole stomach (rare)

- For one or more tumors in the duodenum (the part of the small intestine that connects to the stomach), treatment is usually pancreatoduodenectomy (surgery to remove the head of the pancreas, the gallbladder, nearby lymph nodes and part of the stomach, small intestine, and bile duct).

- If no tumor is found, treatment may include the following:

  - Surgery to cut the nerve that causes stomach cells to make acid and treatment with a drug that decreases stomach acid

- Surgery to remove the whole stomach (rare)
- If the cancer has spread to the liver, treatment may include:
  - Surgery to remove part or all of the liver
  - Radiofrequency ablation or cryosurgical ablation
  - Chemoembolization
- If cancer has spread to other parts of the body or does not get better with surgery or drugs to decrease stomach acid, treatment may include:
  - Chemotherapy
  - Hormone therapy
- If the cancer mostly affects the liver and the patient has severe symptoms from hormones or from the size of tumor, treatment may include:
  - Hepatic arterial occlusion, with or without systemic chemotherapy
  - Chemoembolization, with or without systemic chemotherapy

Insulinoma

Treatment of insulinoma may include the following:

- For one small tumor in the head or tail of the pancreas, treatment is usually surgery to remove the tumor.
- For one large tumor in the head of the pancreas that cannot be removed by surgery, treatment is usually pancreatoduodenectomy (surgery to remove the head of the pancreas, the gallbladder, nearby lymph nodes and part of the stomach, small intestine, and bile duct).
- For one large tumor in the body or tail of the pancreas, treatment is usually a distal pancreatectomy (surgery to remove the body and tail of the pancreas).
- For more than one tumor in the pancreas, treatment is usually surgery to remove any tumors in the head of the pancreas and the body and tail of the pancreas.
- For tumors that cannot be removed by surgery, treatment may include the following:

- Combination chemotherapy

- Palliative drug therapy to decrease the amount of insulin made by the pancreas

- Hormone therapy

- Radiofrequency ablation or cryosurgical ablation

- For cancer that has spread to lymph nodes or other parts of the body, treatment may include the following:

  - Surgery to remove the cancer

  - Radiofrequency ablation or cryosurgical ablation, if the cancer cannot be removed by surgery

- If the cancer mostly affects the liver and the patient has severe symptoms from hormones or from the size of tumor, treatment may include:

  - Hepatic arterial occlusion, with or without systemic chemotherapy

  - Chemoembolization, with or without systemic chemotherapy

Glucagonoma

Treatment may include the following:

- For one small tumor in the head or tail of the pancreas, treatment is usually surgery to remove the tumor.

- For one large tumor in the head of the pancreas that cannot be removed by surgery, treatment is usually pancreatoduodenectomy (surgery to remove the head of the pancreas, the gallbladder, nearby lymph nodes and part of the stomach, small intestine, and bile duct).

- For more than one tumor in the pancreas, treatment is usually surgery to remove the tumor or surgery to remove the body and tail of the pancreas.

- For tumors that cannot be removed by surgery, treatment may include the following:

  - Combination chemotherapy

  - Hormone therapy

  - Radiofrequency ablation or cryosurgical ablation

- For cancer that has spread to lymph nodes or other parts of the body, treatment may include the following:

  - Surgery to remove the cancer

  - Radiofrequency ablation or cryosurgical ablation, if the cancer cannot be removed by surgery

- If the cancer mostly affects the liver and the patient has severe symptoms from hormones or from the size of tumor, treatment may include:

  - Hepatic arterial occlusion, with or without systemic chemotherapy

  - Chemoembolization, with or without systemic chemotherapy

Other Pancreatic Neuroendocrine Tumors (Islet Cell Tumors)

For VIPoma, treatment may include the following:

- Fluids and hormone therapy to replace fluids and electrolytes that have been lost from the body

- Surgery to remove the tumor and nearby lymph nodes

- Surgery to remove as much of the tumor as possible when the tumor cannot be completely removed or has spread to distant parts of the body. This is palliative therapy to relieve symptoms and improve the quality of life.

- For tumors that have spread to lymph nodes or other parts of the body, treatment may include the following:

  - Surgery to remove the tumor

  - Radiofrequency ablation or cryosurgical ablation, if the tumor cannot be removed by surgery

- For tumors that continue to grow during treatment or have spread to other parts of the body, treatment may include the following:

  - Chemotherapy

  - Targeted therapy

For somatostatinoma, treatment may include the following:

- Surgery to remove the tumor

- For cancer that has spread to distant parts of the body, surgery to remove as much of the cancer as possible to relieve symptoms and improve quality of life

- For tumors that continue to grow during treatment or have spread to other parts of the body, treatment may include the following:

  - Chemotherapy

  - Targeted therapy

- Treatment of other types of pancreatic neuroendocrine tumors (NETs) may include the following:

- Surgery to remove the tumor

- For cancer that has spread to distant parts of the body, surgery to remove as much of the cancer as possible or hormone therapy to relieve symptoms and improve quality of life.

- For tumors that continue to grow during treatment or have spread to other parts of the body, treatment may include the following:

  - Chemotherapy

  - Targeted therapy

Recurrent or Progressive Pancreatic Neuroendocrine Tumors (Islet Cell Tumors)

Treatment of pancreatic neuroendocrine tumors (NETs) that continue to grow during treatment or recur (come back) may include the following:

- Surgery to remove the tumor

- Chemotherapy

- Hormone therapy

- Targeted therapy

- For liver metastases:

  - Regional chemotherapy

  - Hepatic arterial occlusion or chemoembolization, with or without systemic chemotherapy

  - A clinical trial of a new therapy

Chapter 45

Liver Cancer

Adult primary liver cancer is a disease in which malignant (cancer) cells form in the tissues of the liver. The liver is one of the largest organs in the body. It has two lobes and fills the upper right side of the abdomen inside the rib cage. Three of the many important functions of the liver are:

- To filter harmful substances from the blood so they can be passed from the body in stools and urine

- To make bile to help digest fat that comes from food

- To store glycogen (sugar), which the body uses for energy

There are two types of adult primary liver cancer. They are:

1. Hepatocellular carcinoma

2. Cholangiocarcinoma (bile duct cancer)

The most common type of adult primary liver cancer is hepatocellular carcinoma. This type of liver cancer is the third leading cause of cancer-related deaths worldwide. Primary liver cancer can occur in both adults and children. However, treatment for children is different than treatment for adults. Having hepatitis or cirrhosis can affect the risk of adult primary liver cancer. Anything that increases your chance of getting a disease is called a risk factor. Having a risk factor

This chapter includes text excerpted from "Adult Liver Cancer Symptoms, Tests, Prognosis, and Stages (PDQ®)—Patient Version," National Cancer Institute (NCI), May 15, 2018.

does not mean that you will get cancer; not having risk factors doesn't mean that you will not get cancer. Talk with your doctor if you think you may be at risk.

The following are risk factors for adult primary liver cancer:

- Having hepatitis B or hepatitis C. Having both hepatitis B and hepatitis C increases the risk even more.

- Having cirrhosis, which can be caused by:

  - hepatitis (especially hepatitis C)

  - drinking large amounts of alcohol for many years or being an alcoholic

- Having metabolic syndrome, a set of conditions that occur together, including extra fat around the abdomen, high blood sugar, high blood pressure, high levels of triglycerides and low levels of high-density lipoproteins in the blood

- Having liver injury that is long-lasting, especially if it leads to cirrhosis

- Having hemochromatosis, a condition in which the body takes up and stores more iron than it needs. The extra iron is stored in the liver, heart, and pancreas.

- Eating foods tainted with aflatoxin (poison from a fungus that can grow on foods, such as grains and nuts, that have not been stored properly)

Signs and Symptoms of Liver Cancer

Signs and symptoms of adult primary liver cancer include a lump or pain on the right side. These and other signs and symptoms may be caused by adult primary liver cancer or by other conditions. Check with your doctor if you have any of the following:

- A hard lump on the right side just below the rib cage

- Discomfort in the upper abdomen on the right side

- A swollen abdomen

- Pain near the right shoulder blade or in the back

- Jaundice (yellowing of the skin and whites of the eyes)

- Easy bruising or bleeding

- Unusual tiredness or weakness

- Nausea and vomiting

- Loss of appetite or feelings of fullness after eating a small meal

- Weight loss for no known reason

- Pale, chalky bowel movements and dark urine

- Fever

Diagnosis of Liver Cancer

Tests that examine the liver and the blood are used to detect (find) and diagnose adult primary liver cancer. The following tests and procedures may be used:

- **Physical exam and history:** An exam of the body to check general signs of health, including checking for signs of disease, such as lumps or anything else that seems unusual. A history of the patient's health habits and past illnesses and treatments will also be taken.

- **Serum tumor marker test:** A procedure in which a sample of blood is examined to measure the amounts of certain substances released into the blood by organs, tissues, or tumor cells in the body. Certain substances are linked to specific types of cancer when found in increased levels in the blood. These are called tumor markers. An increased level of alpha-fetoprotein (AFP) in the blood may be a sign of liver cancer. Other cancers and certain noncancerous conditions, including cirrhosis and hepatitis, may also increase AFP levels. Sometimes the AFP level is normal even when there is liver cancer.

- **Liver function tests:** A procedure in which a blood sample is checked to measure the amounts of certain substances released into the blood by the liver. A higher than normal amount of a substance can be a sign of liver cancer.

- **Computed tomography (CT) scan (CAT scan):** A procedure that makes a series of detailed pictures of areas inside the body, such as the abdomen, taken from different angles. The pictures are made by a computer linked to an X-ray machine. A dye may be injected into a vein or swallowed to help the organs or tissues show up more clearly. This procedure is also called computed tomography, computerized tomography, or computerized axial tomography. Images may be taken at three different times after the dye is injected, to get the best picture of abnormal areas in the liver. This is called triple-phase CT. A spiral or helical CT scan makes a series of very detailed pictures of areas inside the body using an X-ray machine that scans the body in a spiral path.

- **Magnetic resonance imaging (MRI):** A procedure that uses a magnet, radio waves, and a computer to make a series of detailed pictures of areas inside the body, such as the liver. This procedure is also called nuclear magnetic resonance imaging (NMRI). To create detailed pictures of blood vessels in and near the liver, dye is injected into a vein. This procedure is called MRA (magnetic resonance angiography). Images may be taken at three different times after the dye is injected, to get the best picture of abnormal areas in the liver. This is called triple-phase MRI.

- **Ultrasound exam:** A procedure in which high-energy sound waves (ultrasound) are bounced off internal tissues or organs and make echoes. The echoes form a picture of body tissues called a sonogram. The picture can be printed to be looked at later.

- **Biopsy:** The removal of cells or tissues so they can be viewed under a microscope by a pathologist to check for signs of cancer. Procedures used to collect the sample of cells or tissues include the following:

  - **Fine-needle aspiration (FNA) biopsy:** The removal of cells, tissue or fluid using a thin needle.

  - **Core needle biopsy:** The removal of cells or tissue using a slightly wider needle.

  - **Laparoscopy:** A surgical procedure to look at the organs inside the abdomen to check for signs of disease. Small incisions (cuts) are made in the wall of the abdomen and a laparoscope (a thin, lighted tube) is inserted into one of the incisions. Another instrument is inserted through the same or another incision to remove the tissue samples.

A biopsy is not always needed to diagnose adult primary liver cancer. Certain factors affect prognosis (chance of recovery) and treatment options.

The prognosis (chance of recovery) and treatment options depend on the following:

- The stage of the cancer (the size of the tumor, whether it affects part or all of the liver, or has spread to other places in the body)

- How well the liver is working

- The patient's general health, including whether there is cirrhosis of the liver

Stages of Adult Primary Liver Cancer

After adult primary liver cancer has been diagnosed, tests are done to find out if cancer cells have spread within the liver or to other parts of the body. The process used to find out if cancer has spread within the liver or to other parts of the body is called staging. The information gathered from the staging process determines the stage of the disease. It is important to know the stage in order to plan treatment. The following tests and procedures may be used in the staging process:

- Computed tomography (CT) scan (CAT scan)

- Magnetic resonance imaging (MRI)

- Positron emission tomography (PET) scan

The metastatic tumor is the same type of cancer as the primary tumor. For example, if primary liver cancer spreads to the lung, the cancer cells in the lung are actually liver cancer cells. The disease is metastatic liver cancer, not lung cancer. The Barcelona Clinic Liver Cancer (BCLC) staging system may be used to stage adult primary liver cancer. There are several staging systems for liver cancer. The Barcelona Clinic Liver Cancer staging system is widely used and is described below. This system is used to predict the patient's chance of recovery and to plan treatment, based on the following:

- Whether the cancer has spread within the liver or to other parts of the body

- How well the liver is working

- The general health and wellness of the patient

- The symptoms caused by the cancer

The BCLC staging system has five stages:

- Stage 0: Very early

- Stage A: Early

- Stage B: Intermediate

- Stage C: Advanced

- Stage D: End-stage

The following groups are used to plan treatment:

BCLC stages 0, A, and B
Treatment to cure the cancer is given for BCLC stages 0, A, and B.

BCLC stages C and D
Treatment to relieve the symptoms caused by liver cancer and improve the patient's quality of life is given for BCLC stages C and D. Treatments are not likely to cure the cancer.

Recurrent Adult Primary Liver Cancer

Recurrent adult primary liver cancer is cancer that has recurred (come back) after it has been treated. The cancer may come back in the liver or in other parts of the body.

Treatment Option Overview for Liver Cancer

Different types of treatments are available for patients with adult primary liver cancer. Some treatments are standard (the currently used treatment), and some are being tested in clinical trials. A treatment clinical trial is a research study meant to help improve current treatments or obtain information on new treatments for patients with cancer. When clinical trials show that a new treatment is better than the standard treatment, the new treatment may become the standard treatment. Patients may want to think about taking part in a clinical trial. Some clinical trials are open only to patients who have not started treatment.

Patients with liver cancer are treated by a team of specialists who are experts in treating liver cancer.

The patient's treatment will be overseen by a medical oncologist, a doctor who specializes in treating people with cancer. The medical oncologist may refer the patient to other health professionals who have special training in treating patients with liver cancer. These may include the following specialists:

- Hepatologist (specialist in liver disease)

- Surgical oncologist

- Transplant surgeon

- Radiation oncologist

- Interventional radiologist (a specialist who diagnoses and treats diseases using imaging and the smallest incisions possible)

- Pathologist

Seven types of standard treatment are used:

Surveillance

Surveillance for lesions smaller than one centimeter found during screening. Following up every three months is common.

Surgery

A partial hepatectomy (surgery to remove the part of the liver where cancer is found) may be done. A wedge of tissue, an entire lobe, or a larger part of the liver, along with some of the healthy tissue around it is removed. The remaining liver tissue takes over the functions of the liver and may regrow.

Liver Transplant

In a liver transplant, the entire liver is removed and replaced with a healthy donated liver. A liver transplant may be done when the disease is in the liver only and a donated liver can be found. If the patient has to wait for a donated liver, other treatment is given as needed.

Ablation Therapy

Ablation therapy removes or destroys tissue. Different types of ablation therapy are used for liver cancer:

- **Radiofrequency ablation:** The use of special needles that are inserted directly through the skin or through an incision in the abdomen to reach the tumor. High-energy radio waves heat the needles and tumor which kills cancer cells.

- **Microwave therapy:** A type of treatment in which the tumor is exposed to high temperatures created by microwaves. This can damage and kill cancer cells or make them more sensitive to the effects of radiation and certain anticancer drugs.

- **Percutaneous ethanol injection:** A cancer treatment in which a small needle is used to inject ethanol (pure alcohol) directly into a tumor to kill cancer cells. Several treatments may be needed. Usually, local anesthesia is used, but if the patient has many tumors in the liver, general anesthesia may be used.

- **Cryoablation:** A treatment that uses an instrument to freeze and destroy cancer cells. This type of treatment is also called cryotherapy and cryosurgery. The doctor may use ultrasound to guide the instrument.

- **Electroporation therapy:** A treatment that sends electrical pulses through an electrode placed in a tumor to kill cancer cells. Electroporation therapy is being studied in clinical trials.

Embolization Therapy

Embolization therapy is the use of substances to block or decrease the flow of blood through the hepatic artery to the tumor. When the tumor does not get the oxygen and nutrients it needs, it will not continue to grow. Embolization therapy is used for patients who cannot have surgery to remove the tumor or ablation therapy and whose tumor has not spread outside the liver.

The liver receives blood from the hepatic portal vein and the hepatic artery. Blood that comes into the liver from the hepatic portal vein usually goes to the healthy liver tissue. Blood that comes from the hepatic artery usually goes to the tumor. When the hepatic artery is blocked during embolization therapy, the healthy liver tissue continues to receive blood from the hepatic portal vein.

There are two main types of embolization therapy:

- **Transarterial embolization (TAE):** A small incision (cut) is made in the inner thigh and a catheter (thin, flexible tube) is inserted and threaded up into the hepatic artery. Once the catheter is in place, a substance that blocks the hepatic artery and stops blood flow to the tumor is injected.

- **Transarterial chemoembolization (TACE):** This procedure is like TAE except an anticancer drug is also given. The procedure can be done by attaching the anticancer drug to small beads that are injected into the hepatic artery or by injecting the anticancer drug through the catheter into the hepatic artery and then injecting the substance to block the hepatic artery. Most of the anticancer drug is trapped near the tumor and only a small amount of the drug reaches other parts of the body. This type of treatment is also called chemoembolization.

Targeted Therapy

Targeted therapy is a treatment that uses drugs or other substances to identify and attack specific cancer cells without harming normal cells. Adult liver cancer may be treated with a targeted therapy drug that stops cells from dividing and prevents the growth of new blood vessels that tumors need to grow.

Radiation Therapy

Radiation therapy is a cancer treatment that uses high-energy X-rays or other types of radiation to kill cancer cells or keep them from growing. There are two types of radiation therapy:

- External radiation therapy uses a machine outside the body to send radiation toward the cancer. Certain ways of giving radiation therapy can help keep radiation from damaging nearby healthy tissue. These types of external radiation therapy include the following:

  - Conformal radiation therapy: Conformal radiation therapy is a type of external radiation therapy that uses a computer to make a 3-dimensional (3-D) picture of the tumor and shapes the radiation beams to fit the tumor. This allows a high dose of radiation to reach the tumor and causes less damage to nearby healthy tissue.

  - Stereotactic body radiation therapy: Stereotactic body radiation therapy is a type of external radiation therapy. Special equipment is used to place the patient in the same position for each radiation treatment. Once a day for several days, a radiation machine aims a larger than usual dose of radiation directly at the tumor. By having the patient in the same position for each treatment, there is less damage to nearby healthy tissue. This procedure is also called stereotactic external-beam radiation therapy and stereotaxic radiation therapy.

  - Proton beam radiation therapy: Proton-beam therapy is a type of high-energy, external radiation therapy. A radiation therapy machine aims streams of protons (tiny, invisible, positively-charged particles) at the cancer cells to kill them. This type of treatment causes less damage to nearby healthy tissue.

- Internal radiation therapy uses a radioactive substance sealed in needles, seeds, wires, or catheters that are placed directly into or near the cancer.

The way the radiation therapy is given depends on the type and stage of the cancer being treated. External radiation therapy is used to treat adult primary liver cancer.

Chapter 46

Anal Cancer

Anal cancer is a disease in which malignant (cancer) cells form in the tissues of the anus. The anus is the end of the large intestine, below the rectum, through which stool (solid waste) leaves the body. The anus is formed partly from the outer skin layers of the body and partly from the intestine. Two ring-like muscles, called sphincter muscles, open and close the anal opening and let stool pass out of the body. The anal canal, the part of the anus between the rectum and the anal opening, is about 1–1½ inches long. The skin around the outside of the anus is called the perianal area. Tumors in this area are skin tumors, not anal cancer.

Being infected with the human papillomavirus (HPV) increases the risk of developing anal cancer.

Risk factors include the following:

- Being infected with HPV

- Having many sexual partners

- Having receptive anal intercourse (anal sex)

- Being older than 50 years

- Frequent anal redness, swelling, and soreness

- Having anal fistulas (abnormal openings)

- Smoking cigarettes

This chapter includes text excerpted from "Anal Cancer Treatment (PDQ®)—Patient Version," National Cancer Institute (NCI), January 25, 2018.

Signs and Symptoms of Anal Cancer

Signs of anal cancer include bleeding from the anus or rectum or a lump near the anus. These and other signs and symptoms may be caused by anal cancer or by other conditions. Check with your doctor if you have any of the following:

- Bleeding from the anus or rectum

- Pain or pressure in the area around the anus

- Itching or discharge from the anus

- A lump near the anus

- A change in bowel habits

Diagnosis of Anal Cancer

Tests that examine the rectum and anus are used to detect (find) and diagnose anal cancer. The following tests and procedures may be used:

- **Physical exam and history:** An exam of the body to check general signs of health, including checking for signs of disease, such as lumps or anything else that seems unusual. A history of the patient's health habits and past illnesses and treatments will also be taken.

- **Digital rectal examination (DRE):** An exam of the anus and rectum. The doctor or nurse inserts a lubricated, gloved finger into the lower part of the rectum to feel for lumps or anything else that seems unusual.

- **Anoscopy:** An exam of the anus and lower rectum using a short, lighted tube called an anoscope.

- **Proctoscopy:** An exam of the rectum using a short, lighted tube called a proctoscope.

- **Endo-anal or endorectal ultrasound:** A procedure in which an ultrasound transducer (probe) is inserted into the anus or rectum and used to bounce high-energy sound waves (ultrasound) off internal tissues or organs and make echoes. The echoes form a picture of body tissues called a sonogram.

- **Biopsy:** The removal of cells or tissues so they can be viewed under a microscope by a pathologist to check for signs of cancer.

If an abnormal area is seen during the anoscopy, a biopsy may be done at that time.

Certain factors affect the prognosis (chance of recovery) and treatment options. The prognosis (chance of recovery) depends on the following:

- The size of the tumor
- Where the tumor is in the anus
- Whether the cancer has spread to the lymph nodes

The treatment options depend on the following:

- The stage of the cancer
- Where the tumor is in the anus
- Whether the patient has human immunodeficiency virus (HIV)
- Whether cancer remains after initial treatment or has recurred

Stages of Anal Cancer

After anal cancer has been diagnosed, tests are done to find out if cancer cells have spread within the anus or to other parts of the body. The process used to find out if cancer has spread within the anus or to other parts of the body is called staging. The information gathered from the staging process determines the stage of the disease. It is important to know the stage in order to plan treatment. The following tests may be used in the staging process:

- Computed tomography (CT) scan (CAT scan)
- Chest X-ray
- Magnetic resonance imaging (MRI)
- Positron emission tomography (PET) scan
- Pelvic exam

The metastatic tumor is the same type of cancer as the primary tumor. For example, if anal cancer spreads to the lung, the cancer cells in the lung are actually anal cancer cells. The disease is metastatic anal cancer, not lung cancer.

The following stages are used for anal cancer:

Stage 0

In stage 0, abnormal cells are found in the mucosa (innermost layer) of the anus. These abnormal cells may become cancer and spread into nearby normal tissue. Stage 0 is also called high-grade squamous intraepithelial lesion (HSIL).

Stage I

In stage I, cancer has formed and the tumor is two centimeters or smaller.

Stage II

Stage II anal cancer is divided into stages IIA and IIB.

- In stage IIA, the tumor is larger than two centimeters but not larger than five centimeters.
- In stage IIB, the tumor is larger than five centimeters.

Stage III

Stage III anal cancer is divided into stages IIIA, IIIB, and IIIC.

- In stage IIIA, the tumor is five centimeters or smaller and has spread to lymph nodes near the anus or groin.
- In stage IIIB, the tumor is any size and has spread to nearby organs, such as the vagina, urethra, or bladder. Cancer has not spread to lymph nodes.
- In stage IIIC, the tumor is any size and may have spread to nearby organs. Cancer has spread to lymph nodes near the anus or groin.

Stage IV

In stage IV, the tumor is any size. Cancer may have spread to lymph nodes or nearby organs and has spread to other parts of the body, such as the liver or lungs.

Recurrent Anal Cancer

Recurrent anal cancer is cancer that has recurred (come back) after it has been treated. The cancer may come back in the anus or in other parts of the body.

Treatment Option Overview for Anal Cancer

Different types of treatments are available for patients with anal cancer. Some treatments are standard (the currently used treatment), and some are being tested in clinical trials. A treatment clinical trial is a research study meant to help improve current treatments or obtain information on new treatments for patients with cancer. When clinical trials show that a new treatment is better than the standard treatment, the new treatment may become the standard treatment. Patients may want to think about taking part in a clinical trial. Some clinical trials are open only to patients who have not started treatment.

Three types of standard treatment are used:

Radiation Therapy

Radiation therapy is a cancer treatment that uses high-energy X-rays or other types of radiation to kill cancer cells or keep them from growing. There are two types of radiation therapy:

- External radiation therapy uses a machine outside the body to send radiation toward the cancer.

- Internal radiation therapy uses a radioactive substance sealed in needles, seeds, wires, or catheters that are placed directly into or near the cancer.

The way the radiation therapy is given depends on the type and stage of the cancer being treated. External and internal radiation therapy are used to treat anal cancer.

Chemotherapy

Chemotherapy is a cancer treatment that uses drugs to stop the growth of cancer cells, either by killing the cells or by stopping the cells from dividing. When chemotherapy is taken by mouth or injected into a vein or muscle, the drugs enter the bloodstream and can reach cancer cells throughout the body (systemic chemotherapy). When chemotherapy is placed directly into the cerebrospinal fluid, an organ, or a body cavity such as the abdomen, the drugs mainly affect cancer cells in those areas (regional chemotherapy). The way the chemotherapy is given depends on the type and stage of the cancer being treated.

Surgery

- **Local resection:** A surgical procedure in which the tumor is cut from the anus along with some of the healthy tissue around it. Local resection may be used if the cancer is small and has not spread. This procedure may save the sphincter muscles so the patient can still control bowel movements. Tumors that form in the lower part of the anus can often be removed with local resection.

- **Abdominoperineal resection:** A surgical procedure in which the anus, the rectum, and part of the sigmoid colon are removed through an incision made in the abdomen. The doctor sews the end of the intestine to an opening, called a stoma, made in the surface of the abdomen so body waste can be collected in a disposable bag outside of the body. This is called a colostomy. Lymph nodes that contain cancer may also be removed during this operation.

Having the human immunodeficiency virus can affect treatment of anal cancer. Cancer therapy can further damage the already weakened immune systems of patients who have the human immunodeficiency virus (HIV). For this reason, patients who have anal cancer and HIV are usually treated with lower doses of anticancer drugs and radiation than patients who do not have HIV.

Radiosensitizers

Radiosensitizers are drugs that make tumor cells more sensitive to radiation therapy. Combining radiation therapy with radiosensitizers may kill more tumor cells.

Treatment Options by Stage for Anal Cancer
Stage 0

Treatment of stage 0 is usually local resection.

Stage I

Treatment of stage I anal cancer may include the following:

- Local resection
- External-beam radiation therapy with or without chemotherapy. If cancer remains after treatment, more chemotherapy

and radiation therapy may be given to avoid the need for a permanent colostomy.

- Internal radiation therapy
- Abdominoperineal resection, if cancer remains or comes back after treatment with radiation therapy and chemotherapy
- Internal radiation therapy for cancer that remains after treatment with external-beam radiation therapy

Patients who have had treatment that saves the sphincter muscles may receive follow-up exams every three months for the first two years, including rectal exams with endoscopy and biopsy, as needed.

Stage II

Treatment of stage II anal cancer may include the following:

- Local resection
- External-beam radiation therapy with chemotherapy. If cancer remains after treatment, more chemotherapy and radiation therapy may be given to avoid the need for a permanent colostomy
- Internal radiation therapy
- Abdominoperineal resection, if cancer remains or comes back after treatment with radiation therapy and chemotherapy
- A clinical trial of new treatment options

Patients who have had treatment that saves the sphincter muscles may receive follow-up exams every three months for the first two years, including rectal exams with endoscopy and biopsy, as needed.

Stage IIIA

Treatment of stage IIIA anal cancer may include the following:

- External-beam radiation therapy with chemotherapy. If cancer remains after treatment, more chemotherapy and radiation therapy may be given to avoid the need for a permanent colostomy
- Internal radiation therapy
- Abdominoperineal resection, if cancer remains or comes back after treatment with chemotherapy and radiation therapy

- A clinical trial of new treatment options

Stage IIIB

Treatment of stage IIIB anal cancer may include the following:

- External-beam radiation therapy with chemotherapy
- Local resection or abdominoperineal resection, if cancer remains or comes back after treatment with chemotherapy and radiation therapy. Lymph nodes may also be removed.
- A clinical trial of new treatment options

Stage IV

Treatment of stage IV anal cancer may include the following:

- Surgery as palliative therapy to relieve symptoms and improve the quality of life
- Radiation therapy as palliative therapy
- Chemotherapy with radiation therapy as palliative therapy
- A clinical trial of new treatment options

Treatment Options for Recurrent Anal Cancer

Treatment of recurrent anal cancer may include the following:

- Radiation therapy and chemotherapy, for recurrence after surgery
- Surgery, for recurrence after radiation therapy and/or chemotherapy
- A clinical trial of radiation therapy with chemotherapy and/or radiosensitizers

Chapter 47

Gastrointestinal Complications in Cancer Patients

The gastrointestinal (GI) tract is part of the digestive system, which processes nutrients (vitamins, minerals, carbohydrates, fats, proteins, and water) in foods that are eaten and helps pass waste material out of the body. The GI tract includes the stomach and intestines (bowels). The stomach is a J-shaped organ in the upper abdomen. Food moves from the throat to the stomach through a hollow, muscular tube called the esophagus. After leaving the stomach, partly-digested food passes into the small intestine and then into the large intestine. The colon (large bowel) is the first part of the large intestine and is about five feet long. Together, the rectum and anal canal make up the last part of the large intestine and are six to eight inches long. The anal canal ends at the anus (the opening of the large intestine to the outside of the body).

GI complications are common in cancer patients. Complications are medical problems that occur during a disease, or after a procedure or treatment. They may be caused by the disease, procedure, or treatment, or may have other causes. This summary describes the following GI complications and their causes and treatments:

- Constipation

This chapter includes text excerpted from "Gastrointestinal Complications (PDQ®)—Patient Version," National Cancer Institute (NCI), March 2, 2018.

- Fecal impaction

- Bowel obstruction

- Diarrhea

- Radiation enteritis

Treatment of GI complications in children is different than treatment for adults.

Constipation

With constipation, bowel movements are difficult or don't happen as often as usual.

Constipation is the slow movement of stool through the large intestine. The longer it takes for the stool to move through the large intestine, the more it loses fluid and the drier and harder it becomes. The patient may be unable to have a bowel movement, have to push harder to have a bowel movement, or have fewer than their usual number of bowel movements.

Causes

Certain medicines, changes in diet, not drinking enough fluids, and being less active are common causes of constipation.

Constipation is a common problem for cancer patients. Cancer patients may become constipated by any of the usual factors that cause constipation in healthy people. These include older age, changes in diet and fluid intake, and not getting enough exercise. In addition to these common causes of constipation, there are other causes in cancer patients.

Other causes of constipation include:

Medicines

- Opioids and other pain medicines. This is one of the main causes of constipation in cancer patients

- Chemotherapy

- Medicines for anxiety and depression

- Antacids

- Diuretics (drugs that increase the amount of urine made by the body)

- Supplements such as iron and calcium
- Sleep medicines
- Drugs used for anesthesia (to cause loss of feeling for surgery or other procedures)

Diet

- Not drinking enough water or other fluids. This is a common problem for cancer patients.
- Not eating enough food, especially high-fiber food

Bowel Movement Habits

- Not going to the bathroom when the need for a bowel movement is felt
- Using laxatives and/or enemas too often

Conditions That Prevent Activity and Exercise

- Spinal cord injury or pressure on the spinal cord from a tumor or other cause
- Broken bones
- Fatigue
- Weakness
- Long periods of bed rest or not being active
- Heart problems
- Breathing problems
- Anxiety
- Depression

Intestinal Disorders

- Irritable colon
- Diverticulitis (inflammation of small pouches in the colon called diverticula)
- Tumor in the intestine

Muscle and Nerve Disorders

- Brain tumors

- Spinal cord injury or pressure on the spinal cord from a tumor or other cause

- Paralysis (loss of ability to move) of both legs

- Stroke or other disorders that cause paralysis of part of the body

- Peripheral neuropathy (pain, numbness, tingling) of feet

- Weakness of the diaphragm (the breathing muscle below the lungs) or abdominal muscles. This makes it hard to push to have a bowel movement

Changes in Body Metabolism

- Having a low level of thyroid hormone, potassium, or sodium in the blood

- Having too much nitrogen or calcium in the blood

Environment

- Having to go farther to get to a bathroom

- Needing help to go to the bathroom

- Being in unfamiliar places

- Having little or no privacy

- Feeling rushed

- Living in extreme heat that causes dehydration

- Needing to use a bedpan or bedside commode

- Narrow colon

- Scars from radiation therapy or surgery

- Pressure from a growing tumor

Assessment

An assessment is done to help plan treatment.

The assessment includes a physical exam and questions about the patient's usual bowel movements and how they have changed.

The following tests and procedures may be done to help find the cause of the constipation:

- **Physical exam:** An exam of the body to check general signs of health, including checking for signs of disease, such as lumps or anything else that seems unusual. The doctor will check for bowel sounds and swollen, painful abdomen.

- **Digital rectal exam (DRE):** An exam of the rectum. The doctor or nurse inserts a lubricated, gloved finger into the lower part of the rectum to feel for lumps or anything else that seems unusual. In women, the vagina may also be examined.

- **Fecal occult blood test (FOBT):** A test to check stool for blood that can only be seen with a microscope. Small samples of stool are placed on special cards and returned to the doctor or laboratory for testing.

- **Proctoscopy:** An exam of the rectum using a proctoscope, inserted into the rectum. A proctoscope is a thin, tube-like instrument with a light and a lens for viewing. It may also have a tool to remove tissue to be checked under a microscope for signs of disease.

- **Colonoscopy:** A procedure to look inside the rectum and colon for polyps, abnormal areas, or cancer. A colonoscope is inserted through the rectum into the colon. A colonoscope is a thin, tube-like instrument with a light and a lens for viewing. It may also have a tool to remove polyps or tissue samples, which are checked under a microscope for signs of cancer.

- **Abdominal X-ray:** An X-ray of the organs inside the abdomen. An X-ray is a type of energy beam that can go through the body and onto film, making a picture of areas inside the body.

There is no "normal" number of bowel movements for a cancer patient. Each person is different. You will be asked about bowel routines, food, and medicines:

- How often do you have a bowel movement? When and how much?

- When was your last bowel movement? What was it like (how much, hard or soft, color)?

- Was there any blood in your stool?

- Has your stomach hurt or have you had any cramps, nausea, vomiting, gas, or feeling of fullness near the rectum?

643

- Do you use laxatives or enemas regularly?

- What do you usually do to relieve constipation? Does this usually work?

- What kind of food do you eat?

- How much and what type of fluids do you drink each day?

- What medicines are you taking? How much and how often?

- Is this constipation a recent change in your normal habits?

- How many times a day do you pass gas?

Treatment

Treating constipation is important to make the patient comfortable and to prevent more serious problems.

It's easier to prevent constipation than to relieve it. The healthcare team will work with the patient to prevent constipation. Patients who take opioids may need to start taking laxatives right away to prevent constipation.

Constipation can be very uncomfortable and cause distress. If left untreated, constipation may lead to fecal impaction. This is a serious condition in which stool will not pass out of the colon or rectum. It's important to treat constipation to prevent fecal impaction.

Prevention and treatment are not the same for every patient. Do the following to prevent and treat constipation:

- Keep a record of all bowel movements.

- Drink 12 eight-ounce glasses of fluid each day. Patients who have certain conditions, such as kidney or heart disease, may need to drink less.

- Get regular exercise. Patients who cannot walk may do abdominal exercises in bed or move from the bed to a chair.

- Increase the amount of fiber in the diet by eating more of the following:

  - Fruits, such as raisins, prunes, peaches, and apples

  - Vegetables, such as squash, broccoli, carrots, and celery

  - Whole grain cereals, whole grain breads, and bran

- It's important to drink more fluids when eating more high-fiber foods, to avoid making constipation worse. Patients who have had a small or large intestinal obstruction or have had intestinal surgery (for example, a colostomy) should not eat a high-fiber diet.

- Drink a warm or hot drink about one half-hour before the usual time for a bowel movement.

- Find privacy and quiet when it is time for a bowel movement.

- Use the toilet or a bedside commode instead of a bedpan.

- Take only medicines that are prescribed by the doctor. Medicines for constipation may include bulking agents, laxatives, stool softeners, and drugs that cause the intestine to empty.

- Use suppositories or enemas only if ordered by the doctor. In some cancer patients, these treatments may lead to bleeding, infection, or other harmful side effects.

When constipation is caused by opioids, treatment may be drugs that stop the effects of the opioids or other medicines, stool softeners, enemas, and/or manual removal of stool.

Fecal Impaction

Fecal impaction is a mass of dry, hard stool that will not pass out of the colon or rectum.

Fecal impaction is dry stool that cannot pass out of the body. Patients with fecal impaction may not have gastrointestinal (GI) symptoms. Instead, they may have problems with circulation, the heart, or breathing. If fecal impaction is not treated, it can get worse and cause death.

Cause

A common cause of fecal impaction is using laxatives too often.

Repeated use of laxatives in higher and higher doses makes the colon less able to respond naturally to the need to have a bowel movement. This is a common reason for fecal impaction. Other causes include:

- Opioid pain medicines

- Little or no activity over a long period

- Diet changes

- Constipation that is not treated

Certain types of mental illness may lead to fecal impaction.

Symptoms

Symptoms of fecal impaction include being unable to have a bowel movement and pain in the abdomen or back.

The following may be symptoms of fecal impaction:

- Being unable to have a bowel movement

- Having to push harder to have a bowel movement of small amounts of hard, dry stool

- Having fewer than the usual number of bowel movements

- Having pain in the back or abdomen

- Urinating more or less often than usual, or being unable to urinate

- Breathing problems, rapid heartbeat, dizziness, low blood pressure, and swollen abdomen

- Having sudden, explosive diarrhea (as stool moves around the impaction)

- Leaking stool when coughing

- Nausea and vomiting

- Dehydration

- Being confused and losing a sense of time and place, with rapid heartbeat, sweating, fever, and high or low blood pressure

These symptoms should be reported to the healthcare provider.

Assessment

Assessment includes a physical exam and questions like those asked in the assessment of constipation.

The doctor will ask questions similar to those for the assessment of constipation:

- How often do you have a bowel movement? When and how much?

- When was your last bowel movement? What was it like (how much, hard or soft, color)?

- Was there any blood in your stool?

- Has your stomach hurt or have you had any cramps, nausea, vomiting, gas, or feeling of fullness near the rectum?

- Do you use laxatives or enemas regularly?

- What do you usually do to relieve constipation? Does this usually work?

- What kind of food do you eat?

- How much and what type of fluids do you drink each day?

- What medicines are you taking? How much and how often?

- Is this constipation a recent change in your normal habits?

- How many times a day do you pass gas?

The doctor will do a physical exam to find out if the patient has a fecal impaction. The following tests and procedures may be done:

- **Physical exam:** An exam of the body to check general signs of health, including checking for signs of disease, such as lumps or anything else that seems unusual.

- **X-rays:** An X-ray is a type of energy beam that can go through the body and onto film, making a picture of areas inside the body. To check for fecal impaction, X-rays of the abdomen or chest may be done.

- **Digital rectal exam (DRE):** An exam of the rectum. The doctor or nurse inserts a lubricated, gloved finger into the lower part of the rectum to feel for a fecal impaction, lumps, or anything else that seems unusual.

- **Sigmoidoscopy:** A procedure to look inside the rectum and sigmoid (lower) colon for a fecal impaction, polyps, abnormal areas, or cancer. A sigmoidoscope is inserted through the rectum into the sigmoid colon. A sigmoidoscope is a thin, tube-like instrument with a light and a lens for viewing. It may also have a tool to remove polyps or tissue samples, which are checked under a microscope for signs of cancer.

- **Blood tests:** Tests done on a sample of blood to measure the amount of certain substances in the blood or to count different types of blood cells. Blood tests may be done to look for signs of disease or agents that cause disease, to check for antibodies or tumor markers, or to see how well treatments are working.

- **Electrocardiogram (EKG):** A test that shows the activity of the heart. Small electrodes are placed on the skin of the chest, wrists, and ankles and are attached to an electrocardiograph. The electrocardiograph makes a line graph that shows changes in the electrical activity of the heart over time. The graph can show abnormal conditions, such as blocked arteries, changes in electrolytes (particles with electrical charges), and changes in the way electrical currents pass through the heart tissue.

Treatment

A fecal impaction is usually treated with an enema.

The main treatment for impaction is to moisten and soften the stool so it can be removed or passed out of the body. This is usually done with an enema. Enemas are given only as prescribed by the doctor since too many enemas can damage the intestine. Stool softeners or glycerin suppositories may be given to make the stool softer and easier to pass. Some patients may need to have stool manually removed from the rectum after it is softened.

Laxatives that cause the stool to move are not used because they can also damage the intestine.

Bowel Obstruction

A bowel obstruction is a blockage of the small or large intestine by something other than fecal impaction.

Bowel obstructions (blockages) keep the stool from moving through the small or large intestines. They may be caused by a physical change or by conditions that stop the intestinal muscles from moving normally. The intestine may be partly or completely blocked. Most obstructions occur in the small intestine.

Physical Changes

- The intestine may become twisted or form a loop, closing it off and trapping stool.

- Inflammation, scar tissue from surgery, and hernias can make the intestine too narrow.

- Tumors growing inside or outside the intestine can cause it to be partly or completely blocked.

If the intestine is blocked by physical causes, it may decrease blood flow to blocked parts. Blood flow needs to be corrected or the affected tissue may die.

Conditions that affect the intestinal muscle:

- Paralysis (loss of ability to move)

- Blocked blood vessels going to the intestine

- Too little potassium in the blood

The most common cancers that cause bowel obstructions are cancers of the colon, stomach, and ovary.

Other cancers, such as lung and breast cancers and melanoma, can spread to the abdomen and cause bowel obstruction. Patients who have had surgery on the abdomen or radiation therapy to the abdomen have a higher risk of a bowel obstruction. Bowel obstructions are most common during the advanced stages of cancer.

Assessment

Assessment includes a physical exam and imaging tests.

The following tests and procedures may be done to diagnose a bowel obstruction:

- **Physical exam:** An exam of the body to check general signs of health, including checking for signs of disease, such as lumps or anything else that seems unusual. The doctor will check to see if the patient has abdominal pain, vomiting, or any movement of gas or stool in the bowel.

- **Complete blood count (CBC):** A procedure in which a sample of blood is drawn and checked for the following:

  - The number of red blood cells (RBCs), white blood cells (WBCs), and platelets.

  - The amount of hemoglobin (the protein that carries oxygen) in the RBCs.

  - The portion of the blood sample made up of RBCs.

- **Electrolyte panel:** A blood test that measures the levels of electrolytes, such as sodium, potassium, and chloride.

- **Urinalysis:** A test to check the color of urine and its contents, such as sugar, protein, red blood cells, and white blood cells.

- **Abdominal X-ray:** An X-ray of the organs inside the abdomen. An X-ray is a type of energy beam that can go through the body and onto film, making a picture of areas inside the body.

- **Barium enema:** A series of X-rays of the lower gastrointestinal tract. A liquid that contains barium (a silver-white metallic compound) is put into the rectum. The barium coats the lower gastrointestinal tract and X-rays are taken. This procedure is also called a lower GI series. This test may show what part of the intestine is blocked.

Treatment

Treatment is different for acute and chronic bowel obstructions.

Acute Bowel Obstruction

Acute bowel obstructions occur suddenly, may have not occurred before, and are not long-lasting. Treatment may include the following:

- **Fluid replacement therapy:** A treatment to get the fluids in the body back to normal amounts. Intravenous (IV) fluids may be given and medicines may be prescribed.

- **Electrolyte correction:** A treatment to get the right amounts of chemicals in the blood, such as sodium, potassium, and chloride. Fluids with electrolytes may be given by infusion.

- **Blood transfusion:** A procedure in which a person is given an infusion of whole blood or parts of blood.

- **Nasogastric or colorectal tube:** A nasogastric tube is inserted through the nose and esophagus into the stomach. A colorectal tube is inserted through the rectum into the colon. This is done to decrease swelling, remove fluid and gas buildup, and relieve pressure.

- **Surgery:** Surgery to relieve the obstruction may be done if it causes serious symptoms that are not relieved by other treatments.

Patients with symptoms that keep getting worse will have follow-up exams to check for signs and symptoms of shock and to make sure the obstruction isn't getting worse.

Chronic, Malignant Bowel Obstruction

Chronic bowel obstructions keep getting worse over time. Patients who have advanced cancer may have chronic bowel obstructions that cannot be removed with surgery. The intestine may be blocked or narrowed in more than one place or the tumor may be too large to remove completely. Treatments include the following:

- **Surgery:** The obstruction is removed to relieve pain and improve the patient's quality of life.

- **Stent:** A metal tube inserted into the intestine to open the area that is blocked.

- **Gastrostomy tube:** A tube inserted through the wall of the abdomen directly into the stomach. The gastrostomy tube can relieve fluid and air buildup in the stomach and allow medications and liquids to be given directly into the stomach by pouring them down the tube. A drainage bag with a valve may also be attached to the gastrostomy tube. When the valve is open, the patient may be able to eat or drink by mouth and the food drains directly into the bag. This gives the patient the experience of tasting the food and keeping the mouth moist. Solid food is avoided because it may block the tubing to the drainage bag.

- **Medicines:** Injections or infusions of medicines for pain, nausea and vomiting, and/or to make the intestines empty. This may be prescribed for patients who cannot be helped with a stent or gastrostomy tube.

Diarrhea

Diarrhea is frequent, loose, and watery bowel movements. Acute diarrhea lasts more than four days but less than two weeks. Symptoms of acute diarrhea may be loose stools and passing more than three unformed stools in one day. Diarrhea is chronic (long term) when it goes on for longer than two months.

Diarrhea can occur at any time during cancer treatment. It can be physically and emotionally stressful for patients who have cancer.

In cancer patients, the most common cause of diarrhea is cancer treatment.

Causes

Causes of diarrhea in cancer patients include the following:

651

- Cancer treatments, such as chemotherapy, targeted therapy, radiation therapy, bone marrow transplant, and surgery

  - Some chemotherapy and targeted therapy drugs cause diarrhea by changing how nutrients are broken down and absorbed in the small intestine. More than half of patients who receive chemotherapy have diarrhea that needs to be treated.

  - Radiation therapy to the abdomen and pelvis can cause inflammation of the bowel. Patients may have problems digesting food, and have gas, bloating, cramps, and diarrhea. These symptoms may last up to 8–12 weeks after treatment or may not happen for months or years. Treatment may include diet changes, medicines, or surgery.

  - Patients who are having radiation therapy and chemotherapy often have severe diarrhea. Hospital treatment may not be needed. Treatment may be given at an outpatient clinic or with home care. Intravenous (IV) fluids may be given or medicines may be prescribed.

  - Patients who have a donor bone marrow transplant may develop graft-versus-host disease (GVHD). Stomach and intestinal symptoms of GVHD include nausea and vomiting, severe abdominal pain and cramps, and watery, green diarrhea. Symptoms may show up one week to three months after the transplant.

  - Surgery on the stomach or intestines

- The cancer itself

- Stress and anxiety from being diagnosed with cancer and having cancer treatment

- Medical conditions and diseases other than cancer

- Infections

- Antibiotic therapy for certain infections. Antibiotic therapy can irritate the lining of the bowel and cause diarrhea that often does not get better with treatment.

- Laxatives

- Fecal impaction in which the stool leaks around the blockage

- Certain foods that are high in fiber or fat

Assessment

Assessment includes a physical exam, lab tests, and questions about diet and bowel movements.

Because diarrhea can be life-threatening, it is important to find out the cause so treatment can begin as soon as possible. The doctor may ask the following questions to help plan treatment:

- How often have you had bowel movements in the past 24 hours?

- When was your last bowel movement? What was it like (how much, how hard or soft, what color)? Was there any blood?

- Was there any blood in your stool or any rectal bleeding?

- Have you been dizzy, very drowsy, or had any cramps, pain, nausea, vomiting, or fever?

- What have you eaten? What and how much have you had to drink in the past 24 hours?

- Have you lost weight recently? How much?

- How often have you urinated in the past 24 hours?

- What medicines are you taking? How much and how often?

- Have you traveled recently?

Tests and procedures may include the following:

- **Physical exam and history:** An exam of the body to check general signs of health, including checking for signs of disease, such as lumps or anything else that seems unusual. A history of the patient's health habits and past illnesses and treatments will also be taken. The exam will include checking blood pressure, pulse, and breathing; checking for dryness of the skin and tissue lining the inside of the mouth; and checking for abdominal pain and bowel sounds.

- **Digital rectal exam (DRE):** An exam of the rectum. The doctor or nurse inserts a lubricated, gloved finger into the lower part of the rectum to feel for lumps or anything else that seems unusual. The exam will check for signs of fecal impaction. Stool may be collected for laboratory tests.

- **Fecal occult blood test (FOBT):** A test to check stool for blood that can only be seen with a microscope. Small samples of stool are placed on special cards and returned to the doctor or laboratory for testing.

- **Stool tests:** Laboratory tests to check the water and sodium levels in stool, and to find substances that may be causing diarrhea. Stool is also checked for bacterial, fungal, or viral infections.

- **Complete blood count (CBC):** A procedure in which a sample of blood is drawn and checked for the following:

  - The number of red blood cells (RBCs), white blood cells (WBCs), and platelets

  - The amount of hemoglobin (the protein that carries oxygen) in the RBCs

  - The portion of the blood sample made up of RBCs

- **Electrolyte panel:** A blood test that measures the levels of electrolytes, such as sodium, potassium, and chloride.

- **Urinalysis:** A test to check the color of urine and its contents, such as sugar, protein, RBCs, and WBCs.

- **Abdominal X-ray:** An X-ray of the organs inside the abdomen. An X-ray is a type of energy beam that can go through the body and onto film, making a picture of areas inside the body. Abdominal X-rays may also be done to look for a bowel obstruction or other problems.

Treatment

Treatment depends on the cause of the diarrhea. The doctor may make changes in medicines, diet, and/or fluids.

- A change in the use of laxatives may be needed.

- Medicine to treat diarrhea may be prescribed to slow down the intestines, decrease fluid secreted by the intestines, and help nutrients be absorbed.

- Diarrhea caused by cancer treatment may be treated by changes in diet. Eat small frequent meals and avoid the following foods:

  - Milk and dairy products

  - Spicy foods

  - Alcohol

  - Foods and drinks that have caffeine

- Certain fruit juices

- Foods and drinks that cause gas

- Foods high in fiber or fat

- A diet of bananas, rice, apples, and toast (the BRAT diet) may help mild diarrhea.

- Drinking more clear liquids may help decrease diarrhea. It is best to drink up to three quarts of clear fluids a day. These include water, sports drinks, broth, weak decaffeinated tea, caffeine-free soft drinks, clear juices, and gelatin. For severe diarrhea, the patient may need intravenous (IV) fluids or other forms of IV nutrition.

- Diarrhea caused by graft versus host disease (GVHD) is often treated with a special diet. Some patients may need long-term treatment and diet management.

- Probiotics may be recommended. Probiotics are live microorganisms used as a dietary supplement to help with digestion and normal bowel function. A bacterium found in yogurt called *Lactobacillus acidophilus*, is the most common probiotic.

- Patients who have diarrhea with other symptoms may need fluids and medicine given by IV.

Radiation Enteritis

Radiation enteritis is inflammation of the intestine caused by radiation therapy.

Radiation enteritis is a condition in which the lining of the intestine becomes swollen and inflamed during or after radiation therapy to the abdomen, pelvis, or rectum. The small and large intestine are very sensitive to radiation. The larger the dose of radiation, the more damage may be done to normal tissue. Most tumors in the abdomen and pelvis need large doses of radiation. Almost all patients receiving radiation to the abdomen, pelvis, or rectum will have enteritis.

Radiation therapy to kill cancer cells in the abdomen and pelvis affects normal cells in the lining of the intestines. Radiation therapy stops the growth of cancer cells and other fast-growing cells. Since normal cells in the lining of the intestines grow quickly, radiation treatment to that area can stop those cells from growing. This makes it hard for tissue to repair itself. As cells die and are not replaced, gastrointestinal problems occur over the next few days and weeks.

Doctors are studying whether the order that radiation therapy, chemotherapy, and surgery are given affects how severe the enteritis will be.

Symptoms

Symptoms may begin during radiation therapy or months to years later.

Radiation enteritis may be acute or chronic:

- Acute radiation enteritis occurs during radiation therapy and may last up to 8–12 weeks after treatment stops.

- Chronic radiation enteritis may appear months to years after radiation therapy ends, or it may begin as acute enteritis and keep coming back.

The total dose of radiation and other factors affect the risk of radiation enteritis.

Only 5–15 percent of patients treated with radiation to the abdomen will have chronic problems. The amount of time the enteritis lasts and how severe it is depend on the following:

- The total dose of radiation received

- The amount of normal intestine treated

- The tumor size and how much it has spread

- If chemotherapy was given at the same time as the radiation therapy

- If radiation implants were used

- If the patient has high blood pressure, diabetes, pelvic inflammatory disease, or poor nutrition

- If the patient has had surgery to the abdomen or pelvis

Acute and chronic enteritis have symptoms that are a lot alike. Patients with acute enteritis may have the following symptoms:

- Nausea

- Vomiting

- Abdominal cramps

- Frequent urges to have a bowel movement

- Rectal pain, bleeding, or mucus in the stool

- Watery diarrhea

- Feeling very tired

Symptoms of acute enteritis usually go away two to three weeks after treatment ends.

Symptoms of chronic enteritis usually appear 6–18 months after radiation therapy ends. It can be hard to diagnose. The doctor will first check to see if the symptoms are being caused by a recurrent tumor in the small intestine. The doctor will also need to know the patient's full history of radiation treatments.

Patients with chronic enteritis may have the following signs and symptoms:

- Abdominal cramps

- Bloody diarrhea

- Frequent urges to have a bowel movement

- Greasy and fatty stools

- Weight loss

- Nausea

Assessment

Assessment of radiation enteritis includes a physical exam and questions for the patient.

Patients will be given a physical exam and be asked questions about the following:

- Usual pattern of bowel movements

- Pattern of diarrhea:

  - When it started

  - How long it has lasted

  - How often it occurs

  - Amount and type of stools

  - Other symptoms with the diarrhea (such as gas, cramping, bloating, urgency, bleeding, and rectal soreness)

- Nutrition health:
  - Height and weight
  - Usual eating habits
  - Changes in eating habits
  - Amount of fiber in the diet
  - Signs of dehydration (such as poor skin tone, increased weakness, or feeling very tired)
- Stress levels and ability to cope
- Changes in lifestyle caused by the enteritis

Treatment

Treatment depends on whether the radiation enteritis is acute or chronic.

Acute Radiation Enteritis

Treatment of acute enteritis includes treating the symptoms. The symptoms usually get better with treatment, but if symptoms get worse, then cancer treatment may have to be stopped for a while.

Treatment of acute radiation enteritis may include the following:

- Medicines to stop diarrhea
- Opioids to relieve pain
- Steroid foams to relieve rectal inflammation
- Pancreatic enzyme replacement for patients who have pancreatic cancer. A decrease in pancreatic enzymes can cause diarrhea.
- Diet changes. Intestines damaged by radiation therapy may not make enough of certain enzymes needed for digestion, especially lactase. Lactase is needed to digest lactose, which is found in milk and milk products. A lactose-free, low-fat, and low-fiber diet may help to control symptoms of acute enteritis.
- Foods and items to avoid:
  - Milk and milk products, except buttermilk, yogurt, and lactose-free milkshake supplements, such as Ensure
  - Whole-bran bread and cereal

- Nuts, seeds, and coconut
- Fried, greasy, or fatty foods
- Fresh and dried fruit and some fruit juices (such as prune juice)
- Raw vegetables
- Rich pastries
- Popcorn, potato chips, and pretzels
- Strong spices and herbs
- Chocolate, coffee, tea, and soft drinks with caffeine
- Alcohol and tobacco
- Foods to choose:
  - Fish, poultry, and meat that are broiled or roasted
  - Bananas
  - Applesauce and peeled apples
  - Apple and grape juices
  - White bread and toast
  - Macaroni and noodles
  - Baked, boiled, or mashed potatoes
  - Cooked vegetables that are mild, such as asparagus tips, green and waxed beans, carrots, spinach, and squash
  - Mild processed cheese. Processed cheese may not cause problems because the lactose is removed when it is made.
  - Buttermilk, yogurt, and lactose-free milkshake supplements, such as Ensure
  - Eggs
  - Smooth peanut butter
- Helpful hints:
  - Eat food at room temperature
  - Drink about 12 eight-ounce glasses of fluid a day
  - Let sodas lose their fizz before drinking them

- Add nutmeg to food. This helps slow down movement of digested food in the intestines.

- Start a low-fiber diet on the first day of radiation therapy.

Chronic Radiation Enteritis

Treatment of chronic radiation enteritis may include the following:

- Same treatments as for acute radiation enteritis symptoms

- Surgery. Few patients need surgery to control their symptoms. Two types of surgery may be used:

  - **Intestinal bypass:** A procedure in which the doctor creates a new pathway for the flow of intestinal contents around the damaged tissue

  - **Total intestinal resection:** Surgery to completely remove the intestines

Doctors look at the patient's general health and the amount of damaged tissue before deciding if surgery will be needed. Healing after surgery is often slow and long-term tubefeeding may be needed. Even after surgery, many patients still have symptoms.

Part Seven

Food Intolerances and Infectious Disorders of the Gastrointestinal Tract

Chapter 48

Lactose Intolerance

What Is Lactose Intolerance?

Lactose intolerance is a condition in which you have digestive symptoms—such as bloating, diarrhea, and gas—after you consume foods or drinks that contain lactose. Lactose is a sugar that is naturally found in milk and milk products, like cheese or ice cream. In lactose intolerance, digestive symptoms are caused by lactose malabsorption. Lactose malabsorption is a condition in which your small intestine cannot digest, or break down, all the lactose you eat or drink. Not everyone with lactose malabsorption has digestive symptoms after they consume lactose. Only people who have symptoms are lactose intolerant. Most people with lactose intolerance can consume some amount of lactose without having symptoms. Different people can tolerate different amounts of lactose before having symptoms. Lactose intolerance is different from a milk allergy. A milk allergy is an immune system disorder.

How Common Is Lactose Malabsorption?

While most infants can digest lactose, many people begin to develop lactose malabsorption—a reduced ability to digest lactose—after infancy. Experts estimate that about 68 percent of the world's population has lactose malabsorption. Lactose malabsorption is more common

This chapter includes text excerpted from "Lactose Intolerance," National Institute of Diabetes and Digestive and Kidney Diseases (NIDDK), February 2018.

in some parts of the world than in others. In Africa and Asia, most people have lactose malabsorption. In some regions, such as northern Europe, many people carry a gene that allows them to digest lactose after infancy, and lactose malabsorption is less common. In the United States, about 36 percent of people have lactose malabsorption. While lactose malabsorption causes lactose intolerance, not all people with lactose malabsorption have lactose intolerance.

Who Is More Likely to Have Lactose Intolerance?

You are more likely to have lactose intolerance if you are from, or your family is from, a part of the world where lactose malabsorption is more common. In the United States, the following ethnic and racial groups are more likely to have lactose malabsorption:

- African Americans
- American Indians
- Asian Americans
- Hispanics/Latinos

Because these ethnic and racial groups are more likely to have lactose malabsorption, they are also more likely to have the symptoms of lactose intolerance. Lactose intolerance is least common among people who are from, or whose families are from, Europe.

What Are the Complications of Lactose Intolerance?

Lactose intolerance may affect your health if it keeps you from getting enough nutrients, such as calcium and vitamin D. Milk and milk products, which contain lactose, are some of the main sources of calcium, vitamin D, and other nutrients. You need calcium throughout your life to grow and have healthy bones. If you don't get enough calcium, your bones may become weak and more likely to break. This condition is called osteoporosis. If you have lactose intolerance, you can change your diet to make sure you get enough calcium while also managing your symptoms.

What Are the Symptoms of Lactose Intolerance?

If you have lactose intolerance, you may have symptoms within a few hours after you have milk or milk products, or other foods that contain lactose. Your symptoms may include:

- Bloating

- Diarrhea

- Gas

- Nausea

- Pain in your abdomen

- Stomach "growling" or rumbling sounds

- Vomiting

Your symptoms may be mild or severe, depending on how much lactose you have.

What Causes Lactose Intolerance

Lactose intolerance is caused by lactose malabsorption. If you have lactose malabsorption, your small intestine makes low levels of lactase—the enzyme that breaks down lactose—and can't digest all the lactose you eat or drink. The undigested lactose passes into your colon. Bacteria in your colon break down the lactose and create fluid and gas. In some people, this extra fluid and gas causes lactose intolerance symptoms. In some cases, your genes are the reason for lactose intolerance. Genes play a role in the following conditions, and these conditions can lead to low levels of lactase in your small intestine and lactose malabsorption:

- **Lactase nonpersistence.** In people with lactase nonpersistence, the small intestine makes less lactase after infancy. Lactase levels get lower with age. Symptoms of lactose intolerance may not begin until later childhood, the teen years, or early adulthood. Lactase nonpersistence, also called primary lactase deficiency, is the most common cause of low lactase levels.

- **Congenital lactase deficiency.** In this rare condition, the small intestine makes little or no lactase, starting at birth.

Not all causes of lactose intolerance are genetic. The following can also lead to lactose intolerance:

- **Injury to the small intestine.** Infections, diseases, or other conditions that injure your small intestine, like Crohn disease or celiac disease, may cause it to make less lactase.

665

Treatments—such as medicines, surgery, or radiation therapy—for other conditions may also injure your small intestine. Lactose intolerance caused by injury to the small intestine is called "secondary lactose intolerance." If the cause of the injury is treated, you may be able to tolerate lactose again.

- **Premature birth.** In premature babies, or babies born too soon, the small intestine may not make enough lactase for a short time after birth. The small intestine usually makes more lactase as the baby gets older.

What Is the Difference between Lactose Intolerance and Milk Allergies?

Lactose intolerance and milk allergies are different conditions with different causes. Lactose intolerance is caused by problems digesting lactose, the natural sugar in milk. In contrast, milk allergies are caused by your immune system's response to one or more proteins in milk and milk products. A milk allergy most often appears in the first year of life, while lactose intolerance typically appears later. Lactose intolerance can cause uncomfortable symptoms, while a serious allergic reaction to milk can be life threatening.

How Do Doctors Diagnose Lactose Intolerance?

To diagnose lactose intolerance, your doctor will ask about your symptoms, family and medical history, and eating habits. Your doctor may perform a physical exam and tests to help diagnose lactose intolerance or to check for other health problems. Other conditions, such as irritable bowel syndrome (IBS), celiac disease, inflammatory bowel disease (IBD), or small bowel bacterial overgrowth can cause symptoms similar to those of lactose intolerance. Your doctor may ask you to stop eating and drinking milk and milk products for a period of time to see if your symptoms go away. If your symptoms don't go away, your doctor may order additional tests.

Physical Exam

During a physical exam, your doctor may:

- check for bloating in your abdomen
- use a stethoscope to listen to sounds within your abdomen
- tap on your abdomen to check for tenderness or pain

What Tests Do Doctors Use to Diagnose Lactose Intolerance?

Your doctor may order a hydrogen breath test to see how well your small intestine digests lactose.

Hydrogen Breath Test

Doctors use this test to diagnose lactose malabsorption and lactose intolerance. Normally, a small amount of hydrogen, a type of gas, is found in your breath. If you have lactose malabsorption, undigested lactose causes you to have high levels of hydrogen in your breath. For this test, you will drink a liquid that contains a known amount of lactose. Every 30 minutes over a few hours, you will breathe into a balloon-type container that measures the amount of hydrogen in your breath. During this time, a healthcare professional will ask about your symptoms. If both your breath hydrogen levels rise and your symptoms get worse during the test, your doctor may diagnose lactose intolerance.

How Can I Manage My Lactose Intolerance Symptoms?

In most cases, you can manage the symptoms of lactose intolerance by changing your diet to limit or avoid foods and drinks that contain lactose, such as milk and milk products. Some people may only need to limit the amount of lactose they eat or drink, while others may need to avoid lactose altogether. Using lactase products can help some people manage their symptoms.

Lactase Products

Lactase products are tablets or drops that contain lactase, the enzyme that breaks down lactose. You can take lactase tablets before you eat or drink milk products. You can also add lactase drops to milk before you drink it. The lactase breaks down the lactose in foods and drinks, lowering your chances of having lactose intolerance symptoms. Check with your doctor before using lactase products. Some people, such as young children and pregnant and breastfeeding women, may not be able to use them.

How Do Doctors Treat Lactose Intolerance?

Treatments depend on the cause of lactose intolerance. If your lactose intolerance is caused by lactase nonpersistence or congenital lactase deficiency, no treatments can increase the amount of lactase your small intestine makes. Your doctor can help you change your diet to manage your symptoms. If your lactose intolerance is caused by an injury to your small intestine, your doctor may be able to treat the cause of the injury. You may be able to tolerate lactose after treatment. While some premature babies are lactose intolerant, the condition usually improves without treatment as the baby gets older.

How Should I Change My Diet If I Have Lactose Intolerance?

Talk with your doctor or a dietitian about changing your diet to manage lactose intolerance symptoms while making sure you get enough nutrients. If your child has lactose intolerance, help your child follow the dietary plan recommended by a doctor or dietitian. To manage your symptoms, you may need to reduce the amount of lactose you eat or drink. Most people with lactose intolerance can have some lactose without getting symptoms.

Foods That Contain Lactose

You may not need to completely avoid foods and beverages that contain lactose—such as milk or milk products. If you avoid all milk and milk products, you may get less calcium and vitamin D than you need. People with lactose intolerance can handle different amounts of lactose. Research suggests that many people could have 12 grams of lactose—the amount in about one cup of milk—without symptoms or with only mild symptoms.

You may be able to tolerate milk and milk products if you:

- drink small amounts of milk at a time and have it with meals
- add milk and milk products to your diet a little at a time and see how you feel
- try eating yogurt and hard cheeses, like cheddar or Swiss, which are lower in lactose than other milk products
- use lactase products to help digest the lactose in milk and milk products

Lactose-Free and Lactose-Reduced Milk and Milk Products

Using lactose-free and lactose-reduced milk and milk products may help you lower the amount of lactose in your diet. These products are available in many grocery stores and are just as healthy for you as regular milk and milk products.

Calcium and Vitamin D

If you are lactose intolerant, make sure you get enough calcium and vitamin D each day. Milk and milk products are the most common sources of calcium.

Many foods that do not contain lactose are also sources of calcium. Examples include:

- Fish with soft bones, such as canned salmon or sardines

- Broccoli and leafy green vegetables

- Oranges

- Almonds, Brazil nuts, and dried beans

- Tofu

- Products with labels that show they have added calcium, such as some cereals, fruit juices, and soy milk

Vitamin D helps your body absorb and use calcium. Be sure to eat foods that contain vitamin D, such as eggs and certain kinds of fish, such as salmon. Some ready-to-eat cereals and orange juice have added vitamin D. Some milk and milk products also have added vitamin D. If you can drink small amounts of milk or milk products without symptoms, choose products that have added vitamin D. Also, being outside in the sunlight helps your body make vitamin D.

What Foods and Drinks Contain Lactose?

Lactose is in all milk and milk products and may be found in other foods and drinks. Milk and milk products may be added to boxed, canned, frozen, packaged, and prepared foods. If you have symptoms after consuming a small amount of lactose, you should be aware of the many products that may contain lactose, such as:

- Bread and other baked goods, such as pancakes, biscuits, cookies, and cakes

- Processed foods, including breakfast cereals, instant potatoes, soups, margarine, salad dressings, and flavored chips and other snack foods

- Processed meats, such as bacon, sausage, hot dogs, and lunch meats

- Milk-based meal replacement liquids and powders, smoothies, and protein powders and bars

- Nondairy liquid and powdered coffee creamers, and nondairy whipped toppings

You can check the ingredient list on packaged foods to see if the product contains lactose. The following words mean that the product contains lactose:

- Milk

- Lactose

- Hey

- Curds

- Milk by-products

- Dry milk solids

- Nonfat dry milk powder

A small amount of lactose may be found in some prescription and over-the-counter (OTC) medicines. Talk with your doctor about the amount of lactose in medicines you take, especially if you typically cannot tolerate even small amounts of lactose.

Chapter 49

Celiac Disease

What Is Celiac Disease?

Celiac disease is a digestive disorder that damages the small intestine. The disease is triggered by eating foods containing gluten. Gluten is a protein found naturally in wheat, barley, and rye, and is common in foods such as bread, pasta, cookies, and cakes. Many prepackaged foods, lip balms and lipsticks, hair and skin products, toothpastes, vitamin and nutrient supplements, and, rarely, medicines, contain gluten. Celiac disease can be very serious. The disease can cause long-lasting digestive problems and keep your body from getting all the nutrients it needs. Celiac disease can also affect the body outside the intestine.

Celiac disease is different from gluten sensitivity or wheat intolerance. If you have gluten sensitivity, you may have symptoms similar to those of celiac disease, such as abdominal pain and tiredness. Unlike celiac disease, gluten sensitivity does not damage the small intestine. Celiac disease is also different from a wheat allergy. In both cases, your body's immune system reacts to wheat. However, some symptoms in wheat allergies, such as having itchy eyes or a hard time breathing, are different from celiac disease. Wheat allergies also do not cause long-term damage to the small intestine.

This chapter includes text excerpted from "Celiac Disease," National Institute of Diabetes and Digestive and Kidney Diseases (NIDDK), June 2016.

How Common Is Celiac Disease?

As many as 1 in 141 Americans has celiac disease, although most don't know it.

Who Is More Likely to Develop Celiac Disease?

Although celiac disease affects children and adults in all parts of the world, the disease is more common in Caucasians and more often diagnosed in females. You are more likely to develop celiac disease if someone in your family has the disease. Celiac disease also is more common among people with certain other diseases, such as Down syndrome, Turner syndrome, and type 1 diabetes.

What Other Health Problems Do People with Celiac Disease Have?

If you have celiac disease, you also may be at risk for:

- Addison disease
- Hashimoto disease
- Primary biliary cirrhosis
- Type 1 diabetes

What Are the Complications of Celiac Disease?

Long-term complications of celiac disease include:

- Malnutrition, a condition in which you don't get enough vitamins, minerals, and other nutrients you need to be healthy
- Accelerated osteoporosis or bone softening, known as osteomalacia
- Nervous system problems
- Problems related to reproduction

Rare complications can include:

- Intestinal cancer
- Liver diseases
- Lymphoma, a cancer of part of the immune system called the lymph system that includes the gut

In rare cases, you may continue to have trouble absorbing nutrients even though you have been following a strict gluten-free diet. If you have this condition, called refractory celiac disease, your intestines are severely damaged and can't heal. You may need to receive nutrients through an intravenous (IV).

What Are the Symptoms of Celiac Disease?

Most people with celiac disease have one or more symptoms. However, some people with the disease may not have symptoms or feel sick. Sometimes health issues such as surgery, a pregnancy, childbirth, bacterial gastroenteritis, a viral infection, or severe mental stress can trigger celiac disease symptoms. If you have celiac disease, you may have digestive problems or other symptoms. Digestive symptoms are more common in children and can include:

- Bloating or a feeling of fullness or swelling in the abdomen
- Chronic diarrhea
- Constipation
- Gas
- Nausea
- Pale, foul-smelling, or fatty stools that float
- Stomach pain
- Vomiting

For children with celiac disease, being unable to absorb nutrients when they are so important to normal growth and development can lead to:

- damage to the permanent teeth
- delayed puberty
- failure to thrive in infants
- mood changes or feeling annoyed or impatient
- slowed growth and short height
- weight loss

Adults are less likely to have digestive symptoms and, instead, may have one or more of the following:

- Anemia

- A red, smooth, shiny tongue
- Bone or joint pain
- Depression or anxiety
- Dermatitis herpetiformis
- Headaches
- Infertility or repeated miscarriage
- Missed menstrual periods
- Mouth problems such a canker sore or dry mouth
- Seizures
- Tingling numbness in the hands and feet
- Tiredness
- Weak and brittle bones

Adults who have digestive symptoms with celiac disease may have:

- Abdominal pain and bloating
- Intestinal blockages
- Tiredness that lasts for long periods of time
- Ulcers, or sores on the stomach or lining of the intestine

Celiac disease also can produce a reaction in which your immune system, or your body's natural defense system, attacks healthy cells in your body. This reaction can spread outside your digestive tract to other areas of your body, including your:

- Bones
- Joints
- Nervous system
- Skin
- Spleen

Depending on how old you are when a doctor diagnoses your celiac disease, some symptoms, such as short height and tooth defects, will not improve.

Dermatitis Herpetiformis (DH)

Dermatitis herpetiformis (DH) is an itchy, blistering skin rash that usually appears on the elbows, knees, buttocks, back, or scalp. The rash affects about 10 percent of people with celiac disease. The rash can affect people of all ages but is most likely to appear for the first time between the ages of 30 and 40. Men who have the rash also may have oral or, rarely, genital sores. Some people with celiac disease may have the rash and no other symptoms.

Why Are Celiac Disease Symptoms So Varied?

Symptoms of celiac disease vary from person to person. Your symptoms may depend on:

- How long you were breastfed as an infant; some studies have shown that the longer you were breastfed, the later celiac disease symptoms appear

- How much gluten you eat

- How old you were when you started eating gluten

- The amount of damage to your small intestine

- Your age—symptoms can vary between young children and adults

People with celiac disease who have no symptoms can still develop complications from the disease over time if they do not get treatment.

What Causes Celiac Disease

Research suggests that celiac disease only happens to individuals who have particular genes. These genes are common and are carried by about one-third of the population. Individuals also have to be eating food that contains gluten to get celiac disease. Researchers do not know exactly what triggers celiac disease in people at risk who eat gluten over a long period of time. Sometimes the disease runs in families. About 10–20 percent of close relatives of people with celiac disease also are affected. Your chances of developing celiac disease increase when you have changes in your genes or variants. Certain gene variants and other factors, such as things in your environment, can lead to celiac disease.

How Do Doctors Diagnose Celiac Disease?

Celiac disease can be hard to diagnose because some of the symptoms are like symptoms of other diseases, such as irritable bowel syndrome (IBS) and lactose intolerance. Your doctor may diagnose celiac disease with a medical and family history, physical exam, and tests. Tests may include blood tests, genetic tests, and biopsy.

Medical and Family History

Your doctor will ask you for information about your family's health—specifically, if anyone in your family has a history of celiac disease.

Physical Exam

During a physical exam, a doctor most often:

- checks your body for a rash or malnutrition, a condition that arises when you don't get enough vitamins, minerals, and other nutrients you need to be healthy

- listens to sounds in your abdomen using a stethoscope

- taps on your abdomen to check for pain and fullness or swelling

Dental Exam

For some people, a dental visit can be the first step toward discovering celiac disease. Dental enamel defects, such as white, yellow, or brown spots on the teeth, are a pretty common problem in people with celiac disease, especially children. These defects can help dentists and other healthcare professionals identify celiac disease.

What Tests Do Doctors Use to Diagnose Celiac Disease?
Blood Tests

A healthcare professional may take a blood sample from you and send the sample to a lab to test for antibodies common in celiac disease. If blood test results are negative and your doctor still suspects celiac disease, he or she may order more blood tests.

Genetic Tests

If a biopsy and other blood tests do not clearly confirm celiac disease, your doctor may order genetic blood tests to check for certain gene changes or variants. You are very unlikely to have celiac disease if these gene variants are not present. Having these variants alone is not enough to diagnose celiac disease because they also are common in people without the disease. In fact, most people with these genes will never get celiac disease.

Intestinal Biopsy

If blood tests suggest you have celiac disease, your doctor will perform a biopsy to be sure. During a biopsy, the doctor takes a small piece of tissue from your small intestine during a procedure called an upper GI endoscopy.

Skin Biopsy

If a doctor suspects you have dermatitis herpetiformis, he or she will perform a skin biopsy. For a skin biopsy, the doctor removes tiny pieces of skin tissue to examine with a microscope. A doctor examines the skin tissue and checks the tissue for antibodies common in celiac disease. If the skin tissue has the antibodies, a doctor will perform blood tests to confirm celiac disease. If the skin biopsy and blood tests both suggest celiac disease, you may not need an intestinal biopsy.

How Do Doctors Treat Celiac Disease?
A Gluten-Free Diet

Doctors treat celiac disease with a gluten-free diet. Gluten is a protein found naturally in wheat, barley, and rye that triggers a reaction if you have celiac disease. Symptoms greatly improve for most people with celiac disease who stick to a gluten-free diet. Grocery stores and restaurants have added many more gluten-free foods and products, making it easier to stay gluten free.

Your doctor may refer you to a dietitian who specializes in treating people with celiac disease. The dietitian will teach you how to avoid gluten while following a healthy diet. He or she will help you:

- check food and product labels for gluten

- design everyday meal plans

- make healthy choices about the types of foods to eat

For most people, following a gluten-free diet will heal damage in the small intestine and prevent more damage. You may see symptoms improve within days to weeks of starting the diet. The small intestine usually heals in three to six months in children. Complete healing can take several years in adults. Once the intestine heals, the villi, which were damaged by the disease, regrow and will absorb nutrients from food into the bloodstream normally.

Gluten-Free Diet and Dermatitis Herpetiformis

If you have dermatitis herpetiformis—an itchy, blistering skin rash—skin symptoms generally respond to a gluten-free diet. However, skin symptoms may return if you add gluten back into your diet. Medicines such as dapsone, taken by mouth, can control the skin symptoms. People who take dapsone need to have regular blood tests to check for side effects from the medicine.

Dapsone does not treat intestinal symptoms or damage, which is why you should stay on a gluten-free diet if you have the rash. Even when you follow a gluten-free diet, the rash may take months or even years to fully heal—and often comes back over the years.

Avoiding medicines and nonfood products that may contain gluten In addition to prescribing a gluten-free diet, your doctor will want you to avoid all hidden sources of gluten. If you have celiac disease, ask a pharmacist about ingredients in:

- herbal and nutritional supplements

- prescription and over-the-counter (OTC) medicines

- vitamin and mineral supplements

You also could take in or transfer from your hands to your mouth other products that contain gluten without knowing it. Products that may contain gluten include:

- Children's modeling dough, such as Play-Doh

- Cosmetics

- Lipstick, lip gloss, and lip balm

- Skin and hair products

- Toothpaste and mouthwash

- Communion wafers

Medications are rare sources of gluten. Even if gluten is present in a medicine, it is likely to be in such small quantities that it would not cause any symptoms. Reading product labels can sometimes help you avoid gluten. Some product makers label their products as being gluten-free. If a product label doesn't list the product's ingredients, ask the maker of the product for an ingredients list.

What Should I Avoid Eating If I Have Celiac Disease?

Avoiding foods with gluten, a protein found naturally in wheat, rye, and barley, is critical in treating celiac disease. Removing gluten from your diet will improve symptoms, heal damage to your small intestine, and prevent further damage over time. While you may need to avoid certain foods, the good news is that many healthy, gluten-free foods and products are available. You should avoid all products that contain gluten, such as most cereal, grains, and pasta, and many processed foods. Be sure to always read food ingredient lists carefully to make sure the food you want to eat doesn't have gluten. In addition, discuss gluten-free food choices with a dietitian or healthcare professional who specializes in celiac disease.

What Should I Eat If I Have Celiac Disease?

Foods such as meat, fish, fruits, vegetables, rice, and potatoes without additives or seasonings do not contain gluten and are part of a well-balanced diet. You can eat gluten-free types of bread, pasta, and other foods that are now easier to find in stores, restaurants, and at special food companies. You also can eat potato, rice, soy, amaranth, quinoa, buckwheat, or bean flour instead of wheat flour. In the past, doctors and dietitians advised against eating oats if you have celiac disease. Evidence suggests that most people with the disease can safely eat moderate amounts of oats, as long as they did not come in contact with wheat gluten during processing. You should talk with your healthcare team about whether to include oats in your diet.

When shopping and eating out, remember to:

- read food labels—especially on canned, frozen, and processed foods—for ingredients that contain gluten

- identify foods labeled "gluten-free;" by law, these foods must contain less than 20 parts per million (PPM), well below the threshold to cause problems in the great majority of patients with celiac disease

- ask restaurant servers and chefs about how they prepare the food and what is in it

- find out whether a gluten-free menu is available

- ask a dinner or party host about gluten-free options before attending a social gathering

Foods labeled gluten-free tend to cost more than the same foods that have gluten. You may find that naturally gluten-free foods are less expensive. With practice, looking for gluten can become second nature. If you have just been diagnosed with celiac disease, you and your family members may find support groups helpful as you adjust to a new approach to eating.

Chapter 50

Food- and Water-Borne Diseases

Chapter Contents

Section 50.1

Foodborne Illnesses: An Overview

This section includes text excerpted from "Foodborne
Illnesses," National Institute of Diabetes and Digestive and
Kidney Diseases (NIDDK), June 2014. Reviewed September 2018.

What Are Foodborne Illnesses?

Foodborne illnesses are infections or irritations of the gastrointestinal (GI) tract caused by food or beverages that contain harmful bacteria, parasites, viruses, or chemicals. The GI tract is a series of hollow organs joined in a long, twisting tube from the mouth to the anus. Common symptoms of foodborne illnesses include vomiting, diarrhea, abdominal pain, fever, and chills. Most foodborne illnesses are acute, meaning they happen suddenly and last a short time, and most people recover on their own without treatment. Rarely, foodborne illnesses may lead to more serious complications. Each year, an estimated 48 million people in the United States experience a foodborne illness. Foodborne illnesses cause about 3,000 deaths in the United States annually.

What Causes Foodborne Illnesses

The majority of foodborne illnesses are caused by harmful bacteria and viruses. Some parasites and chemicals also cause foodborne illnesses.

Bacteria

Bacteria are tiny organisms that can cause infections of the GI tract. Not all bacteria are harmful to humans. Some harmful bacteria may already be present in foods when they are purchased. Raw foods including meat, poultry, fish and shellfish, eggs, unpasteurized milk, and dairy products, and fresh produce often contain bacteria that cause foodborne illnesses. Bacteria can contaminate food—making it harmful to eat—at any time during growth, harvesting or slaughter, processing, storage, and shipping.

Foods may also be contaminated with bacteria during food preparation in a restaurant or home kitchen. If food preparers do not thoroughly wash their hands, kitchen utensils, cutting boards, and other kitchen surfaces that come into contact with raw foods, cross-contamination—the spread of bacteria from contaminated food to uncontaminated food—may occur.

If hot food is not kept hot enough or cold food is not kept cold enough, bacteria may multiply. Bacteria multiply quickly when the temperature of food is between 40 and 140 degrees. Cold food should be kept below 40 degrees and hot food should be kept above 140 degrees. Bacteria multiply more slowly when food is refrigerated, and freezing food can further slow or even stop the spread of bacteria. However, bacteria in refrigerated or frozen foods become active again when food is brought to room temperature. Thoroughly cooking food kills bacteria. Many types of bacteria cause foodborne illnesses. Examples include:

- *Salmonella*, a bacterium found in many foods, including raw and undercooked meat, poultry, dairy products, and seafood. *Salmonella* may also be present on eggshells and inside eggs.

- *Campylobacter jejuni* (*C. jejuni*), found in raw or undercooked chicken and unpasteurized milk

- *Shigella*, a bacterium spread from person to person. These bacteria are present in the stools of people who are infected. If people who are infected do not wash their hands thoroughly after using the bathroom, they can contaminate food that they handle or prepare. Water contaminated with infected stools can also contaminate produce in the field.

- *Escherichia coli* (*E. coli*), which includes several different strains, only a few of which cause illness in humans. *E. coli O157:H7* is the strain that causes the most severe illness. Common sources of *E. coli* include raw or undercooked hamburger, unpasteurized fruit juices and milk, and fresh produce.

- *Listeria monocytogenes* (*L. monocytogenes*), which has been found in raw and undercooked meats, unpasteurized milk, soft cheeses, and ready-to-eat deli meats and hot dogs

- Vibrio, a bacterium that may contaminate fish or shellfish

- *Clostridium botulinum* (*C. botulinum*), a bacterium that may contaminate improperly canned foods and smoked and salted fish

Viruses

Viruses are tiny capsules, much smaller than bacteria, that contain genetic material. Viruses cause infections that can lead to sickness.

People can pass viruses to each other. Viruses are present in the stool or vomit of people who are infected. People who are infected with a virus may contaminate food and drinks, especially if they do not wash their hands thoroughly after using the bathroom.

Common sources of foodborne viruses include:

- Food prepared by a person infected with a virus
- Shellfish from contaminated water
- Produce irrigated with contaminated water

Common foodborne viruses include:

- Norovirus, which causes inflammation of the stomach and intestines
- Hepatitis A, which causes inflammation of the liver

Parasites

Parasites are tiny organisms that live inside another organism. In developed countries such as the United States, parasitic infections are relatively rare. *Cryptosporidium parvum* and *Giardia intestinalis* are parasites that are spread through water contaminated with the stools of people or animals who are infected. Foods that come into contact with contaminated water during growth or preparation can become contaminated with these parasites. Food preparers who are infected with these parasites can also contaminate foods if they do not thoroughly wash their hands after using the bathroom and before handling food. *Trichinella spiralis* is a type of roundworm parasite. People may be infected with this parasite by consuming raw or undercooked pork or wild game.

Chemicals

Harmful chemicals that cause illness may contaminate foods such as:

- Fish or shellfish, which may feed on algae that produce toxins, leading to high concentrations of toxins in their bodies. Some types of fish, including tuna and mahi-mahi, may be contaminated with bacteria that produce toxins if the fish are not properly refrigerated before they are cooked or served.
- Certain types of wild mushrooms

- Unwashed fruits and vegetables that contain high concentrations of pesticides

Who Gets Foodborne Illnesses?

Anyone can get a foodborne illness. However, some people are more likely to develop foodborne illnesses than others, including:

- Infants and children

- Pregnant women and their fetuses

- Older adults

- People with weak immune systems

These groups also have a greater risk of developing severe symptoms or complications of foodborne illnesses.

What Are the Symptoms of Foodborne Illnesses?

Symptoms of foodborne illnesses depend on the cause. Common symptoms of many foodborne illnesses include:

- Vomiting

- Diarrhea or bloody diarrhea

- Abdominal pain

- Fever

- Chills

Symptoms can range from mild to serious and can last from a few hours to several days. *C. botulinum* and some chemicals affect the nervous system, causing symptoms such as:

- Headache

- Tingling or numbness of the skin

- Blurred vision

- Weakness

- Dizziness

- Paralysis

What Are the Complications of Foodborne Illnesses?

Foodborne illnesses may lead to dehydration, hemolytic uremic syndrome (HUS), and other complications. Acute foodborne illnesses may also lead to chronic—or long lasting—health problems.

Dehydration

When someone does not drink enough fluids to replace those that are lost through vomiting and diarrhea, dehydration can result. When dehydrated, the body lacks enough fluid and electrolytes—minerals in salts, including sodium, potassium, and chloride—to function properly. Infants, children, older adults, and people with weak immune systems have the greatest risk of becoming dehydrated.

Signs of dehydration are:

- Excessive thirst

- Infrequent urination

- Dark-colored urine

- Lethargy, dizziness, or faintness

Signs of dehydration in infants and young children are:

- Dry mouth and tongue

- Lack of tears when crying

- No wet diapers for three hours or more

- High fever

- Unusually cranky or drowsy behavior

- Sunken eyes, cheeks, or soft spot in the skull

Also, when people are dehydrated, their skin does not flatten back to normal right away after being gently pinched and released. Severe dehydration may require intravenous fluids and hospitalization. Untreated severe dehydration can cause serious health problems such as organ damage, shock, or coma—a sleeplike state in which a person is not conscious.

Hemolytic Uremic Syndrome (HUS)

Hemolytic uremic syndrome (HUS) is a rare disease that mostly affects children younger than 10 years of age. HUS develops when

E. coli bacteria lodged in the digestive tract make toxins that enter the bloodstream. The toxins start to destroy red blood cells, which help the blood to clot, and the lining of the blood vessels.

In the United States, *E. coli O157:H7* infection is the most common cause of HUS, but infection with other strains of *E. coli*, other bacteria, and viruses may also cause HUS. A study found that about six percent of people with *E. coli O157:H7* infections developed HUS. Children younger than age five have the highest risk, but females and people age 60 and older also have increased risk.

Symptoms of *E. coli O157:H7* infection include diarrhea, which may be bloody, and abdominal pain, often accompanied by nausea, vomiting, and fever. Up to a week, after *E. coli* symptoms appear, symptoms of HUS may develop, including irritability, paleness, and decreased urination. HUS may lead to acute renal failure, which is a sudden and temporary loss of kidney function. HUS may also affect other organs and the central nervous system. Most people who develop HUS recover with treatment. Research shows that in the United States between 2000 and 2006, fewer than five percent of people who developed HUS died of the disorder. Older adults had the highest mortality rate—about one-third of people age 60 and older who developed HUS died. Studies have shown that some children who recover from HUS develop chronic complications, including kidney problems, high blood pressure, and diabetes.

Other Complications

Some foodborne illnesses lead to other serious complications. For example, *C. botulinum* and certain chemicals in fish and seafood can paralyze the muscles that control breathing. *L. monocytogenes* can cause spontaneous abortion or stillbirth in pregnant women.

Research suggests that acute foodborne illnesses may lead to chronic disorders, including:

- Reactive arthritis

- Irritable bowel syndrome (IBS)

- Guillain-Barré syndrome (GBS)

A study found that adults who had recovered from *E. coli O157:H7* infections had increased risks of high blood pressure, kidney problems, and cardiovascular disease.

When Should People with Foodborne Illnesses See a Healthcare Provider?

People with any of the following symptoms should see a healthcare provider immediately:

- Signs of dehydration
- Prolonged vomiting that prevents keeping liquids down
- Diarrhea for more than two days in adults or for more than 24 hours in children
- Severe pain in the abdomen or rectum
- A fever higher than 101 degrees
- Stools containing blood or pus
- Stools that are black and tarry
- Nervous system symptoms
- Signs of HUS

If a child has a foodborne illness, parents or guardians should not hesitate to call a healthcare provider for advice.

How Are Foodborne Illnesses Diagnosed?

To diagnose foodborne illnesses, healthcare providers ask about symptoms, foods and beverages recently consumed, and medical history. Healthcare providers will also perform a physical examination to look for signs of illness. Diagnostic tests for foodborne illnesses may include a stool culture, in which a sample of stool is analyzed in a laboratory to check for signs of infections or diseases. A sample of vomit or a sample of the suspected food, if available, may also be tested. A healthcare provider may perform additional medical tests to rule out diseases and disorders that cause symptoms similar to the symptoms of foodborne illnesses. If symptoms of foodborne illnesses are mild and last only a short time, diagnostic tests are usually not necessary.

How Are Foodborne Illnesses Treated?

The only treatment needed for most foodborne illnesses is replacing lost fluids and electrolytes to prevent dehydration. Over-the-counter (OTC) medications such as loperamide (Imodium) and bismuth subsalicylate (Pepto-Bismol and Kaopectate) may help stop diarrhea in adults. However, people with bloody diarrhea—a sign of bacterial or parasitic infection—should not use these medications. If diarrhea is caused by bacteria or parasites, OTC medications may prolong the problem. Medications to treat diarrhea in adults can be dangerous for infants and children and should only be given with a healthcare provider's guidance. If the specific cause of the foodborne illness is diagnosed, a healthcare provider may prescribe medications, such as antibiotics, to treat the illness. Hospitalization may be required to treat life-threatening symptoms and complications, such as paralysis, severe dehydration, and HUS.

Eating, Diet, and Nutrition

The following steps may help relieve the symptoms of foodborne illnesses and prevent dehydration in adults:

- Drinking plenty of liquids such as fruit juices, sports drinks, caffeine-free soft drinks, and broths to replace fluids and electrolytes

- Sipping small amounts of clear liquids or sucking on ice chips if vomiting is still a problem

- Gradually reintroducing food, starting with bland, easy-to-digest foods such as rice, potatoes, toast or bread, cereal, lean meat, applesauce, and bananas

- Avoiding fatty foods, sugary foods, dairy products, caffeine, and alcohol until recovery is complete

Infants and children present special concerns. Infants and children are likely to become dehydrated more quickly from diarrhea and vomiting because of their smaller body size. The following steps may help relieve symptoms and prevent dehydration in infants and children:

- Giving oral rehydration solutions such as Pedialyte, Naturalyte, Infalyte, and CeraLyte to prevent dehydration

- Giving food as soon as the child is hungry

- Giving infants breast milk or full strength formula, as usual, along with oral rehydration solutions

Older adults and adults with weak immune systems should also drink oral rehydration solutions to prevent dehydration.

How Are Foodborne Illnesses Prevented?

Foodborne illnesses can be prevented by properly storing, cooking, cleaning, and handling foods.

- Raw and cooked perishable foods—foods that can spoil—should be refrigerated or frozen promptly. If perishable foods stand at room temperature for more than two hours, they may not be safe to eat. Refrigerators should be set at 40 degrees or lower and freezers should be set at zero degrees.

- Foods should be cooked long enough and at a high enough temperature to kill the harmful bacteria that cause illnesses. A meat thermometer should be used to ensure foods are cooked to the appropriate internal temperature:

    - 145 degrees for roasts, steaks, and chops of beef, veal, pork, and lamb, followed by three minutes of rest time after the meat is removed from the heat source

    - 160 degrees for ground beef, veal, pork, and lamb

    - 165 degrees for poultry

- Cold foods should be kept cold and hot foods should be kept hot.

- Fruits and vegetables should be washed under running water just before eating, cutting, or cooking. A produce brush can be used under running water to clean fruits and vegetables with firm skin.

- Raw meat, poultry, seafood, and their juices should be kept away from other foods.

- People should wash their hands for at least 20 seconds with warm, soapy water before and after handling raw meat, poultry, fish, shellfish, produce, or eggs. People should also wash their hands after using the bathroom, changing diapers, or touching animals.

- Utensils and surfaces should be washed with hot, soapy water before and after they are used to prepare food. Diluted bleach— one teaspoon of bleach to one quart of hot water—can also be used to sanitize utensils and surfaces.

Section 50.2

Traveler's Diarrhea

This section includes text excerpted from "Managing Travelers' Diarrhea While Traveling Abroad," Centers for Disease Control and Prevention (CDC), July 24, 2017.

What do you do if you find yourself with a rumbling tummy while traveling overseas? Follow these tips to prevent or treat travelers' diarrhea and still enjoy your international trip.

What Is It?

Travelers' diarrhea is caused by a variety of pathogens but most commonly bacteria found in food and water, often related to poor hygiene practices in local restaurants. An estimated 30–70 percent of travelers experience travelers' diarrhea, depending on where they go and what time of year. Countries are generally divided into three risk groups: high, intermediate, and low.

- Destinations with high risk: Asia, the Middle East, Africa, Mexico, and Central and South America.

- Destinations with intermediate risk: Eastern Europe, South Africa, and some Caribbean islands.

- Destinations with low risk: the United States, Canada, Australia, New Zealand, Japan, and Northern and Western Europe.

Prevention

You can reduce your risk of travelers' diarrhea by staying away from the bacteria that cause it. Adults may also take a bismuth-containing antacid medicine (e.g., Pepto-Bismol*, the equivalent of two 262-mg tabs 4 times a day), which can decrease the incidence of travelers' diarrhea up to 50 percent. However, Pepto-Bismol is not recommended for pregnant women or children aged three years or younger.

* Use of trade names is for identification only and does not imply endorsement by the Centers for Disease Control and Prevention (CDC).

Keep Your Hands Clean

Wash your hands often with soap and water or use an alcohol-based hand sanitizer after using the bathroom and before eating. Good hand hygiene prevents the spread of germs.

Eat and Drink Safely

Stick to safe food and water habits. Some tips include:

- Eat food that is cooked and served hot, fruits and vegetables you have washed in clean water or peeled yourself, and pasteurized dairy products.

- Don't eat food served at room temperature, food from street vendors, or raw or undercooked (rare) meat or fish.

- Drink bottled water that is sealed, ice made with bottled or disinfected water, and bottled or canned carbonated drinks.

- Don't drink tap or well water or drinks with ice made with tap or well water or unpasteurized milk.

Treatment

If you find yourself suffering from travelers' diarrhea, here are some things you can do to manage it.

Mild diarrhea can be tolerated, is not distressing, and does not prevent you from participating in planned activities. To treat mild diarrhea:

- Drink lots of fluids to prevent dehydration.

- Take over-the-counter (OTC) medications such as loperamide (e.g., Imodium) to manage symptoms. These medicines can help decrease the number of times you need to go to the bathroom, making it easier to ride on an airplane or bus. Always consult a healthcare provider before giving OTC medications to infants or children. Pregnant women and children aged three years or younger should avoid medicines containing bismuth, such as Pepto-Bismol or Kaopectate.

Moderate diarrhea is distressing and can interfere with your planned activities. To treat moderate diarrhea:

- Drink lots of fluids to prevent dehydration. Oral rehydration salt is widely available in stores and pharmacies in most countries. Mix as directed in clean water.

- Take OTC medications such as loperamide (Imodium) to manage symptoms. Pregnant women and children aged three years or younger should avoid medicines containing bismuth, such as Pepto-Bismol or Kaopectate.

- Consider taking an antibiotic if your doctor has prescribed you one.

Severe diarrhea is debilitating and completely prevents you from participating in planned activities. To treat severe diarrhea:

- Take antibiotics if prescribed by your doctor.

- You can also take OTC medicines to manage symptoms.

- Stay hydrated by drinking lots of fluids, such as oral rehydration solution.

- Seek healthcare if you are unable to tolerate fluids or if you develop signs of dehydration. It is especially important to look out for signs of dehydration in infants and young children.

Travelers' diarrhea can make international travel unpleasant. Following the treatment advice can help resolve symptoms within just a few days, so you can get back to enjoying your trip.

Section 50.3

Campylobacter *Infections*

This section includes text excerpted from "*Campylobacter* (Campylobacteriosis)—Questions and Answers," Centers for Disease Control and Prevention (CDC), October 2, 2017.

What Is Campylobacter *Infection?*

Campylobacter infection, or campylobacteriosis, is an infectious disease caused by *Campylobacter* bacteria. It is one of the most common causes of diarrheal illness in the United States. The Foodborne Diseases Active Surveillance Network (FoodNet) indicates that about

693

14 cases are diagnosed each year for every 100,000 people. Many more cases go undiagnosed or unreported. The Centers for Disease Control and Prevention (CDC) estimates *Campylobacter* infection affects more than 1.3 million people every year. Most cases are not part of recognized outbreaks, and more cases occur in summer than in winter.

What Are the Symptoms of Campylobacter Infection?

People with *Campylobacter* infection usually have diarrhea (often bloody), fever, and abdominal cramps. The diarrhea may be accompanied by nausea and vomiting. These symptoms usually start within two to five days after exposure and last about a week. Some infected people do not have any symptoms. In people with weakened immune systems, such as people with the blood disorders thalassemia and hypogammaglobulinemia, acquired immune deficiency syndrome (AIDS), or people receiving some kinds of chemotherapy, *Campylobacter* occasionally spreads to the bloodstream and causes a life-threatening infection.

What Kind of Germ Is Campylobacter?

Campylobacter are bacteria that can make people and animals sick. Most human illness is caused by one species, called *Campylobacter jejuni*, but other species also can cause human illness.

How Does Food and Water Get Contaminated with Campylobacter?

Many chickens, cows, and other birds and animals that show no signs of illness carry *Campylobacter*. *Campylobacter* can be carried in the intestines, liver, and giblets of animals and can be transferred to other edible parts of an animal when it's slaughtered. In 2014, the National Antimicrobial Resistance Monitoring System (NARMS) testing found *Campylobacter* on 33 percent of raw chicken bought from retailers. Milk can become contaminated when a cow has a *Campylobacter* infection in her udder or when milk is contaminated with manure. Other foods, such as fruits and vegetables, can be can become contaminated through contact with soil containing feces from cows, birds, or other animals. Animal feces can also contaminate lakes and streams. Pasteurization of milk, washing or scrubbing of fruits and vegetables, and disinfection of drinking water helps prevent illness.

How Do People Get Infected with Campylobacter Bacteria?

Most *Campylobacter* infections are associated with eating raw or undercooked poultry or from contamination of other foods by these items. People can get infected when a cutting board that has been used to cut and prepare raw chicken isn't washed before it is used to prepare foods that are served raw or lightly cooked, such as salad or fruit. People also can get infected through contact with the feces of a dog or cat. *Campylobacter* does not usually spread from one person to another.

Outbreaks of *Campylobacter* infections have been associated most often with poultry, raw (unpasteurized) dairy products, untreated water, and produce.

Campylobacter infection is common in the developing world, and people who travel abroad have a greater chance of becoming infected. About one in five *Campylobacter* infections reported to the FoodNet are associated with international travel.

Even more rarely, people may become infected through contaminated blood during a transfusion.

Is Campylobacter Infection Serious?

Most people with a *Campylobacter* infection recover completely within a week, although they may shed (get rid of) *Campylobacter* bacteria in their stool for several weeks after recovery, which might result in person-to-person transmission. *Campylobacter* infection rarely results in long-term consequences. Some studies have estimated that 5–20 percent of people with *Campylobacter* infection develop irritable bowel syndrome (IBS) for a limited time and one to five percent develop arthritis.

About 1 in every 1,000 reported *Campylobacter* illnesses leads to Guillain-Barré syndrome (GBS). GBS happens when a person's immune system is triggered by an earlier infection, such as *Campylobacter* infection. GBS can lead to muscle weakness and sometimes paralysis that can last for a few weeks to several years, and often requires intensive medical care. Most people recover fully, but some have permanent nerve damage, and some have died of GBS. As many as 40 percent of GBS cases in the United States may be triggered by *Campylobacter* infection.

Section 50.4

Escherichia coli *Infection*

This section includes text excerpted from "*E. coli (Escherichia coli)*—
Questions and Answers," Centers for Disease Control and
Prevention (CDC), February 26, 2018.

Escherichia coli (*E. coli*) bacteria normally live in the intestines of people and animals. Most *E. coli* are harmless and actually are an important part of a healthy human intestinal tract. However, some *E. coli* are pathogenic, meaning they can cause illness, either diarrhea or illness outside of the intestinal tract. The types of *E. coli* that can cause diarrhea can be transmitted through contaminated water or food, or through contact with animals or persons. *E. coli* consists of a diverse group of bacteria. Pathogenic *E. coli* strains are categorized into pathotypes. Six pathotypes are associated with diarrhea and collectively are referred to as diarrheagenic *E. coli*.

- Shiga toxin-producing *E. coli* (STEC)—STEC may also be referred to as Verocytotoxin-producing *E. coli* (VTEC) or enterohemorrhagic *E. coli* (EHEC). This pathotype is the one most commonly heard about in the news in association with foodborne outbreaks.

- Enterotoxigenic *E. coli* (ETEC)

- Enteropathogenic *E. coli* (EPEC)

- Enteroaggregative *E. coli* (EAEC)

- Enteroinvasive *E. coli* (EIEC)

- Diffusely adherent *E. coli* (DAEC)

What Are Escherichia coli *(E. coli)*?

E. coli are a large and diverse group of bacteria. Although most strains of *E. coli* are harmless, others can make you sick. Some kinds of *E. coli* can cause diarrhea, while others cause urinary tract infections, respiratory illness and pneumonia, and other illnesses. Still, other kinds of *E. coli* are used as markers for water contamination—so you might hear about *E. coli* being found in drinking water, which are not themselves harmful, but indicate the water is contaminated. It does get a bit confusing—even to microbiologists.

What Are Shiga Toxin-Producing E. coli (STEC)?

Some kinds of *E. coli* cause disease by making a toxin called Shiga toxin. The bacteria that make these toxins are called "Shiga toxin-producing" *E. coli*, or STEC for short. You might hear these bacteria called verocytotoxic *E. coli* (VTEC) or enterohemorrhagic *E. coli* (EHEC); these all refer generally to the same group of bacteria. The strain of Shiga toxin-producing *E. coli O104:H4* that caused a large outbreak in Europe in 2011 was frequently referred to as EHEC. The most commonly identified STEC in North America is *E. coli O157:H7* (often shortened to *E. coli O157* or even just "O157"). When you hear news reports about outbreaks of "*E. coli*" infections, they are usually talking about *E. coli O157*.

In addition to *E. coli O157*, many other kinds (called serogroups) of STEC cause disease. Other *E. coli* serogroups in the STEC group, including *E. coli O145*, are sometimes called "non-O157 STECs." Currently, there are limited public health surveillance data on the occurrence of non-O157 STECs, including STEC O145; many STEC O145 infections may go undiagnosed or unreported.

Compared with STEC O157 infections, identification of non-O157 STEC infections is more complex. First, clinical laboratories must test stool samples for the presence of Shiga toxins. Then, the positive samples must be sent to public health laboratories to look for non-O157 STEC. Clinical laboratories typically cannot identify non-O157 STEC. Other non-O157 STEC serogroups that often cause illness in people in the United States include O26, O111, and O103. Some types of STEC frequently cause severe disease, including bloody diarrhea and hemolytic uremic syndrome (HUS), which is a type of kidney failure.

Are There Important Differences between E. coli O157 and Other STEC?

Most of what we know about STEC comes from studies of *E. coli O157* infection, which was first identified as a pathogen in 1982. Less is known about the non-O157 STEC, partly because older laboratory practices did not identify non-O157 infections. As a whole, the non-O157 serogroups are less likely to cause severe illness than *E. coli O157*, though sometimes they can. For example, *E. coli O26* produces the same type of toxins that *E. coli O157* produces, and causes a similar illness, though it is typically less likely to lead to kidney problems (called hemolytic uremic syndrome, or HUS).

697

Who Gets STEC Infections?

People of any age can become infected. Very young children and the elderly are more likely to develop severe illness and HUS than others, but even healthy older children and young adults can become seriously ill.

What Are the Symptoms of STEC Infections?

The symptoms of STEC infections vary for each person but often include severe stomach cramps, diarrhea (often bloody), and vomiting. If there is fever, it usually is not very high (less than 101°F/less than 38.5°C). Most people get better within five to seven days. Some infections are very mild, but others are severe or even life-threatening.

What Is Hemolytic Uremic Syndrome (HUS), a Complication of STEC Infections?

Around 5–10 percent of those who are diagnosed with STEC infection develop a potentially life-threatening complication known as hemolytic uremic syndrome (HUS). Clues that a person is developing HUS include decreased frequency of urination, feeling very tired, and losing pink color in cheeks and inside the lower eyelids. Persons with HUS should be hospitalized because their kidneys may stop working and they may develop other serious problems. Most persons with HUS recover within a few weeks, but some suffer permanent damage or die.

How Soon Do Symptoms Appear after Exposure?

The time between ingesting the STEC bacteria and feeling sick is called the "incubation period." The incubation period is usually 3–4 days after the exposure, but may be as short as 1 day or as long as 10 days. The symptoms often begin slowly with mild belly pain or nonbloody diarrhea that worsens over several days. HUS, if it occurs, develops an average of seven days after the first symptoms, when the diarrhea is improving.

Where Does STEC Come From?

STEC live in the guts of ruminant animals, including cattle, goats, sheep, deer, and elk. The major source for human illnesses is cattle. STEC that cause human illness generally do not make animals sick.

698

Other kinds of animals, including pigs and birds, sometimes pick up STEC from the environment and may spread it.

How Do These Infections Spread?

Infections start when you swallow STEC—in other words, when you get tiny (usually invisible) amounts of human or animal feces in your mouth. Unfortunately, this happens more often than we would like to think about. Exposures that result in illness include consumption of contaminated food, consumption of unpasteurized (raw) milk, consumption of water that has not been disinfected, contact with cattle, or contact with the feces of infected people. Some foods are considered to carry such a high risk of infection with *E. coli O157* or another germ that health officials recommend that people avoid them completely. These foods include unpasteurized (raw) milk, unpasteurized apple cider, and soft cheeses made from raw milk. Sometimes the contact is pretty obvious (working with cows at a dairy or changing diapers, for example), but sometimes it is not (like eating an undercooked hamburger or a contaminated piece of lettuce). People have gotten infected by swallowing lake water while swimming, touching the environment in petting zoos and other animal exhibits, and by eating food prepared by people who did not wash their hands well after using the toilet. Almost everyone has some risk of infection.

Where Did My Infection Come From?

Because there are so many possible sources, for most people we can only guess. If your infection happens to be part of the about 20 percent of cases that are part of a recognized outbreak, the health department might identify the source.

How Common Are STEC Infections?

An estimated 265,000 STEC infections occur each year in the United States. STEC O157 causes about 36 percent of these infections, and non-O157 STEC cause the rest. Public health experts rely on estimates rather than actual numbers of infections because not all STEC infections are diagnosed, for several reasons. Many infected people do not seek medical care; many of those who do seek care do not provide a stool specimen for testing, and many labs do not test for non-O157 STEC. However, this situation is changing as more labs have begun using newer, simpler tests that can help detect non-O157 STEC.

How Are STEC Infections Diagnosed and When Should I Contact My Healthcare Provider?

STEC infections are usually diagnosed through laboratory testing of stool specimens (feces). Identifying the specific strain of STEC is essential for public health purposes, such as finding outbreaks. Many labs can determine if STEC are present, and most can identify *E. coli O157*. Labs that test for the presence of Shiga toxins in stool can detect non-O157 STEC infections. However, for the O group (serogroup) and other characteristics of non-O157 STEC to be identified, Shiga toxin-positive specimens must be sent to a state public health laboratory. Contact your healthcare provider if you have diarrhea that lasts for more than three days, or it is accompanied by high fever, blood in the stool, or so much vomiting that you cannot keep liquids down and you pass very little urine.

What Is the Best Treatment for STEC Infection?

Nonspecific supportive therapy, including hydration, is important. Antibiotics should not be used to treat this infection. There is no evidence that treatment with antibiotics is helpful, and taking antibiotics may increase the risk of HUS. Antidiarrheal agents like Imodium® may also increase that risk.

Should an Infected Person Be Excluded from School or Work?

School and work exclusion policies differ by local jurisdiction. Check with your local or state health department to learn more about the laws where you live. In any case, good hand-washing after changing diapers, after using the toilet, and before preparing food is essential to prevent the spread of these and many other infections.

How Can STEC Infections Be Prevented?

- Wash your hands thoroughly after using the bathroom or changing diapers and before preparing or eating food. Wash your hands after contact with animals or their environments (at farms, petting zoos, fairs, even your own backyard).

- Cook meats thoroughly. Ground beef and meat that has been needle-tenderized should be cooked to a temperature of at least 160°F/70°C. It's best to use a thermometer, as color is not a very reliable indicator of "doneness."

- Avoid raw milk, unpasteurized dairy products, and unpasteurized juices (like fresh apple cider).

- Avoid swallowing water when swimming or playing in lakes, ponds, streams, swimming pools, and backyard "kiddie" pools.

- Prevent cross-contamination in food preparation areas by thoroughly washing hands, counters, cutting boards, and utensils after they touch raw meat.

Section 50.5

Salmonellosis

This section includes text excerpted from "Healthy Pets, Healthy People—*Salmonella* Infection," Centers for Disease Control and Prevention (CDC), September 24, 2015.

Salmonella is a group of bacteria that can live in the intestinal tract of many different animals. Salmonellosis is a bacterial disease caused by *Salmonella*.

Although *Salmonella* is most often spread when a person eats contaminated food, the bacteria also can be passed between people and animals. Many different animals and pets can carry these germs. Animals are known to commonly spread *Salmonella* to humans include:

- Reptiles (turtles, lizards, and snakes)
- Amphibians (frogs and toads)
- Poultry (chicks, chickens, ducklings, ducks, geese, and turkeys)
- Other birds (parakeets, parrots, and wild birds)
- Rodents (mice, rats, hamsters, and guinea pigs)
- Other small mammals (hedgehogs)
- Farm animals (goats, calves, cows, sheep, and pigs)
- Dogs
- Cats
- Horses

How Do Animals and People Become Infected?

Animals become infected with *Salmonella* through their environment, by eating contaminated food, or from their mothers before they are even born or hatched. *Salmonella* is naturally in the intestines of many different animals. Animals with *Salmonella* shed the bacteria in their stool which can easily contaminate their body parts (fur, feathers, or scales) and anything in areas where these animals live and roam (terrarium or aquarium, chicken coop, pen or fencing, countertops, sinks, etc.). It is important to know that many animals can carry *Salmonella* and still appear healthy and clean.

People can get a *Salmonella* infection if they do not wash their hands after contact with animals carrying *Salmonella* or their environment, such as their bedding, food, or tank water. For example, some pet products, like pet foods and treats, can be contaminated with *Salmonella* and other germs. Pet food and treats that may be contaminated include dry dog or cat food, dog biscuits, pig ears, beef hooves, and rodents used to feed reptiles (including frozen feeder rodents). Additionally, reptiles and amphibians that live in tanks or aquariums can contaminate the water with *Salmonella*, which can make people sick even if they don't touch the animal.

Who Is Most at Risk for Serious Illness?

Anyone can get sick from *Salmonella*, but some people are more likely than others to get salmonellosis. People who are more likely to get salmonellosis include:

- Infants
- Children five years of age and younger
- Adults aged 65 and older
- People with weakened immune systems, such as people with human immunodeficiency virus (HIV)/acquired immune deficiency syndrome (AIDS), organ transplant patients, and people receiving chemotherapy

What Are the Symptoms of a Salmonella Infection?
People

People infected with *Salmonella* might have diarrhea, vomiting, fever, and abdominal cramps. Infants, the elderly, and people with weak immune systems are more likely than others to develop severe illness.

Pets

Many animals with *Salmonella* have no signs of illness at all and appear healthy. Pets that become sick from *Salmonella* infection typically have diarrhea that may contain blood or mucus. Sick animals may seem more tired than usual and may vomit or have a fever. If your pet has these signs of illness or you are concerned that your pet may have a *Salmonella* infection, please contact your pet's veterinarian.

Since there have been several pet treats recalled due to contamination with *Salmonella*, you should tell your veterinarian if your pet recently consumed a product that has been recalled. Do not feed your pet any more of the recalled product. Throw the product away immediately.

How Can Salmonella Infections Be Diagnosed and Treated?

People

Salmonella infections in people usually resolve within five to seven days, and most do not require treatment other than drinking plenty of fluids. People with severe diarrhea may need to spend time in a hospital getting rehydrated with intravenous fluids. Lab tests are needed to determine if *Salmonella* is the cause of a person's illness.

Pets

If you suspect that your pet has *Salmonella*, see your veterinarian. *Salmonella* infections may require prompt treatment with supportive care and fluids. If your pet is very sick, it may need to be treated with antibiotics or be hospitalized in a veterinary clinic. Your pet's veterinarian is the best source of advice on your pet's health.

How to Prevent Salmonella Infection?

The best way to prevent getting *Salmonella* from animals is to always wash your hands with soap and running water right after contact with these animals, their environments, or their stool.

Do

- Wash your hands thoroughly with soap and water.

  - Right after touching animals.

  - After touching your pet's food (like dry dog or cat food, frozen feeder rodents) or treats (like rawhide bones, pig ears, biscuits).

  - After touching the areas where they live and roam.

- Use running water and soap, if possible.

- Use hand sanitizer if running water and soap are not available.

  - Be sure to wash your hands with soap and water as soon as a sink is available.

  - Adults should always supervise hand washing for young children.

- Use soap or a disinfectant to thoroughly clean any surfaces that have been in contact with animals. Do not let children five years of age and younger do this task. Children six years of age and older can help with cleaning and disinfecting but only if they are supervised by an adult.

- Clean your pet's cage, terrarium, or aquarium and its contents (such as food and water bowls) outdoors, if possible. If you must clean your pet's habitat indoors, use a bathtub or large sink that can be cleaned and disinfected afterward. Avoid using a kitchen sink if possible.

- Use a bleach solution to clean and disinfect.

Do Not

- Do not let children five years of age and younger, the elderly, or people with weakened immune systems handle or touch animals that can spread *Salmonella* (like turtles, water frogs, or poultry). They should also try not to touch the water from the animals' containers or aquariums.

- Avoid keeping live poultry, amphibians, and reptiles in homes and facilities with children five years of age and younger or people with weakened immune systems. A guinea pig eats zucchini.

- Never eat or drink around high-risk animals (like turtles, water frogs, chicks, ducklings), or in areas where they live and roam.

- Keep animals away from areas where food and drinks are prepared, served, or stored, such as kitchens or outdoor patios.

- Do not ask children five years of age and younger, the elderly, or people with weakened immune systems to clean pets' habitats and their contents.

- Persons 65 years of age and older and those with weak immune systems should wear disposable gloves if they have to clean their pet's habitat.

- Once you finish cleaning, throw out the dirty wash water in a toilet or sink that is not used for food preparation or for drinking water.

Section 50.6

Shigellosis

This section includes text excerpted from "Questions and Answers: *Shigella*—Shigellosis," Centers for Disease Control and Prevention (CDC), January 17, 2018.

Shigellosis is a diarrheal disease caused by a group of bacteria called *Shigella. Shigella* causes about 500,000 cases of diarrhea in the United States annually. There are four different species of *Shigella*:

- *Shigella sonnei* (the most common species in the United States)

- *Shigella flexneri*

- *Shigella boydii*

- *Shigella dysenteriae*

S. dysenteriae and *S. boydii* are rare in the United States, though they continue to be important causes of disease in the developing world. *Shigella* dysenteriae type 1 can be deadly.

How Is Shigellosis Spread?

Shigella germs are in the stool (poop) of sick people while they have diarrhea and for up to a week or two after the diarrhea has gone away. *Shigella* germs are very contagious; it takes just a small number of *Shigella* germs to make someone sick. People can get shigellosis when they put something in their mouths or swallow something that has come into contact with the stool of someone else who is sick with shigellosis. People could get sick by:

- Getting *Shigella* germs on their hands and then touching your food or mouth. You can get *Shigella* germs on your hands after:

  - Touching surfaces contaminated with germs from stool from a sick person, such as toys, bathroom fixtures, changing tables or diaper pails

  - Changing the diaper of a sick child or caring for a sick person

- Eating food that was prepared by someone who is sick with shigellosis

- Swallowing recreational water (for example, lake or river water) while swimming or drinking water that is contaminated with stool (poop) containing the germ

- Having exposure to stool during sexual contact with someone who is sick or recently (several weeks) recovered from shigellosis.

What Are the Symptoms of Shigellosis and How Long Do They Last?

Symptoms of shigellosis typically start one to two days after exposure to the germ and include:

- Diarrhea (sometimes bloody)

- Fever

- Stomach pain

- Feeling the need to pass stool [poop] even when the bowels are empty

For most people, symptoms usually last about five to seven days. In some cases, it may take several months before bowel habits (for example, how often someone passes stool and the consistency of their stool) are entirely normal.

Who Is Most Likely to Get Shigellosis?

- Young children are the most likely to get shigellosis, but people of all ages are affected. Many outbreaks are related to child care settings and schools, and illness commonly spreads from young children to their family members and others in their communities because it is so contagious.

- Travelers to developing countries may be more likely to get shigellosis, and to become infected with strains of *Shigella* bacteria that are resistant to important antibiotics. Travelers may be exposed through contaminated food, water (both drinking and recreational water), or surfaces. Travelers can protect themselves by strictly following food and water precautions, and washing hands with soap frequently.

- Gay and bisexual men and other men who have sex with men (MSM)[†] are more likely to acquire shigellosis than the general adult population. *Shigella* passes from feces or soiled fingers of one person to the mouth of another person, which can happen during sexual activity. Many shigellosis outbreaks among MSM have been reported in the United States, Canada, Japan, and Europe since 1999.

- People who have weakened immune systems due to illness (such as human immunodeficiency virus (HIV)) or medical treatment (such as chemotherapy for cancer) can get a more serious illness. A severe shigellosis may involve the infection spreading into the blood, which can be life-threatening.

- Large outbreaks of shigellosis often start in child care settings and spread among small social groups such as in traditionally observant Jewish communities. Similar outbreaks could occur among any race, ethnicity or community social circle because *Shigella* germs can spread easily from one person to another.

Note: The term "men who have sex with men" is used in Centers for Disease Control and Prevention (CDC) surveillance systems because it indicates men who engage in behaviors that may transmit *Shigella* infection, rather than how someone identifies their sexuality.

How Can Shigellosis Be Diagnosed?

Many kinds of germs can cause diarrhea. Knowing which germ is causing an illness is important to help guide appropriate treatment. Healthcare providers can order laboratory tests to identify *Shigella* germs in the stool of an infected person.

How Can Shigellosis Be Treated?

People who have shigellosis usually get better without antibiotic treatment in five to seven days. People with mild shigellosis may need only fluids and rest. Bismuth subsalicylate (for example, Pepto-Bismol) may be helpful, but people sick with shigellosis should not use medications that cause the gut to slow down and interfere with the way the body digests food, such as loperamide (for example, Imodium) or diphenoxylate with atropine (for example, Lomotil).

Healthcare providers may prescribe antibiotics for people with severe cases of shigellosis to help them get better faster. However, some antibiotics are not effective against certain types of *Shigella*. Healthcare providers can order laboratory tests to determine which antibiotics are likely to work. Tell your healthcare provider if you do not get better within a couple of days after starting antibiotics. They can do more tests to learn whether your type of *Shigella* bacteria can be treated effectively with the antibiotic you are taking. If not, your doctor may prescribe another type of antibiotic.

How Can I Reduce My Chance of Getting Shigellosis?

You can reduce your chance of getting sick from *Shigella* by taking these steps:

- Carefully washing your hands with soap and water during key times:
  - Before preparing food and eating
  - After changing a diaper or helping to clean another person who has defecated (pooped)
- If you care for a child in diapers who has shigellosis, promptly throw away the soiled diapers in a covered, lined garbage can. Wash your hands and the child's hands carefully with soap and water right after changing the diapers. Clean up any leaks or spills of diaper contents immediately.

- Avoid swallowing water from ponds, lakes, or untreated swimming pools.

- When traveling internationally, stick to safe eating and drinking habits, and wash hands often with soap and water.

- Avoid having sex (vaginal, anal, and oral) for one week after your partner recovers from diarrhea. Because *Shigella* germs may be in stool for several weeks, follow safe sexual practices, or ideally avoid having sex for several weeks after your partner has recovered.

Section 50.7

Cryptosporidium *Infection*

This section includes text excerpted from "Parasites— *Cryptosporidium* (Also Known as "Crypto")," Centers for Disease Control and Prevention (CDC), November 2, 2010. Reviewed September 2018.

What Is Cryptosporidiosis?

Cryptosporidiosis is a diarrheal disease caused by microscopic parasites, *Cryptosporidium*, that can live in the intestine of humans and animals and is passed in the stool of an infected person or animal. Both the disease and the parasite are commonly known as "Crypto." The parasite is protected by an outer shell that allows it to survive outside the body for long periods of time and makes it very resistant to chlorine-based disinfectants. During the past two decades, Crypto has become recognized as one of the most common causes of water-borne disease (recreational water and drinking water) in humans in the United States. The parasite is found in every region of the United States and throughout the world.

How Is Cryptosporidiosis Spread?

Cryptosporidium lives in the intestine of infected humans or animals. An infected person or animal sheds Crypto parasites in the stool.

Millions of Crypto germs can be released in a bowel movement from an infected human or animal. Shedding of Crypto in the stool begins when the symptoms begin and can last for weeks after the symptoms (e.g., diarrhea) stop. You can become infected after accidentally swallowing the parasite. *Cryptosporidium* may be found in soil, food, water, or surfaces that have been contaminated with the feces from infected humans or animals. Crypto is not spread by contact with blood.

Crypto can be spread:

- By putting something in your mouth or accidentally swallowing something that has come into contact with the stool of a person or animal infected with Crypto

- By swallowing recreational water contaminated with Crypto. Recreational water is water in swimming pools, hot tubs, Jacuzzis, fountains, lakes, rivers, springs, ponds, or streams. Recreational water can be contaminated with sewage or feces from humans or animals.

- By swallowing water or beverages contaminated with stool from infected humans or animals

- By eating uncooked food contaminated with Crypto. Thoroughly wash with uncontaminated water all vegetables and fruits you plan to eat raw.

- By touching your mouth with contaminated hands. Hands can become contaminated through a variety of activities, such as touching surfaces (e.g., toys, bathroom fixtures, changing tables, diaper pails) that have been contaminated by stool from an infected person, changing diapers, caring for an infected person, changing diapers, caring for an infected person, and handling an infected cow or calf.

- By exposure to human feces through sexual contact

What Are the Symptoms of Cryptosporidiosis?

The most common symptom of cryptosporidiosis is watery diarrhea. Other symptoms include:

- Stomach cramps or pain
- Dehydration
- Nausea
- Vomiting

- Fever
- Weight loss

Some people with Crypto will have no symptoms at all. While the small intestine is the site most commonly affected, Crypto infections could possibly affect other areas of the digestive tract or the respiratory tract.

How Long after Infection Do Symptoms Appear?

Symptoms of cryptosporidiosis generally begin 2–10 days (average seven days) after becoming infected with the parasite.

How Long Will Symptoms Last?

In persons with healthy immune systems, symptoms usually last about one to two weeks. The symptoms may go in cycles in which you may seem to get better for a few days, then feel worse again before the illness ends.

Who Is Most at Risk for Cryptosporidiosis?

People who are most likely to become infected with *Cryptosporidium* include:

- Children who attend day care centers, including diaper-aged children
- Child care workers
- Parents of infected children
- People who take care of other people with cryptosporidiosis
- International travelers
- Backpackers, hikers, and campers who drink unfiltered, untreated water
- People who drink from untreated shallow, unprotected wells.
- People, including swimmers, who swallow water from contaminated sources
- People who handle infected cattle
- People exposed to human feces through sexual contact

Contaminated water may include water that has not been boiled or filtered, as well as contaminated recreational water sources (e.g., swimming pools, lakes, rivers, ponds, and streams). Several community-wide outbreaks of cryptosporidiosis have been linked to drinking municipal water or recreational water contaminated with *Cryptosporidium*.

Who Is Most at Risk for Getting Seriously Ill with Cryptosporidiosis?

If you have a severely weakened immune system, talk to your healthcare provider for additional guidance. Although Crypto can infect all people, some groups are likely to develop more serious illness.

- Young children and pregnant women may be more susceptible to the dehydration resulting from diarrhea and should drink plenty of fluids while ill.

- If you have a severely weakened immune system, you are at risk for more serious disease. Your symptoms may be more severe and could lead to serious or life-threatening illness. Examples of persons with weakened immune systems include those with acquired immunodeficiency syndrome (AIDS); cancer and transplant patients who are taking certain immunosuppressive drugs; and those with inherited diseases that affect the immune system.

What Should I Do If I Think I May Have Cryptosporidiosis?

If you suspect that you have cryptosporidiosis, see your healthcare provider.

How Is a Cryptosporidiosis Diagnosed?

Your healthcare provider will ask you to submit stool samples to see if you are infected. Because testing for Crypto can be difficult, you may be asked to submit several stool specimens over several days. Tests for Crypto are not routinely done in most laboratories. Therefore, your healthcare provider should specifically request testing for the parasite.

I Have Been Diagnosed with Cryptosporidiosis; Should I Worry about Spreading the Infection to Others?

Yes, *Cryptosporidium* can be very contagious. Infected individuals should follow these guidelines to avoid spreading the disease to others:

- Wash your hands frequently with soap and water, especially after using the toilet, after changing diapers, and before eating or preparing food.

- Do not swim in recreational water (pools, hot tubs, lakes, rivers, oceans, etc.) if you have cryptosporidiosis and for at least two weeks after diarrhea stops. You can pass Crypto in your stool and contaminate water for several weeks after your symptoms have ended. You do not even need to have a fecal accident in the water. Immersion in the water may be enough for contamination to occur. Water contaminated in this manner has resulted in outbreaks of cryptosporidiosis among recreational water users.

- Avoid sexual practices that might result in oral exposure to stool (e.g., oral or anal contact).

- Avoid close contact with anyone who has a weakened immune system.

- Children with diarrhea should be excluded from child care settings until diarrhea has stopped.

Note: You may not be protected in a chlorinated recreational water venue (e.g., swimming pool, water park, splash pad, and spray park) because *Cryptosporidium* is chlorine-resistant and can live for days in chlorine-treated water.

Section 50.8

Giardiasis

This section includes text excerpted from "Parasites—
Giardia: General Information," Centers for Disease
Control and Prevention (CDC), July 21, 2015.

What Is Giardiasis?

Giardiasis is a diarrheal disease caused by the microscopic parasite *Giardia*. A parasite is an organism that feeds off of another to survive. Once a person or animal (for example, cats, dogs, cattle, deer, and beavers) has been infected with *Giardia*, the parasite lives in the intestines and is passed in feces (poop). Once outside the body, Giardia can sometimes survive for weeks or months. *Giardia* can be found within every region of the U.S. and around the world.

How Do You Get Giardiasis and How Is It Spread?

Giardiasis can be spread by:

- Swallowing *Giardia* picked up from surfaces (such as bathroom handles, changing tables, diaper pails, or toys) that contain feces (poop) from an infected person or animal

- Drinking water or using ice made from water sources where *Giardia* may live (for example, untreated or improperly treated water from lakes, streams, or wells)

- Swallowing water while swimming or playing in water where *Giardia* may live, especially in lakes, rivers, springs, ponds, and streams

- Eating uncooked food that contains *Giardia* organisms

- Having contact with someone who is ill with giardiasis

- Traveling to countries where giardiasis is common

Anything that comes into contact with feces (poop) from infected humans or animals can become contaminated with the *Giardia* parasite. People become infected when they swallow the parasite. It is not possible to become infected through contact with blood.

What Are the Symptoms of Giardiasis?

Giardia infection can cause a variety of intestinal symptoms, which include:

- Diarrhea
- Gas or flatulence
- Greasy stool that can float
- Stomach or abdominal cramps
- Upset stomach or nausea
- Dehydration

These symptoms may also lead to weight loss. Some people with *Giardia* infection have no symptoms at all.

How Long after Infection Do Symptoms Appear?

Symptoms of giardiasis normally begin one to three weeks after becoming infected.

How Long Will Symptoms Last?

In otherwise healthy people, symptoms of giardiasis may last two to six weeks. Occasionally, symptoms last longer. Medications can help decrease the amount of time symptoms last.

Who Is Most at Risk of Getting Giardiasis?

Though giardiasis is commonly thought of as a camping or back-packing-related disease and is sometimes called "beaver fever," anyone can get giardiasis. People more likely to become infected include:

- Children in child care settings, especially diaper-aged children
- Close contacts of people with giardiasis (for example, people living in the same household) or people who care for those sick with giardiasis
- People who drink water or use ice made from places where *Giardia* may live (for example, untreated or improperly treated water from lakes, streams, or wells)
- Backpackers, hikers, and campers who drink unsafe water or who do not practice good hygiene (for example, proper handwashing)

- People who swallow water while swimming and playing in recreational water where *Giardia* may live, especially in lakes, rivers, springs, ponds, and streams
- International travelers
- People exposed to human feces (poop) through sexual contact

What Should I Do If I Think I May Have Giardiasis?

Contact your healthcare provider.

How Is Giardiasis Diagnosed?

Your healthcare provider will ask you to submit stool (poop) samples to see if you are infected. Because testing for giardiasis can be difficult, you may be asked to submit several stool specimens collected over several days.

What Is the Treatment for Giardiasis?

Many prescription drugs are available to treat giardiasis. Although the *Giardia* parasite can infect all people, infants and pregnant women may be more likely to experience dehydration from diarrhea caused by giardiasis. To prevent dehydration, infants and pregnant women should drink a lot of fluids while ill. Dehydration can be life threatening for infants, so it is especially important that parents talk to their healthcare providers about treatment options for their infants.

What Can I Do to Prevent and Control Giardiasis?

To prevent and control infection with the *Giardia* parasite, it is important to:

- practice good hygiene
- avoid water (drinking or recreational) that may be contaminated
- avoid eating food that may be contaminated
- prevent contact and contamination with feces (poop) during sex

Chapter 51

Viral Gastroenteritis

What Is Viral Gastroenteritis ("Stomach Flu")?

Viral gastroenteritis is an infection of your intestines that typically causes watery diarrhea, pain or cramping in your abdomen, nausea or vomiting, and sometimes fever. Viral gastroenteritis is caused by viruses. Viruses invade normal cells in your body. Many viruses cause infections that can be spread from person to person. People commonly call viral gastroenteritis "stomach flu," but the term is not medically correct. Viral gastroenteritis is an infection of the intestines, not the stomach, and it is not caused by influenza (flu) viruses. The flu vaccine does not protect against viral gastroenteritis. Viral gastroenteritis is acute, meaning it happens suddenly and lasts a short time. Most cases of viral gastroenteritis last less than a week, and most people get better on their own without medical treatment. In some cases, viral gastro-enteritis may cause severe symptoms or may lead to dehydration.

How Common Is Viral Gastroenteritis?

Viral gastroenteritis is very common. Norovirus is the most common cause of viral gastroenteritis. In the United States, norovirus causes 19–21 million cases of viral gastroenteritis each year. Other viruses that cause gastroenteritis are less common.

This chapter includes text excerpted from "Viral Gastroenteritis ('Stomach Flu')," National Institute of Diabetes and Digestive and Kidney Diseases (NIDDK), May 2018.

Who Is More Likely to Get Viral Gastroenteritis?

Anyone can get viral gastroenteritis. Some people are more likely to have severe symptoms, including:

- Infants and young children

- Older adults

- People with a weakened immune system

What Are the Complications of Viral Gastroenteritis?

Dehydration is the most common complication of viral gastroenteritis. When viral gastroenteritis causes you to vomit or have diarrhea, your body loses fluids and electrolytes. If you don't replace those fluids and electrolytes, you may become dehydrated. When you are dehydrated, your body doesn't have enough fluids and electrolytes to work properly. Dehydration is especially dangerous in children, older adults, and people with a weakened immune system. Without treatment, dehydration can lead to serious problems such as organ damage, shock, coma, or even death.

What Are the Symptoms of Viral Gastroenteritis?

The symptoms of viral gastroenteritis include:

- Watery diarrhea

- Pain or cramping in your abdomen

- Nausea or vomiting

- Sometimes fever

What Are the Symptoms of Dehydration?

Symptoms of dehydration, the most common complication of viral gastroenteritis, may include the following in adults:

- Extreme thirst and dry mouth

- Urinating less than usual

- Feeling tired

- Dark-colored urine

- Decreased skin turgor, meaning that when a person's skin is pinched and released, the skin does not flatten back to normal right away

- Sunken eyes or cheeks
- Light-headedness or fainting

If you are the parent or caretaker of an infant or young child with viral gastroenteritis, you should watch for the following signs of dehydration:

- Thirst
- Urinating less than usual, or no wet diapers for three hours or more
- Lack of energy
- Dry mouth
- No tears when crying
- Decreased skin turgor
- Sunken eyes or cheeks

Seek Care Right Away

In most cases, viral gastroenteritis is not harmful. However, viral gastroenteritis can become dangerous if it leads to dehydration. Anyone with signs or symptoms of dehydration should see a doctor right away. A person with severe dehydration may need treatment at a hospital. Viral gastroenteritis symptoms may be similar to the symptoms of other health problems. Certain symptoms may suggest that a person has a different health problem. The symptoms listed below may suggest that an adult or child has a severe case of viral gastroenteritis, dehydration, or a more serious health problem instead of viral gastroenteritis.

Adults

Adults with any of the following symptoms should see a doctor right away:

- Change in mental state, such as irritability or lack of energy
- Diarrhea lasting more than two days
- High fever
- Vomiting often
- Six or more loose stools in a day

719

- Severe pain in the abdomen or rectum
- Stools that are black and tarry or contain blood or pus
- Symptoms of dehydration

Adults should also see a doctor if they aren't able to drink enough liquids or oral rehydration solutions—such as Pedialyte, Naturalyte, Infalyte, and CeraLyte—to prevent dehydration or if they do not improve after drinking oral rehydration solutions. Older adults, pregnant women, and adults with a weakened immune system or another health condition should also see a doctor right away if they have any symptoms of viral gastroenteritis.

Infants and Children

If an infant or child has signs or symptoms of viral gastroenteritis, don't hesitate to call a doctor for advice. Diarrhea is especially dangerous in newborns and infants, leading to severe dehydration in just a day or two. A child with symptoms of dehydration can die within a day if left untreated. If you are the parent or caretaker of an infant or child with any of the following signs or symptoms, seek a doctor's help right away:

- Change in the child's mental state, such as irritability or lack of energy
- Diarrhea lasting more than a day
- Any fever in infants
- High fever in older children
- Frequent loose stools
- Vomiting often
- Severe pain in the abdomen or rectum
- Signs or symptoms of dehydration
- Stools that are black and tarry or contain blood or pus

You should also seek a doctor's help right away if a child has signs or symptoms of viral gastroenteritis and the child is an infant, was born prematurely, or has a history of other medical conditions. Also seek a doctor's help right away if the child is not able to drink enough liquids or oral rehydration solutions to prevent dehydration or if the child does not improve after drinking oral rehydration solutions.

What Kinds of Viruses Cause Viral Gastroenteritis?

Many different viruses can cause viral gastroenteritis. The most common causes of viral gastroenteritis include:

- **Norovirus.** Norovirus is the most common cause of viral gastroenteritis. Symptoms usually begin 12–48 hours after you come into contact with the virus and last one to three days.

- **Rotavirus.** Symptoms usually begin about two days after you come into contact with the virus and last for three to eight days. Vaccines can prevent rotavirus infection.

- **Adenovirus.** Symptoms typically begin 3–10 days after you come into contact with the virus and last one to two weeks.

- **Astrovirus.** Symptoms typically begin four to five days after you come into contact with the virus and last one to four days.

Norovirus causes infections in people of all ages. Rotavirus, adenovirus, and astrovirus most often infect infants and young children, but they can also infect adults.

Viruses may cause viral gastroenteritis at any time of the year. In the United States, norovirus, rotavirus, and astrovirus are more likely to cause infections in the winter.

Do Flu Viruses Cause Viral Gastroenteritis ("Stomach Flu")?

Although some people call viral gastroenteritis "stomach flu," influenza (flu) viruses do not cause viral gastroenteritis. Flu viruses cause infections of the respiratory system, while viral gastroenteritis is an infection of the intestines.

Are Viruses the Only Cause of Gastroenteritis?

No. While viruses cause viral gastroenteritis, bacteria, parasites, and chemicals may cause other kinds of gastroenteritis. When gastroenteritis is caused by consuming foods or drinks contaminated with viruses, bacteria, parasites, or chemicals, this is called food poisoning.

How Does Viral Gastroenteritis Spread?

Viral gastroenteritis spreads from person to person through contact with an infected person's stool or vomit. If you have viral gastroenteritis, viruses will be present in your stool and vomit. You may spread the virus in small bits of stool or vomit, especially if you don't wash your hands thoroughly after using the bathroom and:

- touch surfaces or objects used by other people

- prepare or serve foods and drinks for other people

- shake hands with or touch another person

Infected people who do not have symptoms can still spread viruses. For example, norovirus may be found in your stool before you have symptoms and up to two weeks after you recover. Norovirus is especially contagious, meaning that it spreads easily from person to person. Norovirus can live for months on surfaces such as countertops and changing tables. When an infected person vomits, the virus may become airborne and land on surfaces or on another person. Viral gastroenteritis may spread in households, day care centers and schools, nursing homes, cruise ships, restaurants, and other places where people gather in groups. If water comes into contact with stools of infected people, the water may become contaminated with a virus. The contaminated water can spread the virus to foods or drinks, and people who consume these foods or drinks may become infected. People who swim in contaminated water may also become infected.

How Do Doctors Diagnose Viral Gastroenteritis?

Doctors often diagnose viral gastroenteritis based on your symptoms. If your symptoms are mild and last only a short time, you typically won't need tests. In some cases, a medical history, a physical exam, and stool tests can help diagnose viral gastroenteritis. Your doctor may perform additional tests to check for other health problems.

Medical History

Your doctor will ask you about your symptoms, for example:

- What symptoms you have

- How long you have had symptoms

- How often you have had symptoms

Your doctor may also ask you about:

- Recent contacts with other people who are sick

- Recent travel
- Current and past medical conditions
- Prescription and over-the-counter (OTC) medicines you take

Physical Exam

During a physical exam, your doctor may:

- check your blood pressure and pulse for signs of dehydration
- examine you for signs of fever or dehydration
- use a stethoscope to listen to sounds in your abdomen
- tap on your abdomen to check for tenderness or pain

Sometimes, doctors perform a digital rectal exam. Your doctor will have you bend over a table or lie on your side while holding your knees close to your chest. After putting on a glove, the doctor will slide a lubricated finger into your anus to check for blood in your stool. Blood in your stool may be a sign of health conditions other than viral gastroenteritis that may be causing your symptoms.

Stool Tests

A healthcare professional will give you a container for catching and storing the stool. You will receive instructions on where to send or take the container for analysis. Stool tests can show signs of infection, inflammation, and digestive diseases and disorders.

How Can I Treat Viral Gastroenteritis?

In most cases, people with viral gastroenteritis get better on their own without medical treatment. You can treat viral gastroenteritis by replacing lost fluids and electrolytes to prevent dehydration. In some cases, OTC medicines may help relieve your symptoms. Research shows that following a restricted diet does not help treat viral gastroenteritis. When you have viral gastroenteritis, you may vomit after you eat or lose your appetite for a short time. When your appetite returns, you can most often go back to eating your normal diet, even if you still have diarrhea. Find tips on what to eat when you have viral gastroenteritis.

If your child has symptoms of viral gastroenteritis, such as vomiting or diarrhea, don't hesitate to call a doctor for advice.

Replace Lost Fluids and Electrolytes

When you have viral gastroenteritis, you need to replace lost fluids and electrolytes to prevent dehydration or treat mild dehydration. You should drink plenty of liquids. If vomiting is a problem, try sipping small amounts of clear liquids. Most adults with viral gastroenteritis can replace fluids and electrolytes with liquids such as:

- Water
- Fruit juices
- Sports drinks
- Broths

Eating saltine crackers can also help replace electrolytes. If your child has viral gastroenteritis, you should give your child an oral rehydration solution—such as Pedialyte, Naturalyte, Infalyte, and CeraLyte—as directed to replace lost fluids and electrolytes. Oral rehydration solutions are liquids that contain glucose and electrolytes. Talk with a doctor about giving these solutions to your infant. Infants should drink breast milk or formula as usual. Older adults, adults with a weakened immune system, and adults with severe diarrhea or symptoms of dehydration should also drink oral rehydration solutions.

Over-the-Counter (OTC) Medicines

In some cases, adults can take OTC medicines such as loperamide (Imodium) and bismuth subsalicylate (Pepto-Bismol, Kaopectate) to treat diarrhea caused by viral gastroenteritis. These medicines can be unsafe for infants and children. Talk with a doctor before giving your child an OTC medicine.

If you have bloody diarrhea or fever—signs of infections with bacteria or parasites—don't use OTC medicines to treat diarrhea. See a doctor for treatment.

How Do Doctors Treat Viral Gastroenteritis?

Your doctor may prescribe medicine to control severe vomiting. Doctors don't prescribe antibiotics to treat viral gastroenteritis. Antibiotics don't work for viral infections.

In some cases, your doctor may recommend probiotics. Probiotics are live microbes, most often bacteria, that are like the ones you normally have in your digestive tract. Studies suggest that some probiotics may help shorten a case of diarrhea. Researchers are still studying the use of probiotics to treat viral gastroenteritis. For safety reasons, talk with your doctor before using probiotics or any other complementary or alternative medicines or practices. Anyone with signs or symptoms of dehydration should see a doctor right away. Doctors may need to treat people with severe dehydration in a hospital.

How Can I Prevent Viral Gastroenteritis?

You can take several steps to keep from getting or spreading infections that cause viral gastroenteritis. Wash your hands thoroughly with soap and water:

- after using the bathroom

- after changing diapers

- before and after handling, preparing, or eating food

You can clean surfaces that may have come into contact with infected stool or vomit, such as countertops and changing tables, with a mixture of 5–25 tablespoons of household bleach and one gallon of water. If clothes or linens may have come into contact with an infected person's stool or vomit, you should wash them with detergent for the longest cycle available and machine dry them. To protect yourself from infection, wear rubber gloves while handling the soiled laundry and wash your hands afterward.

If you have viral gastroenteritis, avoid handling and preparing food for others while you are sick and for two days after your symptoms stop. People who have viral gastroenteritis may spread the virus to any food they handle, especially if they do not thoroughly wash their hands. Contaminated water may also spread a virus to foods before they are harvested. For example, contaminated fruits, vegetables, and oysters have been linked to norovirus outbreaks. Wash fruits and vegetables before using them, and thoroughly cook oysters and other shellfish. Find tips to help keep food safe. The flu vaccine does not protect against viral gastroenteritis. Although some people call viral gastroenteritis "stomach flu," influenza (flu) viruses do not cause viral gastroenteritis. However, rotavirus vaccines can prevent viral gastroenteritis caused by rotavirus.

Rotavirus Vaccines

Two vaccines, which infants receive by mouth, are approved to protect against rotavirus infections:

- **RotaTeq:** Infants receive three doses, at ages two months, four months, and six months

- **Rotarix:** Infants receive this vaccine in two doses, at ages two months and four months

For the rotavirus vaccine to be most effective, infants should receive the first dose by 15 weeks of age. Infants should receive all doses by eight months of age.

If you have a baby, talk with your baby's doctor about rotavirus vaccination.

What Should I Eat If I Have Viral Gastroenteritis?

When you have viral gastroenteritis, you should drink plenty of liquids to replace lost fluids and electrolytes. You may vomit after you eat or lose your appetite for a short time. When your appetite returns, you can most often go back to eating your normal diet, even if you still have diarrhea. When children have viral gastroenteritis, parents and caretakers should give children what they usually eat as soon as their appetite returns. Parents and caretakers should give infants breast milk or formula as usual.

What Should I Avoid Eating If I Have Viral Gastroenteritis?

Research shows that following a restricted diet does not help treat viral gastroenteritis. Most experts do not recommend fasting or following a restricted diet when you have viral gastroenteritis. For some people, certain food ingredients may make symptoms such as diarrhea worse, including:

- Drinks with caffeine, such as coffee and tea, and some soft drinks

- Foods that are high in fat, such as fried foods, pizza, and fast foods

- Foods and drinks containing large amounts of simple sugars, such as sweetened beverages and some fruit juices

- Milk and milk products, which contain the sugar lactose. Some people recovering from viral gastroenteritis have problems digesting lactose for up to a month or more afterward.

Chapter 52

Rotavirus and Norovirus

Rotavirus

Rotavirus is a contagious virus that can cause gastroenteritis (inflammation of the stomach and intestines). Symptoms include severe watery diarrhea, vomiting, fever, and abdominal pain. Infants and young children are most likely to get rotavirus disease. They can become severely dehydrated and need to be hospitalized and can even die.

Symptoms

Rotavirus disease is most common in infants and young children. However, older children and adults also can get sick from rotavirus. Once a person has been exposed to rotavirus, it takes about two days for symptoms to appear. Children who get infected may have severe watery diarrhea, vomiting, fever, or abdominal pain. Vomiting and watery diarrhea can last three to eight days. Additional symptoms may include loss of appetite and dehydration (loss of body fluids), which can be especially dangerous for infants and young children.

Symptoms of dehydration include:

- Decreased urination

This chapter contains text excerpted from the following sources: Text under the heading "Rotavirus" is excerpted from "Rotavirus," Centers for Disease Control and Prevention (CDC), April 23, 2018; Text under the heading "Norovirus" is excerpted from "Norovirus," Centers for Disease Control and Prevention (CDC), July 16, 2018.

- Dry mouth and throat

- Feeling dizzy when standing up

- Crying with few or no tears and

- Unusual sleepiness or fussiness.

Adults who get rotavirus disease tend to have milder symptoms. Children, even those who are vaccinated, may get infected and sick from rotavirus more than once. That is because neither natural infection with rotavirus nor vaccination provides full protection from future infections. Children who are not vaccinated usually have more severe symptoms the first time they get rotavirus disease. Vaccinated children are less likely to get sick from rotavirus.

Transmission

People who are infected with rotavirus shed the virus in their stool (poop). This is how the virus gets into the environment and can infect other people. People shed rotavirus the most, and are more likely to infect others, when they have symptoms and during the first three days after they recover. People with rotavirus can also infect others before they have symptoms. If you get rotavirus particles in your mouth, you can get sick. This can happen if you:

- Put your unwashed hands that are contaminated with poop into your mouth

- Touch contaminated objects or surfaces then put your fingers in your mouth

- Eat contaminated food

Rotavirus spreads easily among infants and young children. They can spread rotavirus to family members and other people with whom they have close contact. Good hygiene like handwashing and cleanliness are important, but are not enough to control the spread of the disease. Rotavirus vaccination is the best way to protect your child from rotavirus disease. Children are most likely to get rotavirus in the winter and spring (December through June).

Treatment

There is no specific medicine to treat rotavirus infection, but your doctor may recommend medicine to treat the symptoms. Antibiotics will not help because they fight bacteria not viruses. Since rotavirus disease can cause severe vomiting and diarrhea, it can lead to dehydration (loss of body fluids). Infants and young children, older adults, and people with other illnesses are most at risk of dehydration. The best way to protect against dehydration is to drink plenty of liquids. You can get oral rehydration solutions over-the-counter (OTC) in U.S. food and drug stores; these are most helpful for mild dehydration. Severe dehydration may require hospitalization for treatment with intravenous (IV) fluids, which are given to patients directly through their veins. If you or someone you are caring for is severely dehydrated, contact your doctor.

Norovirus

Norovirus is a very contagious virus that causes vomiting and diarrhea. People of all ages can get infected and sick with norovirus. You can get norovirus from:

- Having direct contact with an infected person

- Consuming contaminated food or water

- Touching contaminated surfaces and then putting your unwashed hands in your mouth

You can get norovirus illness many times in your life because there are many different types of noroviruses. Infection with one type of norovirus may not protect you against other types. It is possible to develop immunity to (protection against) specific types. But, it is not known exactly how long immunity lasts. This may explain why so many people of all ages get infected during norovirus outbreaks. Also, whether you are susceptible to norovirus infection is also determined in part by your genes.

Symptoms

The most common symptoms of norovirus are:

- Diarrhea

- Vomiting

- Nausea

- Stomach pain

Other symptoms include:

- Fever

- Headache

- Body aches

A person usually develops symptoms 12–48 hours after being exposed to norovirus. Most people with norovirus illness get better within one to three days.

If you have norovirus illness, you can feel extremely ill, and vomit or have diarrhea many times a day. This can lead to dehydration, especially in young children, older adults, and people with other illnesses.

Symptoms of dehydration include:

- Decrease in urination

- dry mouth and throat

- Feeling dizzy when standing up

Children who are dehydrated may cry with few or no tears and be unusually sleepy or fussy.

Transmission

Norovirus spreads very easily. You can get norovirus by accidentally getting tiny particles of poop or vomit from an infected person in your mouth. This can happen if you

- eat food or drink liquids that are contaminated with norovirus

- touch surfaces or objects contaminated with norovirus then put your fingers in your mouth

- have direct contact with someone who is infected with norovirus, such as by caring for them or sharing food or eating utensils with them

If you get norovirus illness, you can shed billions of norovirus particles that you can't see without a microscope. Only a few norovirus particles can make other people sick. You are most contagious

- when you have symptoms of norovirus illness, especially vomiting

- during the first few days after you recover from norovirus illness

However, studies have shown that you can still spread norovirus for two weeks or more after you feel better.

How Food Can Get Contaminated with Norovirus

Norovirus can easily contaminate food and water because it only takes a very small amount of virus particles to make you sick. Food and water can get contaminated with norovirus in many ways, including when:

- An infected person touches food with their bare hands that have poop or vomit particles on them

- Food is placed on a counter or surface that has poop or vomit particles on it

- Tiny drops of vomit from an infected person spray through the air and land on the food

- The food is grown or harvested with contaminated water, such as oysters harvested from contaminated water, or fruit and vegetables irrigated with contaminated water in the field

How Water Can Get Contaminated with Norovirus

Recreational or drinking water can get contaminated with norovirus and make you sick or contaminate your food. This can happen:

- At the source such as when a septic tank leaks into a well;

- When an infected person vomits or poops in the water; and

- When water isn't treated properly, such as not enough chlorine.

How Surfaces Can Get Contaminated with Norovirus

Surfaces can get contaminated with norovirus in many ways, including when:

- An infected person touches the surface with their bare hands that have poop or vomit particles on them;

- An infected person vomits or has diarrhea that splatters onto surfaces; and

- Food, water, or objects that are contaminated with norovirus are placed on surfaces.

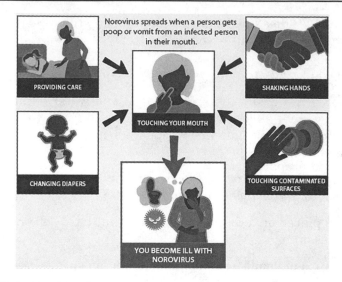

Figure 52.1. *How You Get Norovirus from People or Surfaces*

Prevention

Norovirus spreads very easily from infected people to others, and through contaminated foods and surfaces. There is currently no vaccine to prevent norovirus; although, this is an area of active research. You can help protect yourself and others from norovirus by following these prevention tips.

1. Practice Proper Hand Hygiene

Wash your hands thoroughly with soap and water:

- especially after using the toilet or changing diapers
- always before eating, preparing, or handling food
- before giving yourself or someone else medicine

Norovirus can be found in your vomit or poop even before you start feeling sick. The virus can stay in your poop for two weeks or more after you feel better. It is important to continue washing your hands often during this time. You can use alcohol-based hand sanitizers in addition to hand washing. But, you should not use hand sanitizer as a substitute for washing your hands with soap and water. Hand sanitizers aren't as effective as washing hands with soap and water at removing norovirus particles.

2. Handle and Prepare Food Safely

Carefully wash fruits and vegetables before preparing and eating them. Cook oysters and other shellfish thoroughly before eating them. Be aware that noroviruses are relatively resistant to heat. They can survive temperatures as high as 145°F and quick steaming processes that are often used for cooking shellfish.

Food that might be contaminated with norovirus should be thrown out. Keep sick infants and children out of areas where food is being handled and prepared.

3. When You Are Sick, Do Not Prepare Food or Care for Others Who Are Sick

You should not prepare food for others or provide healthcare while you are sick and for at least two days after symptoms stop. This also applies to sick workers in restaurants, schools, daycares, long-term care facilities, and other places where they may expose people to norovirus.

4. Clean and Disinfect Surfaces

After someone vomits or has diarrhea, always thoroughly clean and disinfect the entire area immediately. Put on rubber or disposable gloves, and wipe the entire area with paper towels, then disinfect the area using a bleach-based household cleaner as directed on the product label. Leave the bleach disinfectant on the affected area for at least five minutes then clean the entire area again with soap and hot water. Finish by cleaning soiled laundry, taking out the trash, and washing your hands.

To help make sure that food is safe from norovirus, routinely clean and sanitize kitchen utensils, counters, and surfaces before preparing food.

You should use a chlorine bleach solution with a concentration of 1000–5000 ppm (5–25 tablespoons of household bleach (5–8%) per gallon of water) or other disinfectant registered as effective against norovirus by the U.S. Environmental Protection Agency (EPA).

5. Wash Laundry Thoroughly

Immediately remove and wash clothes or linens that may be contaminated with vomit or poop. You should:

- handle soiled items carefully without agitating them

735

- wear rubber or disposable gloves while handling soiled items and wash your hands after

- wash the items with detergent and hot water at the maximum available cycle length then machine dry them at the highest heat setting

Treatment

There is no specific medicine to treat people with norovirus illness. Antibiotic drugs will not help because they fight bacteria, not viruses. If you have norovirus illness, you should drink plenty of liquids to replace fluid lost from vomiting and diarrhea. This will help prevent dehydration. Dehydration can lead to serious problems. Severe dehydration may require hospitalization for treatment with fluids given through your vein (intravenous or IV fluids). Watch for signs of dehydration in children who have norovirus illness. Children who are dehydrated may cry with few or no tears and be unusually sleepy or fussy. If you think you or someone you are caring for is severely dehydrated, call the doctor.

Chapter 53

Helicobacter pylori *and Peptic Ulcer*

What Is Helicobacter pylori*?*

Helicobacter pylori (*H. pylori*) is a spiral-shaped bacterium that is found in the gastric mucous layer or adherent to the epithelial lining of the stomach. *H. pylori* causes more than 90 percent of duodenal ulcers and up to 80 percent of gastric ulcers. Before 1982, when this bacterium was discovered, spicy food, acid, stress, and lifestyle were considered the major causes of ulcers. The majority of patients were given long-term medications, such as H2 blockers, and more recently, proton pump inhibitors (PPIs), without a chance for permanent cure. These medications relieve ulcer-related symptoms, heal gastric mucosal inflammation, and may heal the ulcer, but they do NOT treat the infection. When acid suppression is removed, the majority of ulcers, particularly those caused by *H. pylori*, recur. Since we now know that most ulcers are caused by *H. pylori*, appropriate antibiotic regimens can successfully eradicate the infection in most patients, with complete resolution of mucosal inflammation and a minimal chance for recurrence of ulcers.

This chapter includes text excerpted from "*Helicobacter pylori* and Peptic Ulcer Disease—The Key to Cure," Centers for Disease Control and Prevention (CDC), September 28, 2006. Reviewed September 2018.

How Common Is H. pylori *Infection?*

Approximately two-thirds of the world's population is infected with *H. pylori.* In the United States, *H. pylori* is more prevalent among older adults, African Americans, Hispanics, and lower socioeconomic groups.

What Illnesses Does H. pylori *Cause?*

Most persons who are infected with *H. pylori* never suffer any symptoms related to the infection; however, *H. pylori* causes chronic active, chronic persistent, and atrophic gastritis in adults and children. Infection with *H. pylori* also causes duodenal and gastric ulcers. Infected persons have a two- to six-fold increased risk of developing gastric cancer and mucosal-associated-lymphoid-type (MALT) lymphoma compared with their uninfected counterparts. The role of *H. pylori* in nonulcer dyspepsia remains unclear.

What Are the Symptoms of Ulcers?

Approximately 25 million Americans suffer from peptic ulcer disease at some point in their lifetime. Each year there are 500,000–850,000 new cases of peptic ulcer disease and more than one million ulcer-related hospitalizations. The most common ulcer symptom is gnawing or burning pain in the epigastrium. This pain typically occurs when the stomach is empty, between meals and in the early morning hours, but it can also occur at other times. It may last from minutes to hours and may be relieved by eating or by taking antacids. Less common ulcer symptoms include nausea, vomiting, and loss of appetite. Bleeding can also occur; prolonged bleeding may cause anemia leading to weakness and fatigue. If bleeding is heavy, hematemesis, hematochezia, or melena may occur.

Who Should Be Tested and Treated for H. pylori?

Persons with active gastric or duodenal ulcers or documented history of ulcers should be tested for *H. pylori,* and if found to be infected, they should be treated. There has been no conclusive evidence that treatment of *H. pylori* infection in patients with nonulcer dyspepsia is warranted. Testing for and treatment of *H. pylori* infection are recommended following resection of early gastric cancer and for low-grade gastric MALT lymphoma. Retesting after treatment may be prudent for patients with bleeding or otherwise complicated peptic ulcer disease. Treatment recommendations for children have not been formulated. Pediatric patients who require extensive diagnostic work-ups for abdominal symptoms should be evaluated by a specialist.

How Is H. pylori *Infection Diagnosed?*

Several methods may be used to diagnose *H. pylori* infection. Serological tests that measure specific *H. pylori* IgG antibodies can determine if a person has been infected. The sensitivity and specificity of these assays range from 80–95 percent depending upon the assay used. Another diagnostic method is the breath test. In this test, the patient is given either 13C- or 14C-labeled urea to drink. *H. pylori* metabolizes the urea rapidly, and the labeled carbon is absorbed. This labeled carbon can then be measured as CO_2 in the patient's expired breath to determine whether *H. pylori* is present. The sensitivity and specificity of the breath test ranges from 94–98 percent. Upper esophagogastroduodenal endoscopy is considered the reference method of diagnosis.

During endoscopy, biopsy specimens of the stomach and duodenum are obtained and the diagnosis of *H. pylori* can be made by several methods: The biopsy urease test—a colorimetric test based on the ability of *H. pylori* to produce urease; it provides rapid testing at the time of biopsy. Histologic identification of organisms—considered the gold standard of diagnostic tests. Culture of biopsy specimens for *H. pylori*, which requires an experienced laboratory and is necessary when antimicrobial susceptibility testing is desired.

What Are the Treatment Regimens Used for H. pylori Eradication?

Therapy for *H. pylori* infection consists of 10 days to 2 weeks of one or two effective antibiotics, such as amoxicillin, tetracycline (not to be used for children <12 yrs.), metronidazole, or clarithromycin, plus either ranitidine bismuth citrate, bismuth subsalicylate, or a proton pump inhibitor. Acid suppression by the H2 blocker or proton pump inhibitor in conjunction with the antibiotics helps alleviate ulcer-related symptoms (i.e., abdominal pain, nausea), helps heal gastric mucosal inflammation, and may enhance efficacy of the antibiotics against *H. pylori* at the gastric mucosal surface. Eight *H. pylori* treatment regimens are approved by the U.S. Food and Drug Administration (FDA); however, several other combinations have been used successfully. Antibiotic resistance and patient noncompliance are the two major reasons for treatment failure. Eradication rates of the eight

FDA-approved regimens range from 61–94 percent depending on the regimen used. Overall, triple therapy regimens have shown better eradication rates than dual therapy. Longer length of treatment (14 days versus 10 days) results in better eradication rates.

Are There Any Long-Term Consequences of H. pylori Infection?

Studies have shown an association between long-term infection with *H. pylori* and the development of gastric cancer. Gastric cancer is the second most common cancer worldwide; it is most common in countries such as Colombia and China, where *H. pylori* infects over half the population in early childhood. In the United States, where *H. pylori* is less common in young people, gastric cancer rates have decreased since the 1930s.

How Do People Get Infected with H. pylori?

It is not known how *H. pylori* is transmitted or why some patients become symptomatic while others do not. The bacteria are most likely spread from person to person through fecal–oral or oral–oral routes. Possible environmental reservoirs include contaminated water sources. Iatrogenic spread through contaminated endoscopes has been documented but can be prevented by proper cleaning of equipment.

What Can People Do to Prevent H. pylori Infection?

Since the source of *H. pylori* is not yet known, recommendations for avoiding infection have not been made. In general, it is always wise for persons to wash hands thoroughly, to eat food that has been properly prepared, and to drink water from a safe, clean source.

Chapter 54

Clostridium difficile *Infection*

Clostridium difficile (C. *difficile*) is a bacterium that causes inflammation of the colon, known as colitis. People who have other illnesses or conditions requiring prolonged use of antibiotics, and the elderly, are at greater risk of acquiring this disease. The bacteria are found in the feces. People can become infected if they touch items or surfaces that are contaminated with feces and then touch their mouth or mucous membranes. Healthcare workers can spread the bacteria to patients or contaminate surfaces through hand contact.

Symptoms of Clostridium difficile (C. difficile)

Symptoms include:

- Watery diarrhea (at least three bowel movements per day for two or more days)
- Fever
- Loss of appetite
- Nausea
- Abdominal pain/tenderness

This chapter includes text excerpted from "*Clostridium difficile* Infection Information for Patients," Centers for Disease Control and Prevention (CDC), February 24, 2015.

Transmission of C. difficile

Clostridium difficile is shed in feces. Any surface, device, or material (e.g., toilets, bathing tubs, and electronic rectal thermometers) that becomes contaminated with feces may serve as a reservoir for the *Clostridium difficile* spores. *Clostridium difficile* spores are transferred to patients mainly via the hands of healthcare personnel who have touched a contaminated surface or item. *Clostridium difficile* can live for long periods on surfaces.

Treatment of C. difficile *Infection*

Whenever possible, other antibiotics should be discontinued; in a small number of patients, diarrhea may go away when other antibiotics are stopped. Treatment of primary infection caused by *C. difficile* is an antibiotic such as metronidazole, vancomycin, or fidaxomicin. While metronidazole is not approved for treating *C. difficile* infections by the U.S. Food and Drug Administration (FDA), it has been commonly recommended and used for mild *C. difficile* infections; however, it should not be used for severe *C. difficile* infections. Whenever possible, treatment should be given by mouth and continued for a minimum of 10 days.

One problem with antibiotics used to treat primary *C. difficile* infection is that the infection returns in about 20 percent of patients. In a small number of these patients, the infection returns over and over and can be quite debilitating. While the first return of a *C. difficile* infection is usually treated with the same antibiotic used for primary infection, all future infections should be managed with oral vancomycin or fidaxomicin.

Transplanting stool from a healthy person to the colon of a patient with repeat *C. difficile* infections has been shown to successfully treat *C. difficile*. These "fecal transplants" appear to be the most effective method for helping patients with repeat *C. difficile* infections. This procedure may not be widely available and its long-term safety has not been established.

Antibiotic Resistance Threats

Take antibiotics only as prescribed by your doctor. Antibiotics can be life-saving medicines. When a person takes antibiotics, good germs that protect against infection are destroyed for several months. During this time, patients can get sick from *C. difficile* picked up from contaminated surfaces or spread from a healthcare provider's hands. Those most at risk are people, especially older adults, who take antibiotics and also get medical care.

Patients can:

- Take antibiotics only as prescribed by their doctor and complete the prescribed course of treatment. Antibiotics can be lifesaving medicines.

- Tell their doctor if they have been on antibiotics and get diarrhea within a few months

- Wash their hands before eating and after using the bathroom.

- Try to use a separate bathroom if they have diarrhea, or be sure the bathroom is cleaned well if someone with diarrhea has used it.

Part Eight

Additional Help and Information

Chapter 55

Glossary of Gastrointestinal Terms

alanine aminotransferase (ALT): An enzyme released from liver cells.

albumin (ALB): A protein made by the liver to keep body fluids in balance. Low levels can indicate poor health and nutrition or a failing liver.

alkaline phosphatase (alkphos): An enzyme made in the liver's bile ducts and also in bone, kidneys, and intestines. High levels can indicate liver or bone disease.

alpha-fetoprotein (AFP): A protein that can be elevated in liver cancer.

anal fissure: A small tear in the anus that may cause itching, pain or bleeding.

anastomosis: An operation to connect two body parts. An example is an operation in which a part of the colon is removed and the two remaining ends are rejoined.

angiodysplasia: Abnormal or enlarged blood vessels in the gastro-intestinal tract.

This glossary contains terms excerpted from documents produced by several sources deemed reliable.

angiography: An X-ray that uses dye to detect bleeding in the gastrointestinal tract.

anoscopy: A test to look for fissures, fistulae, and hemorrhoids. The doctor uses a special instrument, called an anoscope, to look into the anus.

antacids: Medicines that balance acids and gas in the stomach.

antibodies: Proteins produced by the body as a response to infections.

anticholinergics: Medicines that calm muscle spasms in the intestine.

antiemetics: Medicines that prevent and control nausea and vomiting.

antispasmodics: Medicines that help reduce or stop muscle spasms in the intestines.

anus: The opening of the rectum to the outside of the body.

appendectomy: An operation to remove the appendix.

appendicitis: Reddening, irritation (inflammation), and pain in the appendix caused by infection, scarring, or blockage.

appendix: A four-inch pouch attached to the first part of the large intestine (cecum). No one knows what function the appendix has, if any.

ascending colon: The part of the colon on the right side of the abdomen.

ascites: A buildup of fluid in the abdomen. Ascites is usually caused by severe liver disease such as cirrhosis.

aspartate aminotransferase (AST): An enzyme released from liver and muscle. A blood test that reveals AST levels above normal may indicate liver damage.

atresia: Lack of a normal opening from the esophagus, intestines, or anus.

atrophic gastritis: Chronic irritation of the stomach lining. Causes the stomach lining and glands to wither away.

autoimmune hepatitis: A liver disease caused when the body's immune system destroys liver cells for no known reason.

Barrett esophagus: Peptic ulcer of the lower esophagus. It is caused by the presence of cells that normally stay in the stomach lining.

bezoar: A ball of food, mucus, vegetable fiber, hair, or other material that cannot be digested in the stomach. Bezoars can cause blockage, ulcers, and bleeding.

bile: Fluid made by the liver and stored in the gallbladder. Bile helps break down fats and gets rid of wastes in the body.

bile ducts: Tubes that carry bile from the liver to the gallbladder for storage and to the small intestine for use in digestion.

bilirubin: A bile pigment that is also created by the breakdown of heme pigments. Usually collected by the liver cells, its presence in blood or urine is often a sign of liver damage.

bloating: Fullness or swelling in the abdomen that often occurs after meals.

bulking agents: Laxatives that make bowel movements soft and easy to pass.

cancer: A disease in which cells grow out of control. Cancer cells can invade nearby tissue and spread to other parts of the body.

catheter: A thin, flexible tube that carries fluids into or out of the body.

cecum: The beginning of the large intestine. The cecum is connected to the lower part of the small intestine called the ileum.

celiac disease: Inability to digest and absorb gliadin, the protein found in wheat. Undigested gliadin causes damage to the lining of the small intestine. This prevents absorption of nutrients from other foods.

cholangiography: A series of X-rays of the bile ducts.

cholangitis: Irritated or infected bile ducts.

cholecystectomy: An operation to remove the gallbladder.

chyme: A thick liquid made of partially digested food and stomach juices. This liquid is made in the stomach and moves into the small intestine for further digestion.

cirrhosis: A chronic liver condition caused by scar tissue and cell damage. Cirrhosis makes it hard for the liver to remove poisons (toxins) like alcohol and drugs from the blood.

Clostridium difficile (*C. difficle*)**:** Bacteria naturally present in the large intestine. These bacteria make a substance that can cause a serious infection called pseudomembranous colitis in people taking antibiotics.

colic: Attacks of abdominal pain, caused by muscle spasms in the intestines. Colic is common in infants.

colitis: Irritation of the colon.

collagenous colitis: A type of colitis. Caused by an abnormal band of collagen, a thread-like protein.

colon: The long, coiled, tube-like organ that removes water from digested food. The remaining material, solid waste called "stool," moves through the colon and the rectum and leaves the body through the anus.

colon polyps: Small, fleshy, mushroom-shaped growths in the colon.

colonoscopy: An examination in which the doctor looks at the internal walls of the entire colon through a flexible, lighted instrument called a colonoscope. The doctor may collect samples of tissue or cells for closer examination.

colostomy: An operation that makes it possible for stool to leave the body after the rectum has been removed. The surgeon makes an opening in the abdomen and attaches the colon to it. A temporary colostomy may be done to let the rectum heal from injury or other surgery.

common bile duct: The tube that carries bile from the liver to the small intestine.

computed tomography (CT) scan: An X-ray that produces three-dimensional pictures of the body. Also known as computed axial tomography (CAT) scan.

continence: The ability to hold in a bowel movement or urine.

continent ileostomy: An operation to create a pouch from part of the small intestine. Stool that collects in the pouch is removed by inserting a small tube through an opening made in the abdomen.

corticosteroids: Medicines such as cortisone and hydrocortisone. These medicines reduce irritation from Crohn disease and ulcerative colitis. They may be taken either by mouth or as suppositories.

Crohn disease: A chronic form of inflammatory bowel disease. Crohn disease causes severe irritation in the gastrointestinal tract. It usually affects the lower small intestine (called the ileum) or the colon, but it can affect the entire gastrointestinal tract.

cystic duct: The tube that carries bile from the gallbladder into the common bile duct and the small intestine.

defecography: An X-ray of the anus and rectum to see how the muscles work to move stool. The patient sits on a toilet placed inside the X-ray machine.

dermatitis herpetiformis: A skin disorder associated with celiac disease.

descending colon: The part of the colon where stool is stored. Located on the left side of the abdomen.

dumping syndrome: A condition that occurs when food moves too fast from the stomach into the small intestine. Symptoms are nausea, pain, weakness, and sweating.

duodenum: The first part of the small intestine.

dysphagia: Problems in swallowing food or liquid, usually caused by blockage or injury to the esophagus.

edema: The puffiness that occurs from abnormal amounts of fluid in the spaces between cells in the body, especially just below the skin.

electrocoagulation: A procedure that uses an electrical current passed through an endoscope to stop bleeding in the digestive tract and to remove affected tissue.

electrolytes: Chemicals such as salts and minerals needed for various functions in the body.

encephalopathy: A variety of brain function abnormalities experienced by some patients with advanced liver disease. These most commonly include confusion, disorientation, and insomnia, and may progress to coma.

endoscopic retrograde cholangiopancreatography: A test using an X-ray to look into the bile and pancreatic ducts.

endoscopy: A procedure that uses an endoscope to diagnose or treat a condition.

enema: A liquid put into the rectum to clear out the bowel or to administer drugs or food.

enteroscopy: An examination of the small intestine with an endoscope. The endoscope is inserted through the mouth and stomach into the small intestine.

enzymes: A chemical substance in animals and plants that helps to cause natural processes (such as digestion). Helps chemical changes to take place in the plant or animals.

epithelium: The inner and outer tissue covering digestive tract organs.

Escherichia coli (*E. coli*): Bacteria that cause infection and irritation of the large intestine. The bacteria are spread by unclean water, dirty cooking utensils, or undercooked meat.

esophageal manometry: A test to measure muscle tone in the esophagus.

esophageal pH monitoring: A test to measure the amount of acid in the esophagus.

esophageal stricture: A narrowing of the esophagus often caused by acid flowing back from the stomach. This condition may require surgery.

esophageal varices: Stretched veins in the esophagus that occur when the liver is not working properly. If the veins burst, the bleeding can cause death.

esophagitis: An irritation of the esophagus, usually caused by acid that flows up from the stomach.

esophagogastroduodenoscopy: Exam of the upper digestive tract using an endoscope.

fecal immunochemical test (FIT): A test that uses antibodies to check for blood in a person's stool. Antibodies are proteins made by white blood cells to protect the body from infections.

fecal occult blood test (FOBT): A test to check for hidden blood in stool.

fibrosis: The first stage of scar formation in the liver. Scar tissue is an attempt to contain areas of the liver that have been damaged by alcohol, hepatitis C, or other factors.

flatulence: Excessive gas in the stomach or intestine. May cause bloating.

flexible sigmoidoscopy: Also called proctosigmoidoscopy. A procedure in which the doctor looks inside the rectum and the lower portion of the colon (sigmoid colon) through a flexible, lighted tube called a sigmoidoscope.

gallbladder: The organ that stores the bile made in the liver. Connected to the liver by bile ducts.

gallstones: The solid masses or stones made of cholesterol or bilirubin that form in the gallbladder or bile ducts.

gastrectomy: An operation to remove all or part of the stomach.

gastrin: A hormone released after eating. Gastrin causes the stomach to produce more acid.

gastritis: An inflammation of the stomach lining.

gastroenteritis: An infection or irritation of the stomach and intestines. May be caused by bacteria or parasites from spoiled food or unclean water.

gastroesophageal reflux disease (GERD): Flow of the stomach's contents back up into the esophagus. Happens when the muscle between the esophagus and the stomach (the lower esophageal sphincter) is weak or relaxes when it shouldn't. May cause esophagitis.

gastrointestinal tract: The large, muscular tube that extends from the mouth to the anus, where the movement of muscles and release of hormones and enzymes digest food.

gastroparesis: Nerve or muscle damage in the stomach. Causes slow digestion and emptying, vomiting, nausea, or bloating.

gastrostomy: An artificial opening from the stomach to a hole (stoma) in the abdomen where a feeding tube is inserted.

giardiasis: An infection with the parasite Giardia lamblia from spoiled food or unclean water. May cause diarrhea.

glycogen: A sugar stored in the liver and muscles. It releases glucose into the blood when cells need it for energy. Glycogen is the chief source of stored fuel in the body.

granuloma: A mass of red, irritated tissue in the GI tract found in Crohn disease.

heartburn: A painful, burning feeling in the chest. Heartburn is caused by stomach acid flowing back into the esophagus. Changing the diet and other habits can help to prevent heartburn. Heartburn may be a symptom of GERD.

***Helicobacter pylori* (*H. pylori*):** A spiral-shaped bacterium found in the stomach. *H. pylori* damages stomach and duodenal tissue, causing ulcers. Previously called Campylobacter pylori.

hemochromatosis: A disease that occurs when the body absorbs too much iron. The body stores the excess iron in the liver, pancreas, and other organs. May cause cirrhosis of the liver. Also called iron overload disease.

hemorrhoids: Swollen blood vessels in and around the anus and lower rectum. Continual straining to have a bowel movement causes them to stretch and swell. They cause itching, pain, and sometimes bleeding.

hepatic: Related to the liver.

hepatitis: Irritation of the liver that sometimes causes permanent damage. Hepatitis may be caused by viruses or by medicines or alcohol.

hepatocellular carcinoma (HCC): Cancer stemming from the liver cells. Also called hepatoma.

hernia: The part of an internal organ that pushes through an opening in the organ's wall. Most hernias occur in the abdominal area.

hiatal (hiatus) hernia: A small opening in the diaphragm that allows the upper part of the stomach to move up into the chest. Causes heartburn from stomach acid flowing back up through the opening.

Hirschsprung disease: A birth defect in which some nerve cells are lacking in the large intestine. The intestine cannot move stool through, so the intestine gets blocked. Causes the abdomen to swell.

hydrogen breath test: A test for lactose intolerance. It measures breath samples for too much hydrogen. The body makes too much hydrogen when lactose is not broken down properly in the small intestine.

ileoanal reservoir: An operation to remove the colon, upper rectum, and part of the lower rectum. An internal pouch is created from the remaining intestine to hold stool. The operation may be done in two stages. The pouch may also be called a J-pouch or W-pouch.

ileostomy: An operation that makes it possible for stool to leave the body after the colon and rectum are removed. The surgeon makes an opening in the abdomen and attaches the bottom of the small intestine (ileum) to it.

ileum: The lower end of the small intestine.

inflammatory bowel disease (IBD): Long-lasting problems that cause irritation and ulcers in the GI tract. The most common disorders are ulcerative colitis and Crohn disease.

insulin: A hormone released by the pancreas whose job is to help use or store glucose as glycogen.

intestine: The long, tube-shaped organ in the abdomen, also called the "bowel," that completes the process of digestion. There are both large and small intestines.

irritable bowel syndrome (IBS): A disorder that comes and goes. Nerves that control the muscles in the GI tract are too active. The GI tract becomes sensitive to food, stool, gas, and stress. Causes abdominal pain, bloating, and constipation or diarrhea. Also called spastic colon or mucous colitis.

jaundice: A symptom of many disorders. Jaundice causes the skin and eyes to turn yellow from too much bilirubin in the blood.

jejunostomy: An operation to create an opening of the jejunum to a hole (stoma) in the abdomen.

jejunum: The middle section of the small intestine between the duodenum and ileum.

lactase: An enzyme in the small intestine needed to digest milk sugar (lactose).

laparoscope: A thin tube with a tiny video camera attached. Used to look inside the body and see the surface of organs.

laparoscopic cholecystectomy: An operation to remove the gall-bladder. The doctor inserts a laparoscope and other surgical instruments through small holes in the abdomen. The camera allows the doctor to see the gallbladder on a television screen. The doctor removes the gallbladder through the holes.

laparoscopy: A test that uses a laparoscope to look at and take tissue from the inside of the body.

large intestine: The part of the intestine that goes from the cecum to the rectum. The large intestine absorbs water from stool and changes it from a liquid to a solid form. The large intestine includes the appendix, cecum, colon, and rectum. Also called colon.

laxatives: Medicines to relieve long-term constipation. Used only if other methods fail. Also called cathartics.

liver: The largest organ in the body. The liver carries out many important functions, such as making bile, changing food into energy, and cleaning alcohol and poisons from the blood.

lower gastrointestinal (GI) series: X-rays of the rectum, colon, and lower part of the small intestine. A barium enema is given first. Barium coats the organs so they will show up on the X-ray. Also called barium enema X-ray.

magnetic resonance imaging (MRI): A test that takes pictures of the soft tissues in the body. The pictures are clearer than X-rays.

Mallory-Weiss tear: A tear in the lower end of the esophagus. Caused by severe vomiting. Common in alcoholics.

manometry: Tests that measure muscle pressure and movements in the GI tract.

megacolon: A huge, swollen colon. Results from severe constipation. In children, megacolon is more common in boys than girls.

metabolic syndrome: A medical condition characterized by obesity, insulin resistance, hypertension, and dyslipidemia.

motility: The movement of food through the digestive tract.

mucus: A clear liquid made by the intestines. Mucus coats and protects tissues in the gastrointestinal tract.

necrotizing enterocolitis: A condition in which part of the tissue in the intestines is destroyed. Occurs mainly in underweight newborn babies. A temporary ileostomy may be necessary.

neutropenia: A decreased number of neutrophils. Neutrophils are a type of white blood cells that fights infections in the body. Interferon treatment and chemotherapy can cause neutropenia. Neutropenia can increase risk of infections.

occult bleeding: Blood in stool that is not visible to the naked eye. May be a sign of disease such as diverticulosis or colorectal cancer.

oral dissolution therapy: A method of dissolving cholesterol gallstones. The patient takes the oral medications chenodiol (Chenix) and ursodiol (Actigall). These medicines are most often used for people who cannot have an operation.

ostomy: An operation that makes it possible for stool to leave the body through an opening made in the abdomen. An ostomy is necessary when part or all of the intestines are removed. Colostomy and ileostomy are types of ostomy.

parenteral nutrition: A way to provide a liquid food mixture through a special tube in the chest. Also called hyperalimentation or total parenteral nutrition.

pepsin: An enzyme made in the stomach that breaks down proteins.

peptic ulcer: A sore in the lining of the esophagus, stomach, or duodenum. Usually caused by the bacterium *Helicobacter pylori*. An ulcer in the stomach is a gastric ulcer; an ulcer in the duodenum is a duodenal ulcer.

percutaneous transhepatic cholangiography (PTC): X-rays of the gallbladder and bile ducts. A dye is injected through the abdomen to make the organs show up on the X-ray.

perianal: The area around the anus.

peristalsis: A wavelike movement of muscles in the GI tract. Peristalsis moves food and liquid through the GI tract.

peritoneum: The lining of the abdominal cavity.

peritonitis: Infection of the peritoneum.

polymerase chain reaction (PCR): A test used to determine the number of virus particles in the blood. It is one method to determine the "viral load."

polyp: An abnormal, often precancerous growth of tissue (colorectal polyps are growths of tissue inside the intestine).

polyposis: The presence of many polyps.

porphyria: A group of rare, inherited blood disorders. When a person has porphyria, cells fail to change chemicals (porphyrins) to the substance (heme) that gives blood its color.

portal vein: The large vein that carries blood from the intestines and spleen to the liver.

prescriptions: The number of prescriptions written annually for medications to treat a specific disease.

primary biliary cirrhosis: A chronic liver disease. Slowly destroys the bile ducts in the liver. This prevents release of bile. Long-term irritation of the liver may cause scarring and cirrhosis in later stages of the disease.

primary sclerosing cholangitis (PSC): Irritation, scarring, and narrowing of the bile ducts inside and outside the liver. Bile builds up in the liver and may damage its cells. Many people with this condition also have ulcerative colitis.

proctitis: Irritation of the rectum.

proctocolectomy: An operation to remove the colon and rectum. Also called coloproctectomy.

proctoscope: A short, rigid metal tube used to look into the rectum and anus.

prolapse: A condition that occurs when a body part slips from its normal position.

prothrombin time (PT): A test that measures how long your blood takes to clot. Prothrombin helps the blood to clot, so PT increases if the liver is not making enough of it.

proton pump inhibitors (PPIs): Medicines that stop the stomach's acid pump. Examples are omeprazole (Prilosec) and lansoprazole (Prevacid).

rectal prolapse: A condition in which the rectum slips so that it protrudes from the anus.

rectum: The lower end of the large intestine, leading to the anus.

reflux: A condition that occurs when gastric juices or small amounts of food from the stomach flow back into the esophagus and mouth. Also called regurgitation.

remission: Partial or complete disappearance—or a lessening of the severity—of symptoms of a disease. Remission may happen on its own or occur as a result of a medical treatment.

retching: Dry vomiting.

rotavirus: The most common cause of infectious diarrhea in the United States, especially in children under age two.

Salmonella: A bacterium that may cause intestinal infection and diarrhea.

sarcoidosis: A condition that causes small, fleshy swellings in the liver, lungs, and spleen.

sclerotherapy: A method of stopping upper GI bleeding. A needle is inserted through an endoscope to bring hardening agents to the place that is bleeding.

screening test: Tests used to check, or screen, for disease when there are no symptoms. Recommended screening tests for colorectal cancer include the fecal occult blood test, flexible sigmoidoscopy, and colonoscopy. (When a test is performed to find out why symptoms exist, it is called a "diagnostic")

secretin: A hormone made in the duodenum. Causes the stomach to make pepsin, the liver to make bile, and the pancreas to make a digestive juice.

Shigellosis: Infection with the bacterium *Shigella*. Usually causes a high fever, acute diarrhea, and dehydration.

short bowel syndrome: Problems related to absorbing nutrients after removal of part of the small intestine. Symptoms include diarrhea, weakness, and weight loss. Also called short gut syndrome.

sigmoid colon: The lower part of the colon that empties into the rectum.

sigmoidoscope: A flexible, lighted instrument with a tiny built-in camera that allows the doctor to view the lining of the rectum and lower portion of the colon.

small intestine: Organ where most digestion occurs. It measures about twenty feet and includes the duodenum, jejunum, and ileum.

somatostatin: A hormone in the pancreas. Somatostatin helps tell the body when to make the hormones insulin, glucagon, gastrin, secretin, and renin.

sphincter: A ring-like band of muscle that opens and closes an opening in the body. An example is the muscle between the esophagus and the stomach known as the lower esophageal sphincter.

spleen: The organ that cleans blood and makes white blood cells. White blood cells attack bacteria and other foreign cells.

steatorrhea: A condition in which the body cannot absorb fat. Causes buildup of fat in the stool and loose, greasy, and foul bowel movements.

stool: The waste matter discharged in a bowel movement; feces.

stool test: A test to check for hidden blood in the bowel movement.

stricture: The abnormal narrowing of a body opening. Also called stenosis.

tenesmus: Straining to have a bowel movement. May be painful and continue for a long time without result.

thrombocytopenia: Low level of platelets in the blood caused by cirrhosis and an enlarged spleen and can also be caused by interferon treatment.

transaminase: A term for alanine aminotransferase (ALT) and aminotransferases (AST), the two transaminases.

transverse colon: The part of the colon that goes across the abdomen from right to left.

triglycerides: One of the main fatty substances in the blood that can clog arteries.

triple therapy: Drugs that stop the body from making acid are often added to relieve symptoms.

ulcer: A sore on the skin surface or on the stomach lining.

ulcerative colitis (UC): A serious disease that causes ulcers and irritation in the inner lining of the colon and rectum.

upper GI endoscopy: Looking into the esophagus, stomach, and duodenum with an endoscope.

urea breath test: A test used to detect *Helicobacter pylori* infection. The test measures breath samples for urease, an enzyme *H. Pylori* makes.

vagotomy: An operation to cut the vagus nerve. This causes the stomach to make less acid.

vagus nerve: The nerve in the stomach that controls the making of stomach acid.

varices: Stretched veins such as those that form in the esophagus from cirrhosis.

villi: The tiny, finger-like projections on the surface of the small intestine. Villi help absorb nutrients.

Wilson disease: An inherited disorder. Too much copper builds up in the liver and is slowly released into other parts of the body. The overload can cause severe liver and brain damage if not treated with medication.

Zollinger-Ellison syndrome (ZES): A group of symptoms that occur when a tumor called a gastrinoma forms in the pancreas. The tumor, which may cause cancer, releases large amounts of the hormone gastrin. The gastrin causes too much acid in the duodenum, resulting in ulcers, bleeding, and perforation.

Chapter 56

Resources for Information about Gastrointestinal Conditions

General Information

Academy of Nutrition and Dietetics
120 S. Riverside Plaza
Ste. 2190
Chicago, IL 60606-6995
Toll-Free: 800-877-1600
Phone: 312-899-0040
Website: www.eatrightpro.org
E-mail: cdr@eatright.org

American Academy of Family Physicians (AAFP)
11400 Tomahawk Creek Pkwy
Leawood, KS 66211-2680
Toll-Free: 800-274-2237
Phone: 913-906-6000
Fax: 913-906-6075
Website: www.aafp.org
E-mail: aafp@aafp.org

Resources in this chapter were compiled from several sources deemed reliable; all contact information was verified and updated in September 2018.

American College of Gastroenterology (ACG)
6400 Goldsboro Rd.
Ste. 200
Bethesda, MD 20817
Phone: 301-263-9000
Website: gi.org
E-mail: info@gi.org

American College of Surgeons (ACS)
633 N. Saint Clair St.
Chicago, IL 60611-3295
Toll-Free: 800-621-4111
Phone: 312-202-5000
Fax: 312-202-5001
Website: www.facs.org
E-mail: postmaster@facs.org

American Diabetes Association (ADA)
2451 Crystal Dr.
St. 900
Arlington, VA 22202
Toll-Free: 800-DIABETES
(800-342-2383)
Website: www.diabetes.org

American Gastroenterological Association (AGA)
4930 Del Ray Ave.
Bethesda, MD 20814
Phone: 301-654-2055
Fax: 301-654-5920
Website: www.gastro.org
E-mail: member@gastro.org

American Neurogastroenterology and Motility Society (ANMS)
45685 Harmony Ln.
Belleville, MI 48111
Phone: 734-699-1130
Fax: 734-699-1136
Website: www.motilitysociety.org
E-mail: admin@motilitysociety.org

American Pancreatic Association (APA)
P.O. Box 14906
Minneapolis, MN 55414
Phone: 612-626-9797
Fax: 612-625-7700
Website: www.american-pancreatic-association.org
E-mail: apa@umn.edu

American Porphyria Foundation (APF)
4915 St. Elmo Ave.
Ste. 105
Bethesda, MD 20814
Toll-Free: 866-APF-3635
(866-273-3635)
Phone: 301-347-7166
Fax: 301-312-8713
Website: www.porphyriafoundation.com
E-mail: porphyrus@porphyriafoundation.com

The American Society of Colon and Rectal Surgeons (ASCRS)
One Parkview Plaza
Ste. 800
Oakbrook Terrace, IL 60181
Phone: 847-686-2236
Fax: 847-290-9203
Website: www.fascrs.org
E-mail: ascrs@fascrs.org

American Urogynecologic Society Foundation (AUGS)
1100 Wayne Ave., Ste. 825
Silver Spring, MD 20910
Phone: 301-273-0570
Fax: 301-273-0778
Website: www.augs.org
E-mail: info@augs.org

Association of Gastrointestinal Motility Disorders Inc (AGMD)
AGMD International Corporate Headquarters
12 Roberts Dr.
Bedford, MA 01730
Phone: 781-275-1300
Fax: 781-275-1304
Website: www.agmd-gimotility.org

Department of Genetics and Genomic Sciences
Icahn School of Medicine at Mount Sinai (ISMMS)
One Gustave L. Levy Pl.
New York, NY 10029-5674
Phone: 212-241-6500
Fax: 212-659-6780
Website: icahn.mssm.edu

Digestive Disease National Coalition (DDNC)
507 Capitol Ct. N.E.
Ste. 200
Washington, DC 20002
Phone: 202-544-7497
Fax: 202-546-7105
Website: www.ddnc.org
E-mail: hpayne@hmcw.org

International Foundation for Functional Gastrointestinal Disorders (IFFGD)
P.O. Box 170864
Milwaukee, WI 53217
Toll-Free: 888-964-2001
Phone: 414-964-1799
Fax: 414-964-7176
Website: www.iffgd.org
E-mail: iffgd@iffgd.org

National Organization for Rare Disorders (NORD)
55 Kenosia Ave.
Danbury, CT 06810
Toll-Free: 800-999-6673
Phone: 203-744-0100
Fax: 203-263-9938
Website: www.rarediseases.org

Oley Foundation
Albany Medical Center MC-28
99 Delaware Ave.
Delmar, NY 12054
Toll-Free: 800-776-6539
Phone: 518-262-5079
Fax: 518-262-5528
Website: www.oley.org

763

Pelvic Floor Disorders Network (PFDN)
Data Coordinating Center
Website: pfdnetwork.
azurewebsites.net

Rare Diseases Clinical Research Network (RDCRN)
Office of Rare Diseases Research (ORDR), National Center for Advancing Translational Sciences (NCATS)
Website: www.
rarediseasesnetwork.org

The Simon Foundation for Continence
P.O. Box 815
Wilmette, IL 60091
Toll-Free: 800-23-SIMON
(800-237-4666)
Phone: 847-864-3913
Fax: 847-864-9758
Website: www.simonfoundation.
org

United Ostomy Associations of America (UOAA)
P.O. Box 525
Kennebunk, ME 04043-0525
Toll-Free: 800-826-0826
Website: www.ostomy.org
E-mail: info@ostomy.org

Wound, Ostomy and Continence Nurses Society (WOCN)
1120 Rt. 73, Ste. 200
Mount Laurel, NJ 08054
Toll-Free: 888-224-9626
Fax: 856-439-0525
Website: www.wocn.org
E-mail: info@wocn.org

Government Associations

Centers for Disease Control and Prevention (CDC)
1600 Clifton Rd.
Atlanta, GA 30329-4027
Toll-Free: 800-CDC-INFO
(800-232-4636)
Phone: 404-498-1515
Toll-Free TTY: 888-232-6348
Website: www.cdc.gov
E-mail: cdcinfo@cdc.gov

Eunice Kennedy Shriver *National Institute of Child Health and Human Development (NICHD)*
P.O. Box 3006
Rockville, MD 20847
Toll-Free: 800-370-2943
Toll-Free TTY: 888-320-6942
Toll-Free Fax: 866-760-5947
Website: www.nichd.nih.gov
E-mail: NICHDInformation
ResourceCenter@mail.nih.gov

FoodSafety.gov
U.S. Department of Health and Human Services (HHS)
Web Communications and New Media Division
200 Independence Ave. S.W.
Washington, DC 20201
Website: www.foodsafety.gov

Genetic and Rare Diseases Information Center (GARD)
P.O. Box 8126
Gaithersburg, MD 20898-8126
Toll-Free: 888-205-2311
Phone: 301-251-4925
Toll-Free TTY: 888-205-3223
Fax: 301-251-4911
Website: rarediseases.info.nih.gov

National Cancer Institute (NCI)
9609 Medical Center Dr.
BG 9609 MSC 9760
Bethesda, MD 20892-9760
Toll-Free: 800-4-CANCER (800-422-6237)
Website: www.cancer.gov

National Institute of Allergy and Infectious Diseases (NIAID)
Office of Communications and Government Relations (OCGR)
5601 Fishers Ln.
MSC 9806
Bethesda, MD 20892-9806
Toll-Free: 866-284-4107
Phone: 301-496-5717
Toll-Free TDD: 800-877-8339
Fax: 301-402-3573
Website: www.niaid.nih.gov
E-mail: ocpostoffice@niaid.nih.gov

National Institute of Diabetes and Digestive and Kidney Diseases (NIDDK)
9000 Rockville Pike
Bethesda, MD 20892
Phone: 301-496-3583
Website: www.niddk.nih.gov

National Institute of Neurological Disorders and Stroke (NINDS)
NIH Neurological Institute
P.O. Box 5801
Bethesda, MD 20824
Toll-Free: 800-352-9424
Phone: 301-496-5751
Website: www.ninds.nih.gov

National Institute on Deafness and Other Communication Disorders (NIDCD)
National Institutes of Health (NIH)
31 Center Dr.
MSC 2320
Bethesda, MD 20892-2320
Toll-Free: 800-241-1044
Phone: 301-496-7243
Fax: 301-402-0018
Website: www.nidcd.nih.gov
E-mail: nidcdinfo@nidcd.nih.gov

National Institutes of Health (NIH)
9000 Rockville Pike
Bethesda, MD 20892
Phone: 301-496-4000
TTY: 301-402-9612
Website: www.nih.gov
E-mail: NIHinfo@od.nih.gov

Office on Women's Health (OWH)
U.S. Department of Health and
Human Services (HHS)
200 Independence Ave. S.W.
Washington, DC 20201
Toll-Free: 800-994-9662
Phone: 202-690-7650
Fax: 202-205-2631
Website: womenshealth.gov

U.S. Department of Agriculture (USDA)
1400 Independence Ave. S.W.
Washington, DC 20250
Phone: 202-720-2791
Website: www.usda.gov

U.S. Department of Health and Human Services (HHS)
200 Independence Ave. S.W.
Washington, DC 20201
Toll-Free: 877-696-6775
Website: www.hhs.gov

U.S. Department of Veterans Affairs (VA)
810 Vermont Ave. N.W.
Washington, DC 20420
Toll-Free: 800-273-8255
Website: www.va.gov

U.S. Food and Drug Administration (FDA)
10903 New Hampshire Ave.
Silver Spring, MD 20993
Toll-Free: 888-INFO-FDA
(888-463-6332)
Phone: 301-796-8240
Website: www.fda.gov

Cancer

American Cancer Society (ACS)
250 Williams St. N.W.
Atlanta, GA 30303
Toll-Free: 800-227-2345
Website: www.cancer.org

Celiac Disease

American Celiac Society
Phone: 504-305-2968
Website: www.
americanceliacsociety.org

Beyond Celiac
P.O. Box 544
Ambler, PA 19002
Phone: 215-325-1306
Fax: 215-643-1707
Website: www.beyondceliac.org
E-mail: info@beyondceliac.org

Celiac Disease Foundation (CDF)
20350 Ventura Blvd.
Ste. 240
Woodland Hills, CA 91364
Phone: 818-716-1513
Fax: 818-267-5577
Website: www.celiac.org

Gluten Intolerance Group (GIG)
31214 124th Ave. S.E.
Auburn, WA 98092
Phone: 253-833-6655
Fax: 253-833-6675
Website: www.gluten.org
E-mail: customerservice@gluten.org

National Celiac Association (NCA)
20 Pickering St.
Needham, MA 02492
Toll-Free: 888-4-CELIAC
(888-423-5422)
Phone: 617-262-5422
Website: nationalceliac.org
E-mail: info@nationalceliac.org

Children's Issues

American Pediatric Surgical Association (APSA)
One Parkview Plaza
Ste. 800
Oakbrook Terrace, IL 60181
Phone: 847-686-2237
Fax: 847-686-2253
Website: www.eapsa.org
E-mail: eapsa@eapsa.org

Children's Liver Association for Support Services (CLASS)
25379 Wayne Mills Pl.
Ste. 143
Valencia, CA 91355
Toll-Free: 877-679-8256
Phone: 661-263-9099
Fax: 661-263-9099
Website: www.classkids.org
E-mail: info@classkids.org

North American Society for Pediatric Gastroenterology, Hepatology, and Nutrition (NASPGHAN)
714 N. Bethlehem Pike
Ste. 300
Ambler, PA 19002
Phone: 215-641-9800
Fax: 215-641-1995
Website: www.naspghan.org
E-mail: naspghan@naspghan.org

Crohn Disease

Crohn's & Colitis Foundation
733 Third Ave.
Ste. 510
New York, NY 10017
Toll-Free: 800-932-2423
Website: www.
crohnscolitisfoundation.org
E-mail: info@
crohnscolitisfoundation.org

Cyclic Vomiting Syndrome

Cyclic Vomiting Syndrome Association (CVSA)
P.O. Box 270341
Milwaukee, WI 53227
Phone: 414-342-7880
Fax: 414-342-8980
Website: cvsaonline.org
E-mail: cvsa@cvsaonline.org

Diagnostic Testing

Society of American
Gastrointestinal and
Endoscopic Surgeons
(SAGES)
11300 W. Olympic Blvd., Ste. 600
Los Angeles, CA 90064
Phone: 310-437-0544
Website: www.sages.org

Iron Disorders

American Hemochromatosis
Society (AHS)
P.O. Box 950871
Lake Mary, FL 32795-0871
Toll-Free: 888-655-IRON
(888-655-4766)
Phone: 407-829-4488
Fax: 407-333-1284
Website: www.americanhs.org
E-mail: mail@americanhs.org

Iron Disorders Institute (IDI)
P.O. Box 4891
Greenville, SC 29608
Toll-Free: 888-565-4766
Phone: 864-292-1175
Fax: 864-292-1878
Website: www.irondisorders.org
E-mail: info@irondisorders.org

Liver Disease

Alagille Syndrome Alliance
(ALGSA)
P.O. Box 4216
Wilsonville, OR 97070
Phone: 503-970-1255
Website: alagille.org
E-mail: alagille@alagille.org

American Association for
the Study of Liver Diseases
(AASLD)
1001 N. Fairfax St.
Ste. 400
Alexandria, VA 22314
Phone: 703-299-9766
Fax: 703-299-9622
Website: www.aasld.org

American Liver Foundation
(ALF)
39 Bdwy.
Ste. 2700
New York, NY 10006
Toll-Free: 800-465-4837
Phone: 212-668-1000
Fax: 212-483-8179
Website: www.liverfoundation.
org
E-mail: info@liverfoundation.org

Hepatitis Foundation
International (HFI)
8121 Georgia Ave.
Ste. 350
Silver Spring, MD 20910
Toll-Free: 800-891-0707
Phone: 301-879-6891
Website: hepatitisfoundation.org
E-mail: info@
hepatitisfoundation.org

Wilson Disease Association
(WDA)
1732 First Ave.
Ste. 20043
New York, NY10128
Toll-Free: 866-961-0533
Phone: 414-961-0533
Website: wilsonsdisease.ca
E-mail: info@wilsonsdisease.org

Index

Index